PHYSICAL MEDICINE AND REHABILITATION DIGEST

PHYSICAL MEDICINE AND REHABILITATION DIGEST

Rajesh Pramanik
MBBS MD MRCP (UK)
Associate Professor
Department of Physical Medicine and Rehabilitation
Institute of Post Graduate Medical Education & Research and
Seth Sukhlal Karnani Memorial Hospital
Kolkata, West Bengal, India

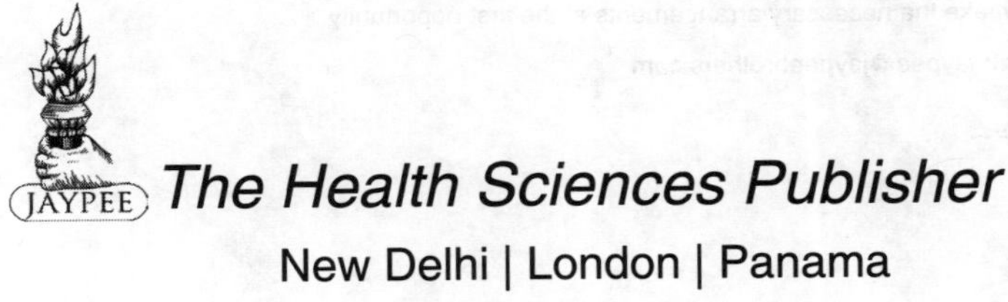

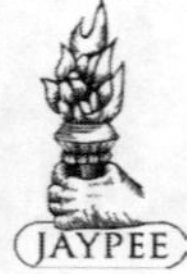

Jaypee Brothers Medical Publishers (P) Ltd

Headquarters

Jaypee Brothers Medical Publishers (P) Ltd
4838/24, Ansari Road, Daryaganj
New Delhi 110 002, India
Phone: +91-11-43574357
Fax: +91-11-43574314
Email: jaypee@jaypeebrothers.com

Overseas Offices

J.P. Medical Ltd
83 Victoria Street, London
SW1H 0HW (UK)
Phone: +44 20 3170 8910
Fax: +44 (0)20 3008 6180
Email: info@jpmedpub.com

Jaypee-Highlights Medical Publishers Inc
City of Knowledge, Bld. 235, 2nd Floor, Clayton
Panama City, Panama
Phone: +1 507-301-0496
Fax: +1 507-301-0499
Email: cservice@jphmedical.com

Jaypee Brothers Medical Publishers (P) Ltd
17/1-B Babar Road, Block-B, Shaymali
Mohammadpur, Dhaka-1207
Bangladesh
Mobile: +08801912003485
Email: jaypeedhaka@gmail.com

Jaypee Brothers Medical Publishers (P) Ltd
Bhotahity, Kathmandu
Nepal
Phone: +977-9741283608
Email: kathmandu@jaypeebrothers.com

Website: www.jaypeebrothers.com
Website: www.jaypeedigital.com

Physical Medicine and Rehabilitation Digest

First Edition: **2017**

ISBN: 978-93-86322-79-1

Printed at Sanat Printers

Dedicated to

My parents
Mr Jagadish Pramanik
and
Mrs Ujjwala Pramanik

Preface

Preparation for postgraduate examination of physical medicine of rehabilitation (PMR) of South-East Asia is really a difficult task for the examinee because there is lack of uniform syllabus, examination pattern and availability of tailor-made book. I faced the same difficulties when I was a postgraduate student 15 years ago. Today, I see my students encountering similar situations. I have noted that students are always trying hard to collect information from several books.

This book comprising of long and short cases, PMR diagnostics, orthosis, prosthesis, instruments, etc. may help the students of PMR, other related specialties like orthopedics, rheumatology, neurology and physiotherapy, occupational therapy, prosthetic orthotics, etc. to prepare themselves for the examinations. Social structures and rehabilitation issues in this part of the world are also different, but there is scarcity of relevant rehabilitation books from South-East Asia. This humble attempt of compilation of *Physical Medicine and Rehabilitation Digest* a tailor-made question-answer format book for oral and practical examinations, may fill the gap in future. Any feedback or constructive criticism will enrich this project further. The first edition of any book is the shape of author's imagination. Incorporation of critic's appraisal will give the real shape of this book.

Rajesh Pramanik

Acknowledgments

I am extremely grateful to my student Dr Saurav Kanti Sinha for his tremendous effort and active contribution to compile this book. I am especially thankful to Dr Rahul Dhar, Surgeon to help me compile the chapter on surgical instruments and Dr Debashis Chakrabarty, Associate Professor, Pathology for providing the photographs in section of PMR specimen. I am taking this opportunity to thank Mr Koushik Mal (Physiotherapist), Mr Akash Das (Occupational Therapist), and Mr Dhruti Sundar Das (Prosthetist) for their great help regarding the respective chapter on PT instruments, OT principles, Prosthesis and Orthosis. I am also grateful to my students Dr Subhasish Pati and Dr Labani Biswas for their hard work and sincere effort to type the manuscript for the last six months. Without the tremendous help and enthusiasms of Dr Sourav Kanti Sinha, Dr Subhasish Pati and Dr Labani Biswas, it was not possible for me to finish this work. I also like to thank my colleagues and Prof R N Haldar for their constant support for this venture. Finally, I would like to extend my sincere heartfelt thanks to M/s Jaypee Brothers Medical Publishers (P) Ltd, New Delhi, India, for their constant support for this project.

Last but not least, I want to express my gratitude to my family (my wife Soumi and my daughter Sonal) for their long suffering without whose forbearance and help the whole venture would not have seen the light of the day.

Contents

Plate 1

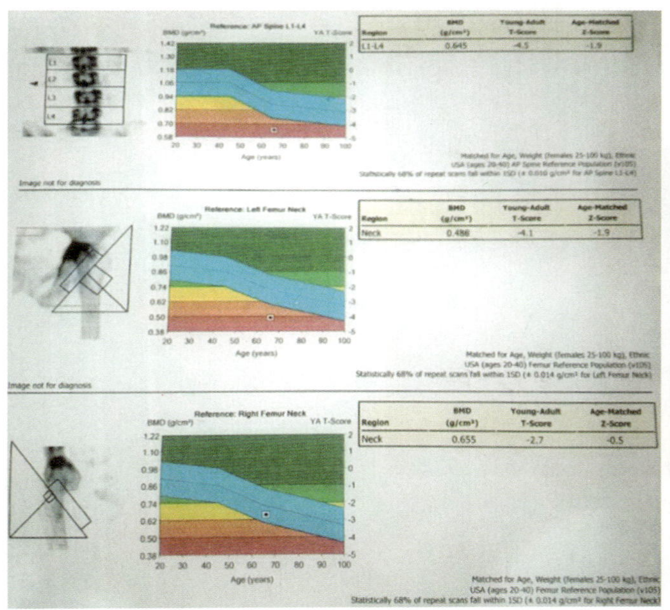

Figure 6.11: DEXA scan report

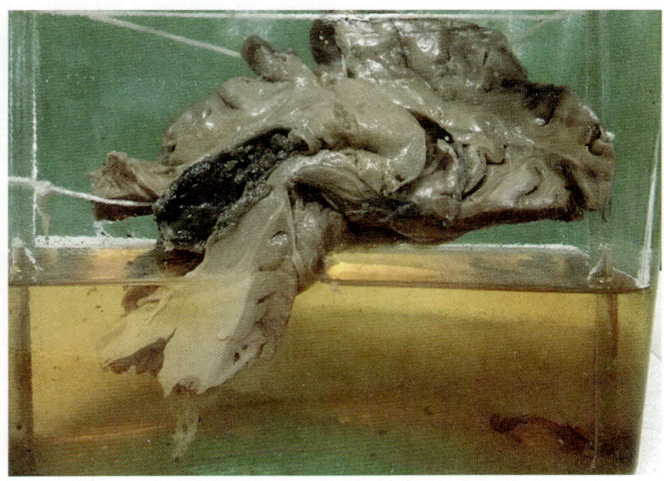

Figure 7.2: Brain hemorrhage

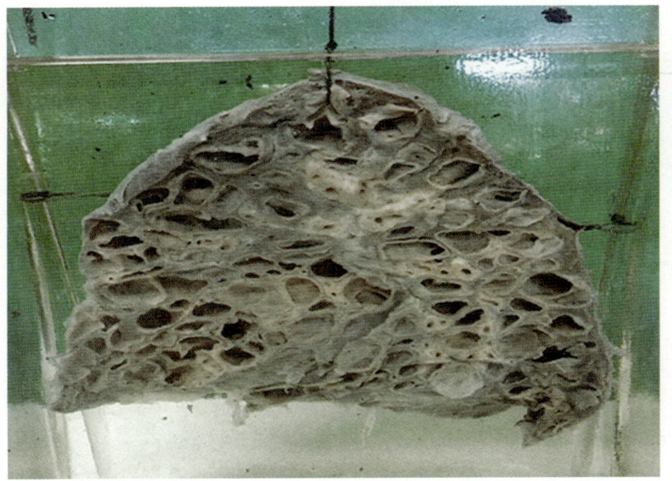

Figure 7.1: Bronchiectasis of lung

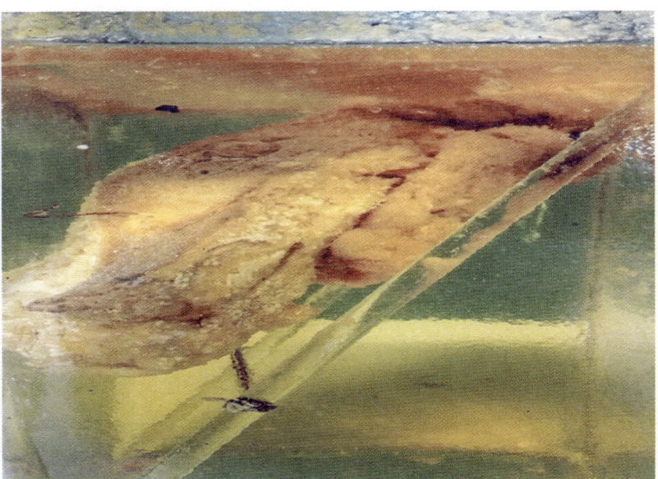

Figure 7.3: Carcinoma breast

Plate 2

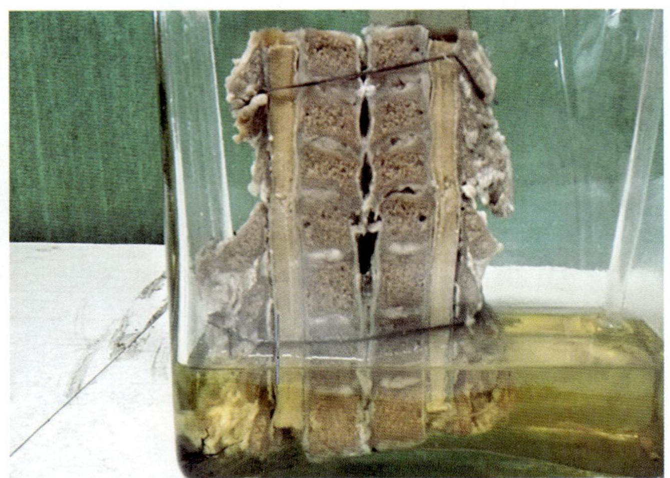

Figure 7.4: Carrie's spine

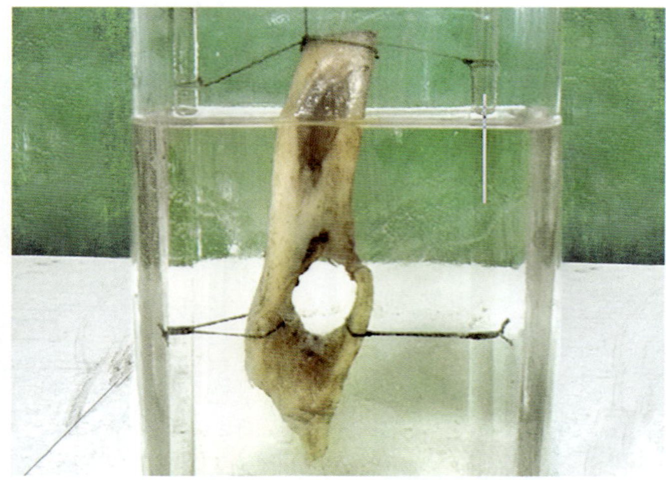

Figure 7.5: Osteomyelitis

1 Chapter

Examination Tips

GENERAL TIPS FOR THE DAY OF EXAMINATION

1. Introduce yourself to the patient.
2. Take the consent from patient or next of kin for examinations.
3. Do not exacerbate or initiate any pain or discomfort to the patient by your examination maneuvers.
4. Maintain patient's privacy.
5. Always ask a chaperon while examining a female patient.
6. Immediately do not go one step forward when the examiner will ask you to do something. Always go one step backward. First think yourself for few seconds, organize the things what you are going to do, then proceed smartly.
7. Show your confidence by your gesture but never be arrogant. Never bluff in examinations.
8. Always observe patients surrounding like any prosthesis, gait aid and other devices that will always give you an extra credit.
9. Better to omit rather than commit any wrong information.
10. Always remember that examiners are experienced physicians. It is very difficult to hide your weakness from them
11. Always start with basic things then proceed systematically. Never jump to higher levels straight way that will invite troubles.
12. If you don't know or forget anything, just confess it. Then you will get another opportunity to face questions. Don't waste your scheduled time. Never be mum during examinations.

TIPS FOR CASE ASSESSMENT

Assessment of Neurological Cases

History of Present illness

- Onset, duration, progression, severity of current symptom, exaggerating factors, relieving factors of current symptoms
- *Never miss to mention:*
  - Weakness or spasticity (motor symptoms)
  - Numbness, paresthesia, tingling tactile alterations (sensory symptoms)
  - Headache, vomiting, loss of consciousness, convulsion, altered sensorium (intracranial pathology)
  - Confusion, delirium, memory deficit (higher functions)
  - Depression, anxiety, sleep deprivation, sleep disorder (mental status)
  - Imbalance, vertigo, dizziness, instability, diplopia (cerebellar signs)
  - Slowness, rigidity, fall, tremor (basal ganglia)
  - Bladder and bowel involvement
  - Swallowing, speech, visual, auditory, taste sensation
- Sexuality issues: Erection, ejaculation, orgasm
- Appetite, sleep (general symptoms)
- Problems with basic ADL (Activities of daily living) like grooming, bathing, eating and IADLs
- Transfer and mobility issues.

History of Past Illness

- Relevant illness

- Risk factors of disease: Example in stroke past history of diabetes, hypertention, dyslipidemia, ischemic heart disease, valvular heart disease, arrhythmia-like atrial fibrillation, previous TIA, stroke, smoking.

History of Allergy

- Please do not forget.

History of Drug Intake

- List of current medications.

Family History

- Relevant illness in the family members
- Cause of death in family members
- Any hereditary disorders like coagulopathy
- Pedigree chart, if possible.

Functional History

- Basic ADLs
- IADLs
- Mobility Aids
- Caregiver: Indoor/Outdoor
  How much time per day or twenty four hours
- Transfer and mobility.

Socioeconomic History

- Home environment and living situation
  - Kutcha/Pucca house
  - Owned/Rented house
  - Elevator access present or not
  - Wheelchair access present or not
  - Bathroom distance
  - Home modification
  - Nearest bus stop, railway station, pitch road
  - Nearest primary center, rehabilitation center
- Family and friend support
  - Family income (financial support)
  - Number of family members (caregiver)
  - Level of assistance from the members
- Substance abuse
  - History of smoking, alcohol, drug abuse (CAGE questioner) (duration of amount of consumption e.g.—pack years).

Sexual History

- Orientation
- Frequency: Previous and after the illness
- Masturbation history
- Erection achievable or not
- Ejaculation achievable or not
- Orgasm achieved or not.

Vocational History

- Previous jobs
- Return to previous jobs: Yes or no: If not why? E.g.: Wheelchair access not present
- Contact with vocational planners.

Finances and Income History

- Lower/Middle/Higher income group
- Monthly family income.

Recreational History

- Music, dance, watching television, games, etc.
- Weekend recreational activities.

Spirituality and Belief

EXAMINATIONS

- FIM: See scales
- GCS: See scales
- Barthel index: See scales.

Important Points in General Survey

- Skin: Pressure sore
- Any palpable lymphnode
- Pulse, blood pressure (specially postural blood pressure), respiratory rate, anemia, JVP, edema.

Systemic Examinations

Higher Mental Status

Mini mental examinations: See charts.

Cranial Nerves

I. Olfactory: Smell sensation (toothpaste, soap).
II. Optic: Visual acuity, visual field, light reflex (direct and consensual), color vision.
III. Occulomotor + IV trochlear +VI abducens: Ptosis, squint, extraocular muscles, pupil size.
V. Trigeminal: Corneal reflex, Jaw jerk, Sensation over face, masseter, pterygoid power.
VII. Facial: Frowning, eye closure, angle of mouth, nasolabial folds.
VIII. Vestibulocochlear: Hearing (watch test, rinnes, webers).

IX. Glossopharyngeal: Soft palate movement, taste sensation posterior one third of tongue.
X. Vagus: Gag reflex.
XI. Spinal Accessory: Power of sternocleidomastoid, trapezius.
XII. Hypoglossal: Power of tongue muscles, atrophy, deviation.

Motor System

Inspection: Wasting, fasciculation
Palpation: Tone (spasticity/flacidity), Power [individual (LMN type)/group (UMN type)].

Sensory

Light touch, pin prick {
- Dermatomal distribution
- Glove and stocking
- Autonomous zone

Reflex

Superficial	**Root values**
• Abdominal	(T7–T12)
• Cremesteric	(T12, L1)
• Planter (Babinisky)	(S1)

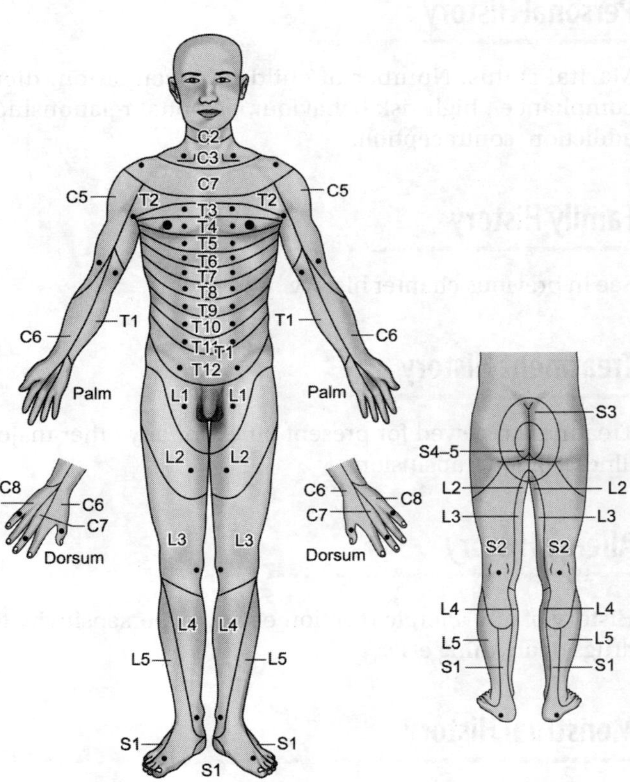

Figure 1: Dermatomal distribution

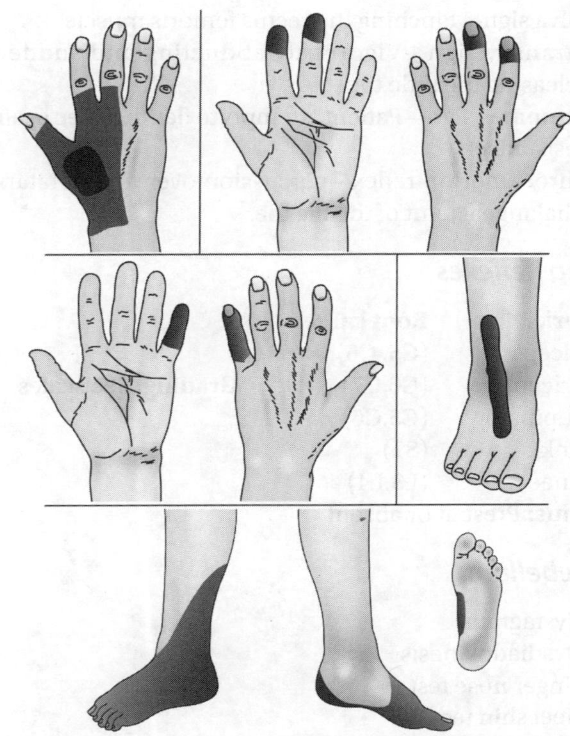

1. Radial nerve: 1st dorsal web space of hand (Anatomical snuff box)
2. Median nerve: Distal phalanx (tip) of index finger (2nd finger)
   - Other: Tip of thumb
3. Ulnar nerve: Distal phalanx (tip) of little finger (5th finger)
4. Common peroneal nerve/Common fibular nerve/External popliteal nerve/Lateral popliteal nerve: Central strip on dorsum of foot
5. Deep peroneal nerve: 1st dorsal web space
6. Posterior tibial nerve: Sole of foot
7. Sciatic nerve: Mixed pattern of common peroneal nerve and posterior tibial nerve

Figure 2: Autonomous zones

Other Planter Reflexes

- **Bing sign**—multiple pinpricks on the dorsum of the foot
- **Cornell sign**—Scratching along the inner side of the extensor hallucis longus tendon
- **Chaddock sign**—Stroking the lateral malleolus
- Gonda sign—Flexing and suddenly releasing the 4th toe
- **Gordon sign**—Squeezing the calf muscle
- Moniz sign—Forceful passive plantar flexion of the ankle
- **Oppenheim sign**—Applying pressure to the medial side of the tibia
- **Schaeffer sign**—Squeezing the Achilles tendon

- Silva sign—Pinching the rectus femoris muscle
- Stransky sign—Vigorously abducting and suddenly releasing the little toe
- Strümpell sign—Patient attempts to flex the knee against resistance
- Throckmorton reflex—percussion over the metatarsophalangeal joint of the big toe.

Deep Reflexes

Jerks	Root values
• Biceps	(C5, C6)
• Triceps	(C6,C7)
• Supinator	(C5,C6)
• Ankle	(S1)
• Knee	(L3,L4)

Grading: See scales

Clonus: Present or absent

Cerebellum

- Nystagmus
- Dysdiadokinesis
- Finger nose test
- Heel shin test.

(Other extrapyramidal examinations: Rigidity, static tremor, glabellar tap).

Position sense: Joint position: Upper limb: Interphalangeal joint of thumb.

Lower limb: Interphalangeal joint of the big toe.

Vibrations: Anterior iliac crest 1st MTP Joint → medial malleolus tibial tuberosity → sternum

Never Ever Miss To Mention GAIT

- Other systems:
  - Cardiovascular: Any murmur, carotid bruit, any arrhythmia
  - Respiratory: Breath sounds, any basal crepitations, adventitious sounds
  - Gastrointestinal: Tender points, peristaltic sounds, organomegaly.

MUSCULOSKELETAL SYSTEM

History of Present Illness

- Onset, severity, duration of symptoms
- Nature of pain, morning stiffness, risk factor, diurnal variation, intensity, fatigue
- Swelling of joints
- Any muscle weakness—proximal or distal
- Number of joints involved
- Involvement—Distal/proximal
- Symmetrical/Asymmetrical sequence of involvement
- Any other system involved
  - Eye: Redness, dryness, itching, congestion, vision
  - Skin: Pigmentation, rash, color changes, photosensitivity, lump/nodule, tightness, hair loss
  - CVS: Palpitation, chest pain
  - GI system: Constipation, diarrhoea, bleeding P/R
  - CNS: Higher mental function, headache, dizziness, sensation, weakness
  - Genitourinary: Burning micturition, frequency of micturition, any dryness, rash or discharge
- Sleep, appetite, bowel, bladder
- Prodromal symptoms like fever, weight loss or gain
- Drug history
- Allergy history
- Exposure to any toxin
- Functional history.

Past History

Past history of relevant sign and symptoms, any major illness like tuberculosis, malaria, jaundice, contact with tuberculosis or any STD, diarrhoea, urinary tract infection.

Personal History

Marital status. Number of children, occupation, diet, compliance , high risk behaviour, personal relationship, addiction, contraception.

Family History

See in previous chapter history.

Treatment History

Treatment received for present illness or any other major illness, blood transfusion.

Allergy History

History of any allergic reaction or any hypersensitivity to drugs or anything else.

Menstrual History

Menarche, any irregularity, quantity of blood loss, amenorrhea, menopause, etc.

Socioeconomic History

See Socioeconomic history in page no 2.

General Survey

- Pulse, BP, respiration, temperature
- Anemia, icterus, cyanosis, clubbing, edema
- Nail changes (Pitting, Beaus line, splinter hemorrhage, half nail)
- Nutrition, built
- Lymph nodes
- Skin rash
- Hair
- Decubitus
- Neck gland, neck vein
- Any lymphadenopathy
- Any gross findings like deformity, swelling.

Systemic

Musculoskeletal System

- Inspection: Deformity, wasting or atrophy, any obvious skin changes, redness or any swelling
- Palpation: Corroborate with inspection findings
  - Superficial: temperature of affected site, joints; tenderness of affected muscle or joints, any lump, nodule; any abnormal sound (click)
  - Deep: Consistency, sensation, etc.
- ROM-affected joints and other joints (especially immediate proximal and distal joints)
- Power: may be required for individual muscle or group of muscle depending upon involvement.
- Spine:
  - ROM
  - SI joint pathology test (Shoebers, Patricks, etc)
  - SLR
  - Femoral nerve stretch test
- Hands:
  - To check deformity
  - Raynauds Phenomenon
  - Heberdons, Bouchards nodules, Tophi
  - Arachinodactyly.
- Foot–any deformities
- Specific tests: Knee
  - Anterior Drawer tests
  - Posterior Drawer tests
  - Pivot shift test
  - Mc Murrays test
  - LachMans test
  - Valgus and Varus stress test.

Other Systems

- Opthalmological: Signs of conjuctivitis, scleritis, episcleritis, excessive dryness
- Respiratory: Signs of interstitial lung disease, other adventitious sounds
- CNS: Higher mental function. Cranium and spine, cranial nerves, tone, jerks, reflexes
- CVS: Any murmur, carotid bruit.

Gait with description of its Phases (Gait Cycle).

2 Chapter

Long Cases

HEMIPLEGIA (STROKE)

Summary

A 65-year-old right-handed diabetic, nonhypertensive, euthyroid literate male from a rural area with low socioeconomic status with previous one episode of TIA without any atrial fibrillation or any other cardiac illness or PVD presented with sudden onset left-sided complete hemiplegia for last 10 days. He didn't have any swallowing or speech abnormality or bladder and bowel incontinence. He is quite depressed because he is currently dependant for his ADL. Although his bed mobility is independent, his transfer is dependant with one person.

On examination he has a regular pulse of 80/min, BP 140/80 without any postural hypotension or carotid bruit. His GCS score is 15/15 and Barthel index is 40/100. He has grade 2 spasticity in left lower limb and grade 1 in left upper limb with gross motor power of 2/5 in proximal and 1/5 in distal UL, and 3/5 in LL. He is not suffering from any hemineglect, aphasia, dysphagia, aspiration, DVT, pressure sore. His left shoulder is slightly subluxated with prominent sulcus sign. He is completely dependent in his transfer.

Provisional Diagnosis

A case of left-sided complete hemiplegia due to anterior circulation stroke secondary to ischemia possibly thrombotic in origin complicated with spasticity and shoulder subluxation in Brunnstrom stage IV of recovery.

DIFFERENTIAL DIAGNOSIS

1. Hemorrhagic stroke (anterior circulation).
2. Intracranial SOL.
3. Demyelinating disease.

Q. What do you mean by complete hemiplegia?

It is hemiplegia with contralateral UMN type facial palsy.

Q. What is stroke ?

It is a nontraumatic brain injury caused by occlusion or rupture of cerebral blood vessels that results in sudden neurologic deficit characterized by loss of motor control, altered sensation, cognitive or language impairment, disequilibrium or coma.

Q. What differentiates ischemic stroke versus hemorrhagic stroke?

Hemorrhagic stroke is sudden-onset weakness associated with headache, recurrent vomiting, convulsions. It develops at height of emotion or excitement and explosive in nature developing over minutes to hours.

Table 2.1: Comparision between hemorrhagic and Ischemic stroke

	Hemorrhagic	*Ischemic*
Frequency	15%	85%
Onset	Sudden	Gradual
Associated signs/ symptoms	Headache, vomiting, convulsion	Weakness
Mortality	High	Low
Disability	Low	High

Q. What is TIA?

- It is a brief episode of neurological dysfunction caused by focal brain or retinal ischemia with clinical symptoms typically lasting less than 1 hour and without any evidence of acute infarction in imaging.

Q. What is RIND?

- RIND stands for "reversible ischemic neurological deficit". This term is not widely used nowadays. Previous description was a stroke that the patient was able to fully recover from within a few weeks.

Q. What are the synergy patterns in stroke?

Upper Limb

- Flexor synergy in upper limb
  - Shoulder: External rotation, abduction, retraction
  - Forearm: Supination
  - Elbow: Flexion
  - Wrist and fingers: Flexion.
- Extensor synergy in upper limb
  - Shoulder: Adduction, protraction
  - Forearm: Pronation
  - Elbow: Extension
  - Wrist: Extension
  - Fingers: Flexion.

Lower Limb

- Flexor synergy in lower limb.
  Hip: Flexion, abduction, external rotation
  Knee: Flexion
  Ankle: Eversion, dorsiflexion
  Toe: Extension.
- Extensor synergy in lower limb
  Hip: Extension, adduction
  Knee: Extension
  Ankle: Inversion, planti flexion
  Toe: Flexion.

Q. What is the pattern of motor recovery?

- Immediately following onset of hemiplegia: There is total loss of voluntary movement and loss or decrease of tendon reflexes
- Within next 48 hour: Increased deep tendon reflexes on the involved side develops
- 1–38 days: Spasticity in the flexors and adductors in the upper extremity (UE) and the extensors and adductors in the lower extremity (LE) on the hemiparetic side
- As spasticity increased, clonus of the ankle plantar flexors appeared
- 6–33 days after the onset of hemiplegia: The first "intentional" movements (shoulder flexion) appear
- In the upper limbs: A flexor synergy pattern develops followed by development of an extensor synergy pattern. Voluntary movement in the lower limb also begins with flexor synergy followed by extensor synergy pattern. With increased voluntary movement, there is a decrease in the spasticity of the muscles involved.

Q. Why is it not posterior circulation?

- Since there is loss of motor function but there is no visual impairment here.

Q. What may be the possible artery involved?

Features:

A. MCA main stem:

- Contralateral hemiplegia,
- Hemianesthesia, hemianopsia
- Head or eye turning toward lesion
- Dysphagia
- Uninhibited neurogenic bladder.

Dominant hemisphere

- Global aphasia
- Apraxia.

Nondominant hemisphere

- Aprosody and affective agnosia
- Visuospatial deficit
- Neglect syndrome

B. Anterior cerebral artery:

- Contralateral hemiplegia (hand more spared than leg and arm)
- Contralateral hemianesthesia
- Head or eye turning toward lesion
- Grasp reflex—groping
- Paratonia (or gegenhalten)
- Disconnection apraxia
- Akinetic mutism (abulia)

C. Posterior cerebral artery:

- Hemisensory deficit
- Visual impairment
- Visual agnosia
- Prosopagnosia
- Dyschromatopsia
- Alexia without agraphia
- Memory deficit

Q.10 What are the brain stem stroke syndromes?

MIDBRAIN

Table 2.2: Different mid brain strokes

Eponym	*Site*	*Cranial nerves involved*	*Tracts involved*	*Signs*
Weber syndrome	Base of midbrain	III	Corticospinal tract	Oculomotor palsy with crossed hemiplegia
Claude syndrome	Tegmentum of midbrain	III	Red nucleus and brachium conjunctivum	Oculomotor palsy with contralateral cerebellar ataxia and tremor
Benedikt syndrome	Tegmentum of midbrain	III	Red nucleus, corticospinal tract, and brachium conjunctivum	Oculomotor palsy with contralateral cerebellar ataxia, tremor, and corticospinal signs
Nothnagel syndrome	Tectum of midbrain	Unilateral or bilateral III	Superior cerebellar peduncles	Ocular palsies, paralysis of gaze, and cerebellar ataxia
Parinaud syndrome	Dorsal midbrain		Supranuclear mechanism for update gaze and other structures in periaqueductal gray matter	Paralysis of upward gaze and accommodation; fixed pupils

PONS

Table 2.3: Pontine strokes

Eponym	*Site*	*Cranial nerves involved*	*Tracts involved*	*Signs*
Millard Gubler syndrome	Pons	VII	Corticospinal tract	Ipsilateral facial palsy Contralateral arm/leg hemiparesis
Foville syndrome	Pons	VII	Paramedian pontine reticular formation Corticospinal tract	Ipsilateral horizontal gaze palsy VII Ipsilateral facial palsy Contralateral arm/leg hemiparesis
Raymond syndrome	Pons	VI	Corticospinal tract	Ipsilateral lateral rectus paresis Contralateral arm/leg hemiparesis
Brissaud	Pons	VII	Corticospinal tract	Ipsilateral facial spasm Contralateral arm/leg hemiparesis
One and a half syndrome	Pons	–	Paramedian pontine reticular formation Medial longitudinal fasciculus	Ipsilateral horizontal gaze palsy Contralateral internuclear ophthalmoplegia
Locked in syndrome	Pons	–	Bilateral corticospinal/corticobulbar tract Bilateral paramedian pontine reticular formation	Tetraplegia with facial palsy (except blinking eyes) Bilateral horizontal gaze palsy

MEDULLA

Table 2.4: Medullary strokes

Syndrome	*Cranial nerves*	*Tracts involved*	*Ipsilateral*	*Contralateral*
Lateral Medullary syndrome	XII	Corticospinal tract Medial leminiscus	Paralysis of one half of tongue	Paralysis of arm and leg, sparing face; impaired tactile and proprioceptive sense over one-half the body
Medial Medullary syndrome	V,VIII, IX, X	Spinothalamic tract Spin cerebellar tract Sympathtic fibers	Pain,numbness, impaired sensation over one-half the face Ataxia of limbs, falling to side of lesion; Nystagmus, diplopia, oscillopsia, vertigo, nausea, vomiting Horner's syndrome Dysphagia, hoarseness, paralysis of palate, paralysis of vocal cord, diminished gag reflex; Loss of taste Numbness of ipsilateral arm, trunk, or leg Weakness of lower face	Impaired pain and thermal sense over half the body, sometimes face

Q. Why is it not a SOL?
- No constitutional symptoms
- No known primary lesion
- No previous history of headache, seizure or loss of consciousness
- Acute in onset
- No bradycardia.

Q. What are the other causes of hemiplegia?
- Traumatic brain injury
- Vasculitis
- Cerebral abscess
- Meningoencephalitis.

Q. What are the causes of stroke in young?
- Cerebral embolism
- AV malformation
- Rupture of berry aneurysm
- Vasculitis (like Takayasu)
- Syphilis
- Collagen vascular disease (like SLE)
- Demyelination (MS)
- Polycythemia, thrombocytosis
- APLA, homocystinuria, Protein C and S deficiency.

Q. How will you manage this patient?

Management
- Counselling of the patient and family
- Patient and family member education
- Goal setting after discussion with patient and family members.

Investigation
- Blood: CBC, CRP, FBS, urea, creatinine, Na^+, K^+, LFT, lipid profile, TSH, T_3, T_4
- In young- ESR, PT, APTT, BT, CT, protein c and S, ANA, APLA, homocysteine, VDRL
- Urine for R/E, M/E, C/S
- ECG: To rule out atrial fibrillation, ischemia
- CXR: To check aspiration (specially right middle lobe)
- CT scan of brain (to confirm)
- Echocardiography (in young/recurrent anterior circulation stroke).

Later on
- MRI (vasculitis/demyelination / SOL)
- MRA (Aneurysm).

Pharmacological
1. Antiplatelet therapy in ischemic stroke
   - Aspirin 75 mg/day—Drug of choice
   - Clopidogrel/ dipyridamole—When aspirin is not tolerated
   - Combined—when patient was already on aspirin.
2. Anticoagulant therapy
   - Low molecular weight heparin (LMWH)—for initial 2 weeks
   - Warfarin—started after 2 weeks if patient has atrial fibrillation.
3. Statins—Now high-dose therapy is preferred.
4. Antihypertensives
   - Perindopril—(PROGRESS trial)
   - Ramipril—(HOPE trial)
   - Calcium channel blockers
   - Avoid diuretics—(causes hyponatremia)
   - *Strict control of blood pressure increases the ischemic perumbra.* That is why use of antihypertensive should be judicious.
5. Antidiabetic
   - Insulin—Sliding scale of insulin followed by regular dose monitoring
   - Oral hypoglycemic agents like sulphonylureas, metformin—After 3–4 weeks.
6. Spasticity medication—later in chapter.
7. Control of other comorbidities.
8. IV Mannitol followed by oral glycerol for cerebral edema in case of massive stroke with midline shift.
9. Antiepileptic drugs.

Table 2.5: Antiepileptics in stroke

Agent	*Dose*	*Administration Rates*	*Serious Adverse Effects*	*Comments*
Phenytoin	20 mg/kg IV Additional 5–10 mg/kg	Up to 50 mg/min IV Additional dose 10 min after load	Arrthythmia Hypotension Purple glove syndrome	IV contains propylene glycol Risk of AEs increases with faster infusion rates Only compatible in NS Therapeutic range 10–20 mcg/mL
Fosphenytoin	15–20 mg PE/kg	100–150 mg PE/min	Hypotension Arrthythmias	Pro-drug of phenytoin May be administered IM or IV
Levetiracetam	1000–3000 mg IV	2.5 mg/min IV		No hepatic metabolism Min drug interactions
Phenobarbital	20 mg/kg IV Additional 5–10 mg/kg	Additional dose 10 min after load	Hypotension Respiratory depression	IV Contains propylene glycol Believed to have higher risk of hypoventilation or hypotension than benzodiazepines of phenytoin

Contd...

Contd...

Agent	*Dose*	*Administration Rates*	*Serious Adverse Effects*	*Comments*
Valproate Sodium	20–40 mg/kg IV Additional 20 mg/kg	3–6 mg/kg/min Additional dose 10 min after load	Hyperammonemia Pancereatitis Thrombocytopenia Hepatotoxic	FDA approved only for slower infusion rates due to adverse effects
Topiramate	200–400 mg/NG/PO	300–1600 mg/day (divided 2–4 times)	Metabolic acidosis	Not available IV
Lacosamide	200–400 mg IV	200 mg over 15 min	Hypotension PR prolongations	Limited experience in SE treatment MIn drug interactions

Nutritional Care

- IV fluids normal saline 12 hourly for 48 hours
  # Avoid 5% dextrose, as it causes brain edema
- NG Tube feeding, maximum till 4 weeks
- If >4 weeks—PEG feeding is ideal.

DVT Prophylaxis

- Compressive stocking
- Ankle pumps
- Anticoagulants
- Foot ankle exercise
  - Nonpharmacological.

Postural Care

Supine

- Foot—against footboard, post. heel—in space between mattress and footboard
- Legs—neutral position with toes upwards
- Knee and hip—in extension (maintained by friction of feet against footboard and cloth roll placed under greater trochanter)
- Shoulder abducted 90 degree and internally rotated slightly and elbow flexed 90 degree
- With forearm pronated partially
  OR
- Shoulder abducted 90 degree and externally rotated full range and elbow flexed 90 degree
  With forearm pronated
  OR
- Shoulder abducted slightly and elbow extended with forearm supinated
- Wrist—extended
- Fingers—partially flexed at MCP and IP joints
- Thumb—abducted, opposed and slight flexion of IP joints.

Side lying

(Most comfortable lying on uninvolved side)

- Top leg—flexion at hip and knee, pillow placed under leg (to avoid contact with lower leg)
- Bottom arm—externally rotated and partially extended, top arm kept away from patients chest.

Prone

(Highly advised if patient tolerates)

- Feet—elevated with roll
- Toes—shouldn't touch footboard
- Hip and knee—extended
- Arm—slightly abducted, extended at elbow, extended and supinated at wrist
- Finger flexion, wrist extn.—handroll, shoulder rolls are used

Physical Therapy

- Exercise
  - ROM exercises
  - Strengthening
  - Mobilization
  - Compensatory techniques
  - Endurance training (e.g. aerobics)
  - Exercise for improving motor control and coordination.

Modalities

- FES for shoulder subluxation and footdrop
- EMG biofeedback
- Robotics.

Occupational Therapy

- Bed mobility
- Sitting balance
- Transfer training
- Standing balance
- Gait training
- ADL/IADL training
  - Robotic training.

Orthotic Support

- Bobath cuff
- Ankle foot orthosis (AFO)

Speech therapy: Not required in this patient.

Vocational therapy: Training for earning livelihood.

Resettlement: Collaboration with government and NGOs. (To assess any other complication and specific management)

Q. What are the indications of thrombolysis?

- Age—18 years or older
- Duration of Stroke—<3 hours
- Patients with measurable neurologic deficits (moderate-to-severe stroke symptoms)
- Head CT negative for hemorrhage.

Q. What are the contraindications of thrombolysis?

- Minor stroke symptoms/TIA (symptoms rapidly improving)
- Head CT positive for blood
- BP >185/100 despite medical treatment
- Coagulopathy/patient on anticoagulants (warfarin, heparin)
  - PT >15 seconds or INR >1.7
  - Patient received heparin within 48 hours prior with elevated PTT
  - Patient taking warfarin
- Platelet count <100,000
- Blood sugar <50 or >400
- History of stroke or severe head injury in past 3 months
- History of ICH, AVM, or aneurysm
- History of gastrointestinal (GI) or genitourinary (GU) bleeding within past 21 days
- Pregnancy or lactation within past 30 days
- Major surgery within past 14 days
- Seizure at onset of stroke
- Acute myocardial infarction.

Q. What are the surgical indication of stroke?

- Large hematoma
- AV malformation
- >70% stenosis in carotid artery.

Q. Describe the different techniques of antispasticity exercise?

Proprioceptive neuromuscular facilitation—This technique uses spiral and diagonal components of movement rather than the traditional movements in cardinal planes of motion. Goal of facilitating movement patterns that will have more functional relevance than the traditional technique of strengthening individual group of muscles.

Bobath approach/neurodevelopmental technique (NDT)—The goal of NDT is to normalize tone, to inhibit primitive patterns of movement and to facilitate automatic, voluntary reactions as well as subsequent normal movement patterns.

- It suppresses abnormal muscle patterns before normal patterns introduced
- Mass synergies are avoided although they may strengthen weak, unresponsive muscles because it reinforce abnormally increased tonic reflexes and spasticity
- Abnormal patterns modified at proximal key points of control
- It is just opposite to the Brunnstrom approach.

Brunnstrom approach/movement therapy—Uses primitive synergistic patterns in training in an attempt to improve motor control through central facilitation.

Sensorimotor approach/rood approach— Modification of muscle tone and voluntary motor activity can be done by using cutaneous sensorimotor stimulation. Facilitatory or inhibitory inputs through the use of sensorimotor stimuli including quick stretch, icing, fast brushing, slow stroking, tendon tapping, vibration, and joint compression, etc promote contraction of proximal muscles and reduce spasticity.

Constrain induced motor technique (CIMT).

Q. What are the prerequisites to start CIMT and its regimen?

- Patient is required to have at least 10 degrees of active wrist extension, at least 10 degrees of thumb abduction/extension, and at least 10 degrees of extension in at least 2 additional digits
- It is a 2 weeks program which utilizes CIMT in 90% waking hours of the patient including 6 hours per day of institutional-based therapy. The forced use of the impaired upper limb is the key component of the regimen.

Q. What specific upper limb occupational therapy should you prescribe for this patient?

- Hand-based activity
- Table top activity
- Integration to normal task activities
- ADL (Activities of daily living) (Basic and Instrumental)
- Training for fine hand function .

Q. What are the different OT regimens according to stages of recovery in upper limbs?

STAGE 1 – 2:

- Pro synergy positioning
- Facilitation technique to facilitate tone
- Bed mobility
- Transfer training.

STAGE 3:

- Movement deviating from synergy
- Inhibition technique to reduce hyperplasticity
- Weight bearing activities
- Bobath's approach
- Functional stretching of tight muscles
- Antisynergy positioning and splinting.

STAGE 4:

- Hand-based activity
- Table top activity
- Integration to normal task activities

- ADL (activities of daily living) (Basic and Instrumental)
- Training for fine hand function.

STAGE 5:

- Strengthening activities
- Strengthening protocol
- Compensatory approach
- Assistive and adaptive device.

Q. What are the poor prognostic factors of stroke recovery?

- No measureable grasp strength by 4 weeks
- Severe proximal spasticity
- Prolonged flaccidity
- Late return of proprioceptive facilitation
- Late return of proximal traction response.

Q. What are the main hindrances of rehabilitation in this patient?

- Spasticity
- Weakness
- Poor socioeconomic status
- Shoulder sublaxation.

Q. How will you assess spasticity?

- Modified asworth scale (MAS)
- Modified Tardeau scale (other scales not applicable here).

Q. Which is the choice of antispastic medication here and why?

- Preference is based on individual patients and condition.

Table 2.6: Antispasticity drugs

Drug	*Dosage*	*Mechanism of action*	*Side effects*	*Uses*
Baclofen	Start 5 mg BID or TID; increase dose by 5 mg q3–5 days up to 80 mg/day	Oral GABA-mimetic agent which acts as a GABA agonist at GABA/B receptors	Sedation/Drowsiness, lowered seizure threshold, weakness, symptoms, tremor, insomnia, confusion	*Spinal forms of spasticity and MS* (also used in acquired brain injury, but no literature has demonstrated benefit) #Studies suggest greater effect on lower extremity tone than on upper extremity tone
Diazepam	Start 25 mg BID up to a total dose of 400 mg/d (100–200 mg/d usually appropriate). Usual dose BID or TID	Does not substitute for GABA, but rather facilitates GABA's effects on the GABAA receptor subtype; overall effect results in membrane hyperpolarization and decreased neuronal firing	Sedation (most sedating of commonly used oral spasticity medications) Memory impairment Decreased REM sleep	Demonstrated benefit in SCI and MS spasticity
Dantrolene sodium	Start 25 mg BID up to a total dose of 400 mg/d (100–200 mg/d usually appropriate). Usual dose BID or TID	Acts peripherally in the striated muscle by blocking the release of Ca++ from the sarcoplasmic reticulum	Liver toxicity in ~1% of patients. (Highest risk in females over 30 yr, on high doses (> 300mg), for >2 months) : Risk of Hepatonecrosis, drowsiness (mild to moderate), less central effects, weakness fatigue, parasthesia, nausea, vomiting	Classically preferred drug for spasticity of cerebral origin (stroke, CP, head injury) (also used to treat malignant hyperthermia, neuroleptic malignant syndrome, and hyperthermia due to baclofen withdrawal)
Clonidine	Oral: Start with 0.05 mg PO BID, may increase up to 0.4 mg/day	Central acting alpha2-adrenergic agonist with effects in locus ceruleus. In the spinal cord, provides presynaptic inhibition of sensory afferents	Hypotension/Syncope, nausea, sedation, depression, dry mouth, ankle edema	Largely studied in treatment of SCI related spasticity Reported useful in treatment of supraspinal (brainstem) spasticity
Tizanidine	Start at 2–4 mg/d, usually at bed time • May increase dose and frequency up to max 36 mg/d depending on patient tolerance	Central acting alpha-2 adrenergic agonist, chemically related to clonidine • Binds to alpha-2 receptors both spinally and supraspinally	Sedation/Drowsiness, noted in up to 50% of patients, potential for liver damage, hypotension, dry mouth, bradycardia, dizziness	Spasticity due to SCI, MS, or acquired brain injury *(clinical trials show tizanidine to be as effective as oral baclofen or diazepam with a better overall tolerability)*

Q. What are the other modalities for treatment of spasticity?

- Electrical stimulation to antagonist muscle
- Cryotherapy
- Vibration therapy.

Q. What are the other interventions effective for Spasticity?

- Chemoneurolysis by phenol or alcohol
- Botulinum toxin.

Q. Which one will you prefer?

Based on individual case.

Comparison of efficacy:

Table 2.7: Comparison between phenol and botox

	Phenol	*Botulinum toxin*
Effectiveness	+++	+++
Evidence of efficacy	Lower limb	Upper limb
Ease of administration	+	+++
Onset	+++	+
Duration	+++	+
Pain and adverse events	+++	+
Cost	+	++++

Q. What are the common chemoneurolysis done in lower limb spasticity?

- Obturator nerve block for adductor spasticity
- Posterior tibial nerve block for ankle plantar flexor spasticity.

Q. Outline the steps of obturator and posterior tibial nerve block?

Obturator nerve block

- The patient was placed in supine position with legs abducted
- A mark was made on the skin 1–2 cm, medial to the femoral artery just below the inguinal ligament
- The adductor longus tendon was then identified near its insertion site at the pubis. The teflon coated needle was attached to an out syringe which contained 5% aqueous phenol, introduced behind the adductor longus tendon and directed laterally with a slight posterior and superior inclination toward the skin mark
- The needle was advanced until adductor muscle contraction was elicited with a nerve stimulator. Then the needle was manipulated to a point where maximum contraction was visible with minimum current.

Posterior tibial nerve block

- The knee was flexed to allow palpation of the superior popliteal fossa borders and identification of the skin crease behind the knee joint
- The Teflon coated needle was attached to an out syringe which contained 5% aqueous phenol, and inserted just above the crease line in the middle of the popliteal fossa
- The stimulating needle was advanced towards femur perpendicularly till contraction of gastrosoleus was visible
- Then the needle was manipulated to a point where maximum contraction was visible with minimum current
- After negative aspiration, phenol solution was injected.

Q. What is the maximum dose of phenol?

- 20 mL of 5% aqueous phenol.

Q. How much of botulinum toxin will you inject?

- 1 - 3 U/kg/muscle in upper limb
- 3 - 6 U/kg/muscle in lower limb
- Maximum dose 400 to 600 U.

Q. What are the usual sites of botulinum toxin in limbs?

- Upper limbs: Flexor digitorum superficialis and profundus and pronators
- Lower limbs: Gastrocnemius and soleus.

Q. What botulinum toxin is commonly used?

Toxin A is commonly used (Toxin B is also available).

Q. What are the beneficial effects of spasticity?

- Decreases edema
- Decreases osteoporosis
- Decreases atrophy
- Decreases DVT and PE
- Aids in standing, transfer, ambulation
- Assists ADL.

Q. What are the harmful effects of spasticity?

- Contracture
- Difficulty in transfer
- Difficulty in maintaining perineal hygiene (hip adductor spasticity)
- Pressure sore
- Difficulty in standing (Hamstring spasticity)
- Gait deviation.

Q. What worsens spasticity?

- Emotional stress
- Retention of urine
- Impacted stool
- Infections
- Pressure ulcer
- Ingrowing toe nail
- Any other noxious stimulations

Q. What is the role of functional electric stimulation (FES) in hemiplegia?
- Shoulder subluxation
- Foot drop.

Q. How FES works in foot drop?

Open loop systems:
- Feedback is provided manually
- Stimulation is activated by switches.

Example: Therapist triggers a heel switch to activate anterior tibialis during gait cycle.

Closed loop systems:
- More sophisticated system utilizing more complex automated technology
- Electrodes activated by computer generated patterns of stimulation to cause functional movement
- Feedback provided automatically through movement sensors
- **EMG-FES**: EMG sensor triggers FES once threshold is reached; FES triggers desired movement.

Q. What are the gait abnormalities seen in hemiplegia?
- Persistence of ankle plantar flexion in swing and stance phase
- Persistence of knee extension in swing phase
- Inadequate knee extension in stance phase
- This leads to typical circumduction gait.

Q. How can you correct this?

Orthotic support—
- AFO (for weak dorsiflexors and plantiflexors)
- PLS (for weak dorsiflexors but strong plantiflexors with power 3/5)
- Robotics
- BWSTT (body weight supported treadmill training).

Q. What are the swallowing difficulties in stroke?

Oral Phase
- Drooling
- Facial asymmetry
- Pocketing food in the cheek
- Poor tongue movement
- Inability to close lips tightly, with resulting leakage of food or fluid from the mouth.

Pharyngeal Phase
- Nasal regurgitation
- Inability to swallow
- Coughing when eating or drinking
- Wet sounding voice or cough
- Complaints of food catching in the throat.

Esophageal Phase
- Burping or indigestion
- Globus sensation: "Lump in the throat"
- Complaints about a bad taste in the mouth on awakening.

Q. What is the management?
- Cognitive stimulation
- ROM and strengthening exercise
- Compensatory techniques
- Diet modification.

Q. What is dysphagia diet?

A dysphagia diet is one that features different textures of foods and liquids. It is used with people who have problems with chewing and swallowing.

Q. Types of dysphagia diet?
- NPO—Indicated in patients with high aspiration risk. It is disadvantageous because swallowing itself is the best exercise for recovery
- Mechanical soft—Requires little chewing and are easy to control in mouth, e.g. banana, ground meat with gravy, used in patients who cant tolerate liquids
- Pureed—Requires no chewing, smooth, soft, blenderized foods, e.g. apple sauce, whipped potato, given in patients who have difficulty in forming cohesive bolus.
- Thick liquids—Honey thick followed by nectar thick these are liquids that have body, are easier to control in the mouth.
- Thin liquids—Clear with little or no body (water, tea, juice, milk). It can be given when nectar thick liquids are tolerated
- Regular—No texture restriction are allowed if patient can tolerate the above mentioned consistencies. Solid food in regular diet may be chopped to dice size.

Q. What are the different rehab techniques for swallowing?

Table 2.8: Rehabilitation of swallowing

Problems		*Rehabilitation techniques*
Oral cavity Oral motor control exercises (jaw, tongue, lip)	→	Jaw opening and closing Tongue rotation, lateralization, protrusion, retraction Lip protrusion, lateralization, and opening-closing
Relaxation and range of motion (jaw, tongue, lip)	→	Stretching and increasing range of motion

Contd...

Contd...

Problems		*Rehabilitation techniques*
Resistance exercise (jaw, tongue, lip)	→	Opening-closing the jaw against resistance Pushing the tongue against resistance
Pharynx Laryngeal elevation exercise	→	Volitonal laryngeal elevation by saying a high-pitched 'ee'
Vocal cord adduction exercise	→	Pushing wall or table, uttering 'ah' simulaneously
Masako maneuver	→	Swallowing with the tongue tip held anteriorly outside the month
Sensory stimulation	→	Tactile stimulation of the faucial arches with cold or sour stimuli
Upper esophageal sphincter opening Shaker exercise	→	Active head raising (neck flexion) in the supine position
Upper esophageal sphincter dilatation	→	Expansion of a balloon catheter in the upper esophageal sphincter

Q. What maneuver will you prescribe for the following?

Table 2.9: Different swallowing maneuvers

Problems		*Maneuvers*
Reduced oral control with aspiration before or during the swallow	→	Chin tuck
Impaired oral bolus propulsion	→	Neck extension
Unilatral pharyngeal weakness with retertion after swallowing	→	Head trun (to week side)
Unilateral oral and pharyngeal weekness	→	Head tilt (to week side)
Pharyngeal weakness with retention and overflow aspiration after swallowing	→	Reclining position
Inadequate or delayed vocal fold closure	→	Supraglottic swallow
Inadequate or delayed closure of laryngeal aditius (entrance)	→	Supersupraglottic swallow
Poor tongue base ratraction	→	Effortful swallow
Inadequate upper esophageal sphincter opening	→	Mendelsohn maneuver
Impaired oral bolus propulsion	→	Syringe feeding
Retention in the pharynx after swallowing	→	Double swallow
Retention in the pharynx after swallowing	→	Alternating solids and liquids

Q. What are the speech abnormalities?

- Aphasia
- Aprosody.

Q. How will you classify dysphasia?

Table 2.10: Classification of dysphasia

Fluent				*Nonfluent*			
+ Comprehension		– Comprehension		+ Comprehension		– Comprehension	
REPETITION		REPETITION		REPETITION		REPETITION	
+	–	+	–	+	–	+	–
Naming	Conduction	Transcortical Sensory	Wernicke's	Transcortical motor	Broca's	Mixed transcortical	Global
+	–						
Normal	Anomia						

(For other questions see short case on dysphasia)

Q. What is hemineglect?

A neuropsychological condition characterized by inability to process and perceive stimuli on one side of the body or environment that is not due to lack of sensation, resulting from damage to contralateral cerebral hemisphere.

Q. How will you assess hemineglect?

- Collide with objects on the neglected side
- Fails to eat food on the one half of plate
- If asked to draw a clock might show 12 and 1–6 but the other side will be distorted or blank
- When asked to write there is a tendency to leave unusually wide margin on left
- Fail to read left half of sentences
- Line cancellation test
- Monothematic delusion/anosognosia: Deny ownership of contralesional limb/body half
- Extinction: Detected by simultaneous bilateral stimulation
- Problem with "interior" left information
- Ignore left side of dreams and hallucination.

Q. How will you manage a patient of hemineglect?

- Constrained induced therapy: To encourage use of contralesional limb by keeping the good limb in a sling (patient must have active control of wrist and elbow extension)
- Prismatic adaptation: To pull the vision towards left

- Eye patching over the good eye
- Neck muscle vibration: On contralesional post. Neck muscle can be utilized to induce diversion of gaze
- Vestibular caloric stimulation: Induces brief remission in some cases
- Trunk rotation therapy: Improves postural disorders and balance deficit
- Visual scanning training
- Mental imagery training
- Video feedback training.

Q. What is apraxia?

This is inability to perform skilled movement in the absence of motor, sensory or cognitive impairment. It is most commonly seen in left hemispheric strokes and affects left nonhemiplegic limb.

Q. Is this patient suffering from apraxia?

It is too early to comment. The left hand is involved hence, chances are less as right hemisphere is involved.

Q. What are the types of apraxia?

- Ideational apraxia
- Ideomotor apraxia (# Constructional apraxia, dressing apraxia are not true apraxia but visuospatial defects).

Q. What are the causes of post stroke shoulder pain?

- Adhesive capsulitis
- Subluxation
- Impingement syndrome
- Rotator cuff injury
- Bicipital tendinitis
- Complex regional pain syndrome type 1
- Brachial plexopathy
- Axillary neuropathy
- Suprascapular neuropathy
- Myofascial pain
- Spasticity
- Soft tissue contracture.

Q. What are the bladder problems in stroke?

- Loss of supra sacral inhibition
- Initialy acute retention (cause not known)
- Impaired awareness (urge incontinence)
- Urodynamics - Detrussor overactivity with uninhibited bladder contraction.

Q. How will you manage?

See page number 23.

CEREBELLAR STROKE

Salient Features: Ipsilateral

- Dyssynergia
- Dysdiadochokinesia
- Diplopia
- Dysmetria
- Past pointing
- Heel shin test positive
- Skewed deviation of eyes
- Dysarthria
- Hypotonia
- Ataxia
- Pendular knee jerk
- Nystagmus
  (NO MOTOR DEFICIT)

Differential Diagnosis

- Multiple sclerosis
- Cerebellar SOL
- Paraneoplastic syndrome
- Friedreich's ataxia.

Investigations

Same as above but MRI brain should be done as first line of investigation because CT scan will be inconclusive.
No need to investigate source of emboli by ECHO.

Management

- Focus on ataxia: Frenkel's exercise
- Gait training.

Final Goal

- Integration with the family, society and work environment.

SPECIAL ISSUES IN TBI

- Post-traumatic seizure/epilepsy
- Paroxysmal autonomic instability and dystonia (PAID)
- Post-traumatic hydrocephalus
- Cranial nerve injuries
- Post-traumatic agitation
- Hypothalamic pituitary dysfunction

- SIADH
- Cerebral salt wasting syndrome
- Diabetes insipidus
- Cognitive dysfunction.

PARAPLEGIA (SPINAL CORD INJURY)

Summary

This 40-years-old illiterate right-handed, mansion worker, married male patient from lower socioeconomic status presented with sudden onset lower limb weakness and decreased sensation below the chest after a fall from height of approximately 24 feet since 6 months. Following the incident patient was transferred to a local secondary care hospital by untrained persons and received initial care with IV injections for few hours. After that there was slight improvement and was transferred to tertiary care rehab setting for further management. He is bed ridden since then with slight improvement of muscle strength, catheterized but continent bowel. There is a pressure ulcer on his buttocks but there is no feature suggesting DVT. During his stay he developed episodes of flushing and sweating on the upper half of the body which was relieved after bladder wash. He performs most of his upper limb activities of daily livings by himself. He is now independent in transfer and is able to stand with HKAFO. He is sexually active and achieves errection and ejaculation but has difficulty in maintaining sexual postures due to spasticity in lower limbs which is also creating difficulty in perineal care of this patient. He is quite depressed but fully conscious with FIM score of 86.

P/D: A case of post-traumatic spinal cord injury with NLI at D6 in AIS Stage B complicated with pressure ulcer spasticity and autonomic dysreflexia.

Q. What are the causes of paraplegia?

UMN Type:

1. Cerebral causes: Diplegic CP, superior saggital venous thrombosis, ACA thrombosis, parasaggital meningioma.
2. Spinal causes:
   a. Compressive:
      i. Intramedullary:
         - Glioma
         - Ependyomoma
         - Chordoma.
      ii. Extramedullary:
         - Intradural
           - Meningioma
           - Neurofibroma
           - AV malformation
           - Patchy arachnoditis
         - Extradural
           - Caries spine
           - Multiple myeloma
           - Metastasis
           - PIVD
           - Patchy meningitis
           - Spondylolysthesis
           - Abcess.
   b. Noncompressive:
      i. Motor neuron disease.
      ii. Multiple sclerosis.
      iii. Subacute cord degeneration.
      iv. Syringomyelia.
      v. Hereditary spastic paraparesis.
      vi. Anterior spinal artery thrombosis.
      vii. Acute transverse myelopathy.
      v iii Radiating myelopathy.

LMN Type: (Causes of Paraparesis Only)

1. UMN in shock stage.
2. Ante horn cell/peripheral nerves lesion
   i. Poliomyelitis.
   ii. GB syndrome.
   iii. Progressive muscular atrophy (PMA).
   iv. Cauda equine syndrome.
   v. Peripheral neuropathy.
   vi. Tabes Dorsalis.
3. Myoneural junction:
   Myasthenia gravis.
   Periodic paralysis.
4. Myopathy.
5. Hysterical.

Q. What is compressive myelopathy?

It is a type of myelopathy due to external compression of the cord.

Q. What are the difference between compressive and noncompressive myelopathy?

Table 2.11: Difference between compressive and non-compressive myelopathy

	Compressive	*Noncompressive*
Spinal deformity	May be present	Absent
Spinal tenderness	May be present	Absent
Girdle-like sensation	May be present	Absent
Upper level of sensory loss	May be present	Absent
Zone of hyperesthesia	May be present	Absent
Root pain	May be present	Absent
Onset and progress	Gradual	May be acute
Presence of symmetry	Asymmetrical	Symmetrical
Flexor spasm	Common	Absent

Contd...

Contd...

	Compressive	*Noncompressive*
Pattern of neurodeficit	U shaped	Bilaterally symmetrical
Bladder and bowel involvement	Early	Late
Classical examples	Caries spine	Transverse myelitis

Q. What is complete and incomplete SCI?

- Complete SCI is a type of SCI with no sensory or motor function present in sacral segments S4 and S5
- Incomplete SCI: If any of the above is present.

Q. What are the different types of incomplete SCI?

The different types of incomplete SCI are as follows:

1. ***Brown sequard syndrome:***
   - 2–4% of all traumatic SCI
   - Results from a lesion that causes a relative hemisection of the cord
   - Associated classically with stabbing but can occur from other causes also.

   Features:

   At the level of the injury:

   a. Ipsilateral loss of all sensory modalities.
   b. Ipsilateral motor loss (flacid paralysis).
   c. Contralateral sensory normal.
   d. Contralateral motor normal.

   Below the level:

   a. Ipsilateral loss of position and vibration sense.
   b. Contralateral loss of pain and temperature sensation.
   c. Ipsilateral motor loss (spasticity).

   Overall patients present with ipsilateral motor and proprioceptive loss and contralateral loss of pain and temperature.
2. ***Central cord syndrome:***
   - Most common incomplete SCI (9%)
   - Sacral sensory sparing
   - Upper limbs more weak than lower limbs
   - Variable loss of sensation, bowel, and bladder function.

   May occur at any age, most common in older age patients with cervical spondylosis who sustained hyperextension injury.
3. ***Anterior cord syndrome:***
   - Lesions affecting anterior 2/3rd of the spinal cord
   - Causes: Flexion injury, direct injury to anterior spinal cord, retro pulsed disk, anterior spinal artery lesion
   - Variable loss of motor and pain and temperature sensation
   - Preservation of proprioception and light touch and deep pressure sensation
   - Recovery: 10–20% chance of muscle recovery.
4. ***Posterior cord syndrome:***

   Least frequent syndrome.

   Injury to posterior column results in proprioceptive loss in muscle strength.

   (pain and temperature spared)

   Poor ambulation due to proprioceptive loss.

Q. What are the differences between conus medullaris and cauda equina syndrome?

Table 2.12: Comparison between conus medullaris and cauda equina

	Conus medullaris syndrome	*Cauda equina syndrome*
Location	T12–L1–2 vertebral level injury of sacral cord and lumbosacral nerve roots	Below L1–L2 to sacrum vertebral level injury of lumbosacral nerve roots
Causes	T12–L1 fracture Tumors, gliomas Vascular injury Spina bifida, tethering of the cord	Fracture at L1–L2 or below Sacral fractures Fracture of pelvic ring Can be associated with spondylosis
Signs and symptoms	1. Normal motor function of lower extremities unless S1–S2 motor involvement (since only involves S1–S5). Lower motor neuron lesion (LMN) results with lumbar root involvement 2. *Saddle distribution sensory loss (touch is spared)* 3. *Pain not a significant factor* 4. Symmetric abnormalities 5. *Bowel, bladder, and sexual dysfunction* 6. If a high conus lesion, bulbocavernosus reflex may be present 7. May be *hyperreflexic*	1. Flaccid paralysis of lower extremities of involved lumbosacral nerve roots Results in a LMN Lesion Areflexia in muscle groups affected 2. *Sensory loss in root distribution* 3. *Pain is a more significant feature* 4. Abnormalities may predominate on one side (asymmetric) 5. High cauda equina lesions (lumbar roots) Sparing bowel and bladder Lower lesions (S3–S5) causes areflexic bowel, bladder, and sexual dysfunction 6. *Bulbocavernosus reflex is absent (in low cauda equina [sacral] lesions)* 7. *Hyopreflexia or areflexia in affected muscle groups*
EMG	Normal EMG (except for external sphincter or S1, S2 involvement)	Findings show multiple root level involvement (Prognosis: Good)

Q. What is the importance of prehospital care in SCI?

Spinal immobilizations consisting of cervical collar, supports on either side of the head, the long and short backboards with associated straps to attach and immobilize the entire body to the board.

These are the core component of prehospital care.

Q. How will you manage an acute SCI in tertiary care set up?

- Immobilization of spine
- Input output maintainance
- Intravenous steroid
- Stabilization of spine if required
- Further rehab care.

Q. What is spinal instability?

It is the loss of the ability of the spine under physiological loads to maintain its pattern of displacement so that there is no initial or additional neurological deficit or no major deformity and no incapacitating pain.

Q. When is surgery considered for spinal instability?

- More than two spinal segments are affected
- Loss of vertebral height >50%
- Complete destruction of vertebra.

Q. What are the different surgical approaches?

There are mainly two types of approaches:

- Anterior approach.
- Posterior approach.

Q. Which approach is preferred when and why?

- Cervical spine: Anterior approach apparently preferable (But increased complication of recurrent laryngeal nerve palsy).
- Orthosis to be used for 3 months.
- Lumbar spine: Lower lumbar region: Anterior approach with thoracotomy or thoracoabdominal approach.
- Upper lumber region: Posterior approach.

Q. How will you manage this patient with SCI?

- Counselling and patient education
- Goal setting after discussion with patient and family
- Nutritional care
- Pharmacological management
  - Analgesics—Gabapentine, NSAID
  - Supportive—Multivitamin like methylcobalamine, L carnitine
  - Medication for complication:
    1. Orthostatic hypotension—NacL 1g BD, mineralocorticoid along with pressure garments.
    2. Heterotrophic ossification—NSAID, bisphosphonates, Radiation, surgery.
    3. Pneumonia—Antibiotics, bronchodilators.
    4. Autonomic dysreflexia—Antihypertensives, Removal of noxious stimuli.
    5. Reflux—PPI, H2 blockers, antacids, prokinetics.
    6. Impaired bowel evacuation—Laxatives, enemas.
    7. Spasticity—Baclofen, tizanidine, chemical neurolysis, botulinum toxin.
    8. DVT—Low molecular weight heparin (LMWH), warfarin
    9. Depression - SSRI
- Nonpharmacological management
  - Postural care:
    1. Positioning in bed
       - Patients at risk of developing pressure ulcers should be turned and repositioned every 2 hrs (when lying on side: 30 degrees laterally inclined position)
       - Prone position better if patient can tolerate
       - Positioning devices like pillow may be used
    2. Positioning in wheelchair
       - Must be re-positioned every hour
       - If possible patient should raise themselves from seat for 15 s every 30 mins
       - Anterior weight shift—Patients bend forward at waist
       - Lateral weight shift—Patient removes arm rest on one side and lean to that side and support with hand
       - Press up weight shift—Lifts his body with support of wrist and elbow.
  - DVT stocking
  - PT management:

    Exercise:
    1. PROM of all 4 limbs.
    2. Stretching of TA and Hamstrings.
    3. Deep breathing exercise.
    4. Stretching of the spastic muscles.
    5. Trunk muscle strengthening.
    6. Crutch muscle strengthening.
  - Modalities:
    1. TENS—For localized pain
    2. No other modalities required.
  - Robotics:
    1. Body weight supported treadmill training (BWSTT)
    2. Tilt table training.
  - Occupational therapy:
    1. Sitting balance.
    2. Transfer training.

3. Weight shifting.
4. Standing balance.
5. Wheelchair training.
6. Gait training.
7. ADL training.
8. IADL training.

- Orthotic support:
  As per the NLI level like.

Table 2.13: Orthosis as per NLI

NLI (Complete)	*Orthosis And Mobility Aids*
T4 – T6	Standing table THKAFO
T9 – T12	HKAFO KAFO with crutches
L2, 3, 4	KAFO with crutches
L4, 5	AFO with crutches

Q. What are the different approaches to occupational therapy according to the phases of SCI?

Acute phase:
- Stabilizing spine
- Splinting.

Active phase:
- AROM maintenance
- Prevention of elbow and wrist contracture
- Initiation of weight bearing
- Focus on strengthening elbow extensors (wheelchair, trunk elevation)
- Hand function retraining
- Bed mobility
- Wheelchair transfer technique
- Wheelchair modification
- Training of sexual position.

Extended rehab phase:
- Wheelchair evaluation
- Modification of home, work place, etc.
- Psychological support
- Use of assistive device.

Q. What are the crutch muscles?
- Shoulder depressors, extensors, adductors and abductors
- Elbow and wrist extensors
- Finger flexors.

Q. What are the different types of electronic wheelchair?

A. Power assisted:
   - Power source external
   - Add on device
   - Less cost than fully powered
   - Less weight.

B. Power wheelchair
   - Conventional power wheelchair
   - Folding and transporting power wheelchair
   - Combination indoor and outdoor power wheelchair
   - Heavy duty indoor and outdoor power wheelchair.

Q. What are the different types of base selection in power wheelchair?

1. Rear wheel drive.
   - Large drive wheel in the rear
   - Small pivoting casters in front
   - Naturally tracks straight
   - Preferred for those using special input device
   - Large turning radius
   - Difficulty in climbing small obstacles
2. Front wheel drive
   - Large drive wheel in front
   - Small pivoting casters in front
   - Stable for uneven and hilly areas
   - Medium turning radius
   - Tendency to fish tail in high speeds
3. Medium wheel drive
   - Drive wheel in center
   - Turns on center
   - Increased maneurvality
   - Suspended anterior tip wheels clears obstacles
   - Possibility to get stuck on front and rear wheels in uneven surface.

Q. What are the various input methods?

A. Proportional control continuous adjustment of speed and direction requires fine motor skill.

B. Switch control
   - Responds to discreet position of joy stick
   - Speed not directly controllable
   - For those with limited motor control
   - Can be operated by chin, head, shoulders, elbows, arms, knee, foot.

C. Integrated control.

Q. What are the types proportional control?
- Position sensing: Proportional to deflection from neutral.
- Force sensing: For people with tremor, spasm and decreased range of motion.

Q. What is the indication of steroid and dose of steroid in SCI?
- Ideally started within 3 hours of trauma. Dose—30 mg/kg bolus dose followed by 5.4mg/kg/h. for 23 hours

- If started between 3–8 hours. Same but should be continued for 48 hours.

Q. Which antispastic medicine would you prefer?
- Baclofen
- Tizanidine
  See Page number 12.

Q. Is there any other method/drug-delivery system for control of intractable spasticity?
- Liquid baclofen delivered from a pump, known as baclofen pump
- In lower abdominal wall, through a catheter tunneled around to the spine and then into the intrathecal space through the lumbar spinal canal up to T10 vertebral level.

Q. What are the advantages and disadvantages of baclofen pump?
- Advantages:
  - Increase in potency
  - Excellent spasticity control
  - Decreased side effects
- Disadvantages:
  - Invasive nature
  - Increased cost
  - Increased complications.

Q. What are the complications of baclofen pump?
- Kinking
- Chemical meningitis
- Leakage
- Pump failure
- Displacement
- Fracture pump.

Q. What is the dose of intrathecal baclofen pump in management of SCI?
- Trial dose of 50\microgram
- Evaluated for 6 hours
- If MAS improved by 2 then it can be considered significant
- If there is no improvement, dose is increased to 75 microgram
- Dosage is twice the value the patient responded over 24 hours, or thrice the value the patient responded for 8 hours.

Q. What are the different delivery systems of baclofen pump?

Table 2.14: Different types of baclofen pump

Electronic	*Mechanical*
Programmable	Not programmable
Dosing can be changed	To change the dose the concentration of baclofen is changed
Requires programmer	No programmer is required
Requires battery	No battery is required
Requires regular charging	Better for geographically isolated areas

Q. Why flushing and sweating occurred in this patient?
Due to autonomic dysreflexia.

Q. What is autonomic dysreflexia?
- Autonomic dysreflexia is a potentially dangerous clinical syndrome that develops in individuals with spinal cord injury resulting in acute, uncontrolled hypertension
- It develops in individuals with a neurologic level of SCI at or above T6 due to an imbalanced reflex sympathetic discharge, leading to potentially life-threatening hypertension.

Q. What are the signs and symptoms of autonomic dysreflexia?
- Symptoms:
  Severe headache, blurred vision, spots in visual fields, nasal congestion, anxiety, sense of impending doom, goosebumps
- Signs:
  Rapid rise BP 20–40 mmHg above patient's baseline, bradycardia, cardiac arrhythmias, profuse diaphoresis, piloerection, flushing of skin.

Q. What are the risk factors for it?
- Bladder distention
- Urinary tract infection
- Calculus
- Cystoscopy/instrumentation
- Epididymitis or scrotal compression
- Blocked catheter
- Bowel distention
- Bowel impaction
- Bowel instrumentation
- Invasive testing
- Hemorrhoids

- Appendicitis or other intra-abdominal pathology/ trauma
- Anal fissure
- Pressure ulcers
- Ingrown toenail
- Burns or sunburn
- Blisters
- Insect bites
- Contact with hard or sharp objects
- Temperature fluctuations
- Constrictive clothing, shoes, or appliances
- Menstruation
- Pregnancy—Especially labor and delivery
- Vaginitis
- Sexual intercourse
- Ejaculation
- Deep vein thrombosis
- Heterotopic bone
- Fractures or other skeletal trauma.

Q. What is the management of this condition?

- Locate and remove stimuli
- Antihypertensive medications
- Look for complications.

Q. What antihypertensives will you use?

- GTN: 1 spray of GTN (400mcg), or ½ tab sublingual (300mcg), or 5 mg /24 hr transdermal patch. *The dose can be repeated if no effect after 5–10 mins. Up to 3 dose can be given in 30 mins*
- Captopril: Administered sublingually as 25mg effectively lowers BP within 15 minutes of administration
- Nifedepine: Chew and swallow 1 nifedipine 10mg tablet (not slow release tablet) with water
- Other agents hydralazine, clonidine,terazosin can be used
- **Parenteral therapy:**
  - *Labetolol:* 20 mg IV over 2 minutes, may be repeated after 10 min, (maximum dose 300mg)
  - *Esmolol:* 250–500 mvg/kg bolus iv over 1–3 min followed by 50mcg/kg/min for 4 min
  - *Phentolamine:* Bolus 5–20 mg iv every 5 min followed by continuous 0.2–0.5 mg iv per min
  - *Nitroprusside*: 0.3-0.5 mcg/kg/min infusion.

Q. What is pressure sore and how will u grade it?

It is defined as localized injury to the skin and/or underlying tissue, usually over a bony prominence as a result of pressure or pressure combined with shear and/or friction.

Gradings given in Chapter 11, Page no. 260.

Q. What are the preventive strategies used in pressure sore?

- Two hourly positional change
- Air/Water mattress
- Avoiding friction and shear
- Weight shifts in wheelchair
- Reclining wheelchair
- Tilt in space wheelchair.

Q. What are the risk factors of pressure ulcer?

Extrinsic

- Applied pressure
- Surface shear
- Friction
- Local microenvironment
- Psychological.

Intrinsic

- Anemia
- Impaired nutritional status
- Impaired vascular status
- Muscle atrophy
- Impaired mobility and sensation.

Q. How will you manage pressure ulcer?

- Removal of risk factors
- Proper nutrition
- Regular dressing (avoid iodine and hydrogen peroxide except for infected and necrotic debris)
- Wet to dry dressing
- Keeping area moistened with hydrocolloidal substances
- Modalities—Infrared radiation, UST, SWD
- Surgeries.

Q. What are the corrective surgeries done?

- Primary direct closure
- Skin grafting—
  - Partial thickness or split- thickness skin graft
  - Full thickness skin graft
- Skin flaps
- Free flaps
- Musculocutaneous flaps and fasciocutaneous flaps
- Amputation and fillet procedures.

Q. What is the bowel management in this patient of SCI?

As it is a UMN lesion, the following management is done

- Dietary fiber—15g/day
- Fluid—40mL/kg/day + 500mL
- Use of gastrocolic reflex (started 20 min after meal)

- Use of rectocolic reflex (digital stimulation)
- Use of laxatives and stool softeners
- Empty bladder before starting
- Setting up padded commode or side lying
- Cleaning stool from rectum and inserting enema
- Followed by digital stimulation.

Q. How will you manage bladder problems in SCI? What is the ideal target in management?

An ideal bladder should have

- A low pressure drainage
- Continence
- Synergia between sphincter and bladder
- No renal functional deterioration.

Q. How will you manage this patient with a UMN bladder?

- Behavioral—Timed voiding, limited fluid intake
- Pharmacological—Anticholinergics
- Supportive—Clean intermittent catheterization (CIC)
- Surgical—Urinary diversion, augmentation.

Q. What are the steps for CIC?

- Setting up instruments
- Washing hands
- Inserting catheter with 2% lignocaine gel
- Maintaining resistance while inserting
- Bladder evacuation
- Washing the catheter with soap water
- Drying in gunny bag/glass container.

Q. What are the advantages of CIC?

- Increased self image
- Conducive for sexual activity
- Decreased incidence of UTI, bladder stones
- Decreased incidence of cancer.

Q. When will you prefer indwelling catheter over CIC?

- Poor hand skill
- High fluid intake
- Cognitive impairment
- No caregiver
- Low bladder capacity
- Increased detrussor pressure
- Temporary management of vesicouteric reflex

Q. How will you screen your patient for renal dysfunction?

- Blood for urea, creatinine
- Urine for R/E, M/E, C/S.
- Renal sonogram every 2 year
- Cystoscope every 2 year
- UDS to monitor pressure.

Q. What do you mean by balanced bladder?

- Low pressure storage
- Continence
- Minimizing risk of infection
- Minimizing upper tract deterioration.

Q. What are the advantages of indwelling suprapubic catheter?

- Catheter can be changed without undressing
- Tube less likely to be kinked
- No interference with sexual activity
- Much comfortable and easier to clean
- Decreased urethral stricture, irritation and epididymitis.

Q. What are the sexual issues in SCI?

- Erection
- Copulation
- Ejaculation
- Fertilization.

Q. How can you help this patient maintain an adequate erection?

- Topical erectogenic medicine
- PDE5 inhibitors
- Vaccum and ring devices
- Intracorporeal prostaglandin injections
- Penile implants.

Q. What are the various methods of ejaculation?

- Autonomic ejaculation
- Somatic ejaculation
- Vibratory ejaculation
- Electro ejaculation.

Q. What are the different methods of fertilization?

- In vitro fertilization
- Gametocyte intrafallopian transfer (GIFT)
- Intracytoplasmic sperm injection (ICSI)
- Intrauterine insemination.

Q. What are the complications in SCI?

- Thromboembolic disorders
- Pneumonia
- Respiratory failure
- Sleep apnea
- Orthostatic hypotension
- Autonomic dysreflexia
- Immobilization hypercalcemia

- GI complications—Stress ulcer, adynamic ileus, superior mesentric artery syndrome, gall stones
- GU complications—UTI, bladder stones, renal stones
- Osteoporosis
- Fracture
- Heterotrophic ossification
- Impaired thermoregulation (above T6)—automomic dysreflexia
- Anemia
- Pressure ulcer
- Spasticity
- Pain.

Q. Mention the causes of death in SCI patient?

- Tetraplegia—Pneumonia
- Paraplegia—Heart disease > Septicemia > Suicide.

Q. How does occupational therapist help patients of SCI?

See page 19.

Q. What are the tendon transfer surgeries done in SCI patient?

Table 2.15: Tendon surgeries commonly done in SCI

NLI	*Tendon transfered*	*Function acheived*
C5	BR to ECRB Deltoid to triceps	Wrist extension Elbow extension
C6	BR to FPL Post deltoid to triceps	Lat pinch and grasp Elbow extension
C7	BR to FPL ECRL/FCU to FDP	Lat pinch and grasp Hook
C8	Not required	

Abbreviations: BR, brachioradialis; ECBR, extensor carpi radialis brevis; FPL, flexor pollicis longus; ECRL, extensor carpi radialis longus; FDP, flexor digitorum profundus; FCU, flexor carpi ulnaris

Q. What are the good prognostic criterias in SCI?

- Incomplete injury
- Initial better muscle power
- Lower NLI.

Q. What are the features of prolonged immobilization?

- Muscle:
  - Strength declines 1–3%/day
  - 10–25% per week (plateaus at 35–50% in 3–5 wks)
  - Greater in antigravity muscles (quadriceps, back extensors, plantar flexors)
  - Type 1 (slow twitch, oxidative) muscles are more affected
  - ↓ glycogen, ↓ oxidative enzyme, ↓ mitochondrial function.
  - Decreased size of muscle fibers and reduction of muscle mass
  - Reduction of muscle protein synthesis
  - Reduction of the synthesis of collagen fibers
  - Increase titin
- Contracture:
  - Myogenic contracture: A shortening of resting muscle length
  - Arthrogenic contracture: Pathologic process involving joint components, or synovial inflammation
  - Soft-tissue contracture: Cutaneous, subcutaneous and loose connective tissue around the joint may become contracted
- Bone:
  - Osteoporosis
  - Immobilization hypercalcemia
- Cardiovascular system:
  - Increase resting heart rate
  - Increase heart rate response to submaximal exercise
  - Orthostatic hypotension
  - Decrease stroke volume and cardiac output
  - Decrease VO2 max
  - NO CHANGE in systolic and mean blood pressure
  - Deep vein thrombosis
- Respiratory system:
  - Decrease diaphragmatic and chest wall movement
  - Weakness of respiratory and abdominal muscles
  - Contracture of chest wall
  - Potential decrease in lung volumes and impaired cough
  - Risk for atelectasis and pneumonia
- Gastrointestinal system:
  - Loss of appetite
  - Slow rate of absorption
  - Increased transit time in esophagus, stomach and small bowel
  - Constipation
- Genitourinary system:
  - Diuresis
  - Urinary retention
  - Bladder or renal stone, UTI
  - Hypercalciuria

- Central nervous system:
  - Alteration in mental concentration, orientation to space and time and other intellectual function
  - Restlessness, anxiety, decrease pain tolerance, irritability, insomnia and depression
  - Lack of judgment, problem solving and learning ability, psychomotor skills and memory.

Q. What is post-traumatic syringomyelia?

In traumatic SCI, syringomyelic changes occur after months to decades initiated by cord hematoma, residual stenosis or kyphotic changes. The cyst extends both cranially and caudally compressing the structures from inside to outwards.

Q. What are its clinical features?

- Ascending sensory loss
- Dissociated sensory loss
- Ascending loss of deep tendon reflex
- Radiating pain
- Worsening or decrease in spasticity
- Worsening of orthostatic hypotension.

Q. Will you be worried if your patient suddenly has a decrease in spasticity without any intervention with ascending sensory loss and loss of DTRs? If so, why?

Yes, it may be due to post-traumatic syringomyelia.

Q. What is dissociated sensory loss? Why it occurs?

- Impaired pain and temperature sensation but intact touch, position, and vibration sense
- This is because the ascending fibers of the lateral spinothalamic tract (pain and temperature) are earlier involved in the syrinx.

Q. What is its management?

Investigations

Imaging: MRI to confirm

Conservative treatment:

- Close monitoring
- Pain control
- Activity restrictions include avoiding maneuvers that increase intra-thoracic/abdominal pressure, avoid high-force exercise like valsalva, Crede, and quad coughing
- Avoiding anterior weight reliefs and weight lifting.

Surgical treatment:

- Shunting (syringo-subarachnoid, syringo-pleural, or syringo-peritoneal)
- Reconstructing the subarachnoid space with dissection of arachnoiditis/meningeal scarring and duraplasty, and cordectomy.

Q. What are long segment myelitis? Mention its etiology?

When demyelination extends in more than three segments of spinal cord it is called long segment myelitis.

Causes are:

- Neuromyelitis optica (NMO)
- Transverse myelitis complete form
- MS (generally short segment)

Q. What is transverse myelitis?

Acute transverse myelitis may be defined as an idiopathic inflammatory disorder causing symmetric spinal cord dysfunction below a specific level of cord function.

Q. Mention the diagnostic features? What are the investigations to be done and management?

Signs and symptoms:

- Very often following a viral illness
- Onset is acute or subacute
- Girdle-like sensation but absence of root pain, spinal deformity
- Early bladder involvement.

Investigation:

- Blood—CBC, CRP, LFT, urea, creatinine, ANA, and other autoantibodies
- Urine—R/E, M/E, C/S
- CSF study
- MRI—Brain and spinal cord.

Management:

- Steroids
- Plasma exchange
- IV immunoglobulin
- Rituximab
- Azathioprine
- Cyclophosphamide.

Rehabilitation: As described in SCI.

Q. What are the assessments done in wheelchair?

See Chapter 4, page number 145

Q. Measurement of wheelchair?

See Chapter 4, page number 145

Q. What are the orthosis used to stabilize the spine?

See Chapter 4, page number 131

Q. If the patient improves, what are the orthotic support to be used?

See Chapter 4, Page number 131

Q. What are components of PWD Act?

PWD act

Chapter I Preliminary
Chapter II The Central Coordination Committee
Chapter III The State Coordination Committee
Chapter IV Prevention And Early Detection Of Disabilities
Chapter V Education
Chapter VI Employment
Chapter VII Affirmative Action
Chapter VIII Non-discrimination
Chapter IX Research And Manpower Development
Chapter X Recognition Of Institutions For Persons With Disabilities
Chapter XI Institution For Persons With Severe Disabilities
Chapter XII The Chief Commissioner And Commissioners For Persons With Disabilities
Chapter XIII Social Security
Chapter XIV Miscellaneous

QUADRIPARESIS (GB SYNDROME)

A 14-years-old boy from lower socioeconomic class presented with sudden-onset flaccid quadraparesis for last two weeks with gradual progression which was ascending in nature. This episode was preceeded by a febrile illness asscociated with cough and coryza. This boy became very sick with associated facial weakness and little bit of respiratory difficulty and urinary incontinence. He was shifted to pediatric ICU, where he received intravenous injections for few days. There after his weakness improved a little bit. There after he has been shifted to rehabilitative ward for further care. Now his bladder and bowel is continent and respiration and feeding has been established. He is the only child of his parents. His family lives in a remote village in a pucca house with bathroom to living room distance of 10 feet and a staircase in the entrance of their house. Currently he studies in class IX and is worried about his board exam in next year. On examinations his GCS is 15/15, FIM Score of 80/126. Cranial nerves are within normal limits with hyporeflexia and flexor planter. Gross motor power is 1/5 in both upper limb and 2/5 in both lower limb without any sensory deficit. There is no tendo achilis or hamstring tightness at present. He is enjoying games lying on his bed.

P/D: Acute onset polyneuropathy probably AIDP with FIM score of 80/126

D/D:
1. AMAN variety of GBS.
2. Pure motor polyneuropathy.

Q. What are the etiopathogenesis of pure motor variety of polyneuropathy?

- Carcinomatosis
- Lead
- Porphyria
- Diptheria
- Charcot Marie Tooth disease.

Q. Most common causes of peripheral neuropathy in adults?

1. Diabetes mellitus.
2. Carcinomatosis.
3. Vit B12 deficiency (SCD).
4. Alcoholism.
5. Drugs:
   - INH
   - Nitrofurantoin
   - Amidarone
   - Vinblastin
   - Ethambutol
   - Chloramphenicol.

Other rare causes:
- Polyarthritis nodusa.
- Rheumatoid arthritis.
- Amyloidosis.

Q. Definition of GBS?

GBS is a progressive, symmetrical weakness of the limbs, with hyporeflexia or areflexia, with or without sensory abnormalities with maximum weakness occuring within 4 weeks, although typically peaks by 2 weeks. Two thirds of patients have an antecedent infection with three weeks of onset of weakness and most commonly identified infectious agent is *Campylobacter jejuni*.

Q. How did the name GBS come?

Based on mane of French neurologists Guillain, Barré, and Strohl.

Q. Different Types of GBS?

Table 2.16: Types of GBS

Types	*Clinical Features*	*Incidence*	*Antibodies*	*NCS/EMG*
Acute inflammatory demyelinating polyradiculoneuropathy (AIDP)	• Symmetrical weakness of all limbs • Hyporeflexia, • Areflexia • Mild sensory symptoms • Respiratory involvement • Facial nerve palsy	Most common in Europe and US (90%)	Anti-GM1	Demyelination NCS SNAP: Abnormal CMAP: Abnormal, Temporal Dispersion:Increased F wave: Abnormal—(first electrodiagnostic sign) EMG Normal
Axonal (AMAN, ASMAN)	Symmetrical weakness Reflexes may be normal or increased Variable sensory symptoms Respiratory involvement	Around 5 % but in ASIA its around 30% of all cases	Anti-GM1, GD1a, Ga1Nac GD1a	Axonal NCS SNAP: Normal CMAP: Abnormal EMG Abnormal activity (fibrillation potentials) ASMAN : SNAP Abnormal Rest Same
Miller Fisher	Ophthalmoplegia Ataxia Areflexia Minimal weakness		Anti-GQ1b	Demyelinating NCS SNAP: normal CMAP: normal Facial & trigeminal axonopathy *(Brainstem auditory evoked potential study -peripheral auditory and brainstem involvement)*

Q. What investigations do you suggest in a case of GBS?

1. Rotine blood test.
2. Urine RE/ME/CS.
3. Chest Xray.
4. CSF study: Albuminocytologic dissociation.
5. NCS (Demylenating polyneuropathy).

Q. What is albuminocytologic dissociation?

An elevated CSF protein with normal white blood cell (WBC) count (<5 to 10 × 10_6 cells/L) is referred to as albuminocytologic dissociation.

Q. How will you manage a case of GBS?

- Counseling
- Education of patient party and family
- Nutritional care
- Investigations: As described above
- Management:

A. Pharmacological.
B. Nonpharmacological.

A. Pharmacological:

1. Intravenous immunoglobulin/Plasmapheresis.
2. Antibiotics.
3. Supportive therapy: 25% cases will require ventilatary support.

B. Nonpharmacological.

PT:

Exercise:

- PROM of all limbs with power 0/5
- AAROM of other limbs
- Deep breathing exercise
- Postural care
- TA and Hamstring stretching
- Care of pressure sore (if any)
- Bladder and bowel care.

Modalities:

Electric stimulations to affected limbs after 2 weeks.

OT: Acute stage

- Positioning in anticontracture position
- Maintenance of normal ROM.
- Sub acute stage
- Initiation of AROM in gravity eliminated plain to normal ROM.
- Initiation of sitting balance and weight bearing of joints.

After AROM is achieved strengthening protocol of all major muscles initiated

- Hand function training started and ADL training started
- Sitting balance to standing balance started
- When independent standing is achieved gait training initiated with assistive device to independent walking and staircase climbing started
- Strengthening protocol is maintained and return to work protocol initiated after proper work evaluation.

PO:
- AFO
- PLS (see orthosis section).

Recreational therapy.
Vocational training .

Q. Describe the dose and durations of IVIG?

It is administered at 0.4 g/kg daily for five consecutive days.

Q. What is the role of oral steroid in GBS?

No role in GBS. [But has role in CIDP (described later)].

Q. Why modalities should be started after 2 weeks?

1. To give time for spontaneous recovery.
2. To prevent abnormal sprouting.
   (Wallarian degenation completed by 2 weeks period)

Q. What is the recovery pattern in GBS?

Recovery pattern is from distal to proximal.

Q. Mention the prognostic factors in GBS?

- Prognosis of GBS is generally good
- *Persistent disability* is seen in 20% of patients. Those remain nonambulatory or require an assistive device to walk at 6 months
- *Poor outcome* is seen with patients of advanced age, male gender, axonal involvement, antecedent diarrhea, and CMV infection *(Relapse rate is 3–5%).*

Q. Name the possible complications in GBS?

- Deep venous thrombosis
- Cardiac arrhythmias
- Neuropathic pain
- Pressure ulcers
- Contractures
- Swallowing difficulty
- Respiratory failure.

Q. What are the types of neuropathy based on distributions?

- Polyneuropathy: Wide spread and symmetrical dysfunction of peripheral nerves
- Mononeuropathy: Involves single peripheral nerve
- Multiple mononeuropathy (mononeuropathy multiplex): Multifocal involvement of individual peripheral nerves
- Plexopathies: Multiple peripheral nerves in asymmetric fashion.

Q. Name some predominantly motor neuropathy ?

- Inflammatory/demyelinating
  - GBS or CIDP with motor predominance (common)
  - Multifocal neuropathy with persistent conduction block (includes multifocal motor neuropathy).
- *Infection-associated*
  - Diphtheria
  - Metabolic
  - Porphyria
- *Hypoglycemia-associated neuropathy*
- *Toxic*
  - Lead, mercury
  - Dapsone
  - Delayed neurotoxicity after organophosphate poisoning.
- *Neoplasm-associated*
  - Lymphoma-associated motor neuropathy
  - Paraprotein-associated motor neuropathy
  - POEMS syndrome.
- Genetically determined
  - CMT-1, CMT-2 (sensory features often overshadowed by motor involvement).

Q. Name some predominantly sensory neuropathy?

Inflammatory
- Idiopathic Inflammatory polyganglionopathy (IPG) not associated with malignancy
- Sjogren's syndrome (can be associated with IPG).

Neoplasia-associated
- Paraneoplastic sensory ganglionopathy
- Paraprotein associated
- Infiltration with lymphoma/leukemia
- Early amyloid neuropathy (small fiber).

Infection-associated
- HIV distal predominantly sensory neuropathy (DPSN)
- Leprosy (some)
- Lyme disease (some).

Endocrine
- Diabetes (small fiber, large fiber, or both)
- Hypothyroidism (some).

Organ dysfunction
- Uremia (early)
- Liver disease (including primary biliary cirrhosis).

Nutritional
- B12 deficiency
- Pyridoxine excess
- Thiamine deficiency (atypical cases)
- Strachans syndrome/Cuban neuropathy (multinutrient deficiency)
- Vitamin E deficiency
- Malaborption associated with Celiac disease (without evident vitamin deficiency).

Toxins
- Cis-platinum
- Chloramphenicol
- Metronidazole
- Isoniazid, ethionamide
- Nitrous oxide (produces a B12 deficiency state)
- Thalidomide, ethylene oxide
- Chlorpyrifos (organophosphate insecticide), Taxol
- Vacor.

Genetically determined
- Associated with spinocerebellar degeneration, especially Friedreich's ataxia
- Hereditary sensory and autonomic neuropathies (several types)
- Fabry's disease
- Tangier disease (pleomorphic clinical features)
- Familial amyloid neuropathy (early)
- Some mitochondrial diseases.

Q. Mention the causes of death of GBS?

Mortality rate is 10%. *The main causes are infections, pulmonary embolus, and cardiac arrhythmia.*

Q. What is CIDP?

It is an acronym for chronic inflammatory demyelinating polyneuropathy.

Q. What are the clinical features of CIDP?

- Over a period of 2 months motor symptoms generally predominate, and both proximal and distal muscles are affected
- As CIDP is mainly demyelinating disorder, muscle atrophy is uncommon
- Reflexes are reduced or absent
- Cranial involvement is seen in 10–20% of cases, with a small number of patients having painful dysesthesias
- Sensory involvement is typically seen in large fiber nerves, affecting vibration and proprioception mainly. Sensory symptoms generally shows progression from distal to proximal with hand involvement is often perceived earlier than feet
- The classic course of CIDP is recurrence and remittance (polyphasic), mainly in younger patients
- Older adults are more likely to have a progressive form of CIDP (monophasic).

Q. What are the investigations generally done in CIDP?

- Electrodiagnostic studies are needed for confirmation of CIDP. NCS shows primary demyelination in multiple segments mainly conduction block (*conduction slowing that is greater than can be explained by axon loss, prolonged F wave and H reflex latencies, and temporal dispersion of CMAP between proximal and distal stimulation points)*
- Sural nerve biopsy can show demyelination and to rule out other pathology but is rarely done
- Lumbar puncture shows albuminocytologic dissociation in 90% of patients
- Magnetic resonance imaging (MRI) with gadolinium of the brachial and lumbar plexi and cauda equina can reveal enhancing or enlarged nerves.

Q. What is the treatment of CIDP?

Mainly IVIG and plasma exchange is used. Most patients require repeated treatment at 2–6 weeks to prevent relapse.

Corticosteroids are useful in preventing relapse but Should not be used in pure motor variety.

Q. What are the types of descending polyneuropathy?

- Polio
- Botulinum
- Diptheria.

Q. What is autonomic neuropathy?

Autonomic neuropathies are a collection of syndromes and diseases affecting autonomic neurons, may be parasympathetic, sympathetic, or both. It can be hereditary or acquired in nature.

Etiology

A. Inherited autonomic neuropathies

- Familial amyloid polyneuropathy
- Hereditary sensory autonomic neuropathy
- Fabry disease
- Acute intermittent porphyria and variegate porphyria.

B. Acquired autonomic neuropathies

- Primary acquired autonomic neuropathies
  - Pandysautonomia:
  - Idiopathic distal small-fiber neuropathy
  - Holmes-Adie syndrome and Ross syndrome:
  - Chronic idiopathic anhidrosis.
  - Amyloid neuropathy
  - Postural orthostatic tachycardia syndrome.
- **Secondary acquired autonomic neuropathies**
  - Diabetes mellitus
  - Uremic neuropathy
  - Hepatic disease–related neuropathy
- Deficiency of vitamin B_{12} neuropathy
- Toxic and drug-induced
  - Vincristine, cisplatin, carboplatin, vinorelbine, paclitaxel, and suramin
  - Alcohol.
- **Infectious diseases**
  - Lyme disease
  - HIV infection
  - Chagas disease
  - Botulism
  - Diphtheria.
- **Others**
  - Leprosy
  - Celiac disease
  - Sjögren syndrome
  - Rheumatoid arthritis, systemic lupus erythematosus
  - Guillain-Barré syndrome
  - Lambert-Eaton myasthenic syndrome
  - Paraneoplastic autonomic neuropathy
  - Inflammatory bowel disease.

Q. What is mononeuritis multiplex and its etiology?

Mononeuritis multiplex is a painful, asymmetrical, asynchronous sensory and motor peripheral neuropathy involving isolated damage to at least two separate areas of same nerve.

Etiologies:

- Diabetes mellitus
- Vasculitis
- Amyloidosis
- Direct tumor involvement—Lymphoma, leukemia
- Polyarteritis nodosa
- Rheumatoid arthritis
- Systemic lupus erythematosus
- Paraneoplastic syndromes.

QUADRIPLEGIA (CEREBRAL PALSY)

Summary

This 7-year-old boy born of nonconsanguineous marriage from upper socioeconomic status with risk factors of preterm delivery and low birth weight, presented with weakness of all for limbs with lower limbs more involved than upper limbs and delayed developmental mile stones since birth. Just after birth he became little bit bluish and he received oxygen supplementation for one day and was discharged on day 5. Then his parents noticed the gradual onset weakness of all four limbs associated with floppy neck even after 6 months of age. The child was not able to sit or stand till 3 years of age and had toilet control at age of 6 years. His immunization history is up to date. He is currently ambulatory only in house and cannot go out and is studying at home. He had past history of seizure for which he has been taking anticonvulsants regularly. Previously he had received botulinum toxin injections to control spasticity in both the lower limbs. His FIM score is 100/126.

On examination he is alert and playful with good built and nutrition. He has spasticity in all four limbs with lower limbs involved greater than upper limbs. He has a crouch gait. His intelligence level is normal. He has tightness of ITB. His planter is extensor with exaggerated jerks in all four limbs. Upper limb power is 5/5 but lower limb could not be assessed due to spasticity. Sensory system is within normal limits.

P/D: Cerebral palsy (CP) with FIM Score 100/126.

D/D: Hypoxic ischemic encephalopathy.

Q. What is CP?

Cerebral palsy describes a group of permanent disorders of the development of movement and posture, causing activity limitation, that are attributed to non-progressive disturbances that occurred in the developing fetal or infant brain. The motor disorders of CP are often accompanied by disturbances of sensation, perception, cognition, communication, and behavior, by epilepsy, and by secondary musculoskeletal problems.

Q. Who coined the term CP?

The term cerebral palsy was first used in 1843 by English orthopedic surgeon William Little in a series of lectures entitled 'deformities of the human frame'.

Q. What is the other name of CP?

CP was known for many years as 'Little's disease'

Q. What are the types of CP?

Based on distribution/involvement of limbs

- **Hemiplegic CP:** A unilateral upper and lower limb distribution (with upper limb involvement > lower limbs)
- **Quadriplegic CP or tetraplegic CP:** Bilateral upper and lower limb distribution (all limbs equally involved)
- **Diplegic CP:** Bilateral lower extremity distribution. (upper limb can be involved but << lower limbs)
- **Triplegic CP:** Used to state when bilateral lower limb with asymmetrical involvement of upper limb.
- Based on tone:
  - Spastic
  - Dyskinetic
  - Athetoid
  - Choreiform
  - Ballistic
  - Ataxic.
- Hypotonic
- "Mixed".

Q. Difference between CP and HIE?

Hypoxic-ischemic encephalopathy, or HIE, is the brain injury caused by oxygen deprivation to the brain, also commonly known as intrapartum asphyxia. It may result into CP in 9% cases.

Q. What are the etiologies of CP?

There are mainly five types of risk factors.

Preconception

- Maternal seizures
- Intellectual disability
- Thyroid disorders
- History of still birth or neonatal death
- Maternal age >40
- Low socioeconomic status.

Antenatal

- Birthdefects
- Small for gestational age
- Low birth weight
- Placental abnormalities
- Maternal disease during pregnancy
- Abnormalities in fluid volume
- Maternal bleeding in 2nd and 3rd trimester
- Hypertension
- Preeclampsia
- Chorioamnionitis.

Postnatal

- Stroke
- Abusive head trauma
- Bacterial meningitis.

Intrapartum

- Birth hypoxia
- Meconium staining
- Meconium aspiration
- Abnormal duration of labor
- Fetal presentation.

Neonatal

- Seizures
- Respiratory distress
- Hypoglycemia
- Infections
- Jaundice.

Q. What are the other causes of spastic quadriparesis in young boy?

- Cervical injury
- Malignancy at cervical level
- Hereditary spastic paresis
- Tumors at cervical level.

Q. What are the primitive reflexes?

- Primitive reflexes are body postures dictated by head position
- Seen at birth, more elicitable in the first 2–3 months
- Start to fade by 4–6 months
- The ability to obtain the reflex on every attempt or the infant's persistence in the reflex posture more than 30 seconds considered abnormal at any age.

Q. Mention the types of primitive reflexes?

Table 2.17: Types of Primitive reflexes

	Purpose	*Appears at*	*Integrate by*	*Sign of retention*
Moro reflex	Primitive fight or flight reaction	at birth	2–4 months	Hypersensitivity, hyper reactivity, poor impulse control, sensory overload, social and emotional immaturity
Rooting reflex	Automatic response to turn towards food	at birth	3–4 months	
Palmar reflex	Automatic flexing of fingers to grab	at birth	5–6 months	Difficulty with fine motor skills, poor manual dexterity, messy handwriting

Contd...

Contd...

	Purpose	*Appears at*	*Integrate by*	*Sign of retention*
Asymmetric tonic neck reflex	To assist baby through birth canal and develop cross pattern movements	at birth	6 months	
Spinal gallant reflex	Assist baby with birth process	at birth	3–9 months	Unilateral or bilateral postural issues, fidgetting, bedwetting, poor concentration, poor short-term memory
Tonic labyrinthine reflex	Basis for head management and postural stability using major muscle group	in utero	31/2 years	Poor muscle tone, tendency to walk on toes, poor balance, motion sickness, spatial orientation problem
Landau reflex	Assist with posture development	4–5 months	1 year	Poor motor development
Symmetric tonic neck reflex	Preparation of crawling	6–9 months	9–11 months	Tendency to slamp while sitting, poor muscle tone, poor eye hand coordination, inability to sit still and concentrate
Parachute reflex	To protect itself	6 months	Persist lifelong	

Q. What are the normal developmental mile stone?

Table 2.18: Normal developmental milestones

Physical	*Cognitive*	*Social*
Newborn: rough, random, uncoordinated, reflexive movement	sensori-motor: physically explores environment to learn about it; repeats movements to master them, which also stimulates brain cell development	Attachment: baby settles when parent comforts; toddler seeks comfort from parent, safe-base exploration
3 months: head at 90 degree angle, uses arms to prop; visually track through midline	4-5 months: coos, curious and interested in environment	
5 months: purposeful grasp; roll over; head lag disappears; reaches for objects; transfer objects from hand to hand; plays with feet; exercises body by stretching, moving; touch genitals, rock on stomach for pleasure		5 months: responsive to social stimuli; facial expressions of emotion
7 months: sits in "tripod"; push head and torso up off the floor; support weight on legs; "raking" with hands	6 months: babbles and imitates sounds	
9 months: gets to and from sitting; crawls, pulls to standing; stooping and recovering; fingerthumb opposition; eyehand coordination, but no hand preference	9 months: discriminates between parents and others; trial and error problem solving	9 months: socially interactive; plays games (i.e., pattycake) with caretakers
12 months: walking	12 months: beginning of symbolic thinking; points to pictures in books in response to verbal cue; object permanence; some may use single words; receptive language more advanced than expressive language	11 months: stranger anxiety; separation anxiety; solitary play
15 months: more complex motor skills	15 months: learns through imitating complex behaviors; knows objects are used for specific purposes	
2 yrs: learns to climb up stairs first, then down	2 yrs: 2 word phrases; uses more complex toys and understands sequence of putting toys, puzzles together	2 yr: imitation, parallel and symbolic, play

Q. What are the complications of CP?

Following complications can take place in CP:

Feeding, growth, and nutrition

- Dysphagia
- Malnutrition
- Growth disturbances

- Increased infection rates
- Skin breakdown
- Osteopenia
- Decreased life expectancy.

Pulmonary
- Sleep-disordered breathing
- Increased risk of aspiration.

Neurologic issues
- Seizures
- Intellectual disability
- Sensorineural hearing loss.

Genitourinary
- Urinary incontinence.

Gastrointestinal
- Gastroesophageal reflux disease (GERD)
- Constipation.

Musculoskeletal:
- Pain and osteopenia.

Q. What are the hindrances in management of this case?
- Inability to sit at even 3 years of age is poor prognostic factor
- History of seizures
- Spasticity
- Inability to walk
- Nutritional support.

Q. What is the management in this case?

Counseling of patient and patient's parents.

Goal setting after discussion with patient's family.

Investigations
- Routine blood
- CT brain
- MRI brain (when indicated)
- VEP
- BERA
- EEG.

Pharmacological
- Antispasticity
- Nutritional support
- Anticonvulsant
- Calcium.

Nonpharmacological
- Antispasticity approaches:
  - Neuro facilitatory techniques
  - Bobath (NDT)—To inhibit primitive reflexes and to facilitate automatic reactions and normal movement patterns
  - Rood (sensorimotor)—Sensory stimulation to activate motor responses, eg tapping, brushing, icing, etc.
  - Vojta—Trigger reflex locomotive zones to encourage movement patterns, eg reflex crawling .

PO: Tone inhibiting orthosis
- Gait aids
- Reciprocal walker
- ***School: Recreational therapy and sports activity***
- ***Resettlement***
- ***Home modification.***

Q. Name the different types of anticonvulsants used in CP?

Table 2.19: Choice of anticonvulsants in CP

	1st choice	*2nd choice*
Generalized tonic clonic	Valproate	Carbamazepine, phenytoin, topiramate
Absence	Ethosuximide, lamotrigine, valproate	Topiramate, zonisamide
Myoclinic	Valproate	Clonezepam, zonisamide
Tonic	Lamotrigine, valproate	Phenytoin, topiramate
Atonic	Lamotrigine, valproate	Topiramate

Q. What will you do if patient develops status epilepticus?
- **0–5 min**: Monitor pulse, BP, respiration, temparature, ECG, EEG.

Insert oral airway + oxygen + suction.

Check glucose, electrolyte, BUN, CBC, level of antiepileptics
- **6–9 min**: NS + bolus 50% glucose (2 mL/kg)
- **10–30 min**: IV Lorazepam (0.1mg/kg) rate 1–2 mg/min
- **31–59 min**: IV phenytoin (18–20 mg/kg) rate 50 mg/min repeat phenytoin (10mg/kg) bolus phenobarbital (20 mg/kg) at a rate of 50 mg/min
- **60 min**: Midazolam loading 0.15 mg/kg followed by continuous infusion 1-2\microgm/kg/min for 12–48 hours
- **80 min**: General anaesthesia with halothane and neuromuscular blockage.

Q. Relevant questions on spasticity (see SCI)

See page number 21.

Q. What are the chances of bladder and bowel involvement in CP?

There is delayed bowel and bladder control but once its maintained no further regression takes place.

Q. What is tone inhibiting orthosis?

These are orthosis given to exert prolonged stretch to inhibit or decrease tone.

Q. Mention the mechanism of action and duration of wearing?

- Decreasing muscle spasticity by increasing muscle length through providing a prolonged stretch and exerting an inhibitory effect through sensory stimulation
- Breaking up mass patterns of movement
- Improving biomechanics and improving stability

Duration of wearing: Maximum time except during toileting, gradually increased in hours.

Q. What is reverse walker?

- Facilitate extension posture as is designed to be positioned behind the child.

It has the following advantages:

- Child has more upright position
- Decreases double support time
- Increases walking speed
- It shows better gait characteristics than anterior walker
- No studies have been done on energy consumption

- Commonly used in spastic CP.

Q. What is difference between true equinus and false equinus?

- True equinus: Its due to gastrocnemius and soleus spasticity or contracture
- False equinus: Due to hip and knee flexors spasticity.

Q. Question regarding phenol and botox.... See chapter SCI

See Page number 13.

Q. When can they be repeated ?

- Phenol after 6 months
- Botulinum toxin after 3 months.

Q. What are the surgeries in CP and there indications?

The types of surgeries done are as follows:

- Soft Tissue Procedure
  - Transfer
  - Lengthening
  - Release
  - Recession
- Bony Procedures
  1. Oseotomy
     a. Derotational.

Q. Name the gait deviations in CP?

Table 2.20: Gait deviations in CP

Gait deviation surgical	*Description*	*Causes*	*Comments*
Scissoring gait	Excessive lower extremity adduction	Femoral anteversion medial hamstring spasticity Hip adductor spasticity	May coexist with crouch and jump gait
Jump gait	Excessive hip and knee flexion and **ankle equinous**	Multifactorial: Hamstring, psoas, rectus femoris, and gastrocnemius contractures Weakness Bony rotational deformities (lever arm dysfunction [LAD])	Most common diplegic gait pattern in young children Jump gait may be a precursor to crouch gait
Equinus	Gastrocnemius contracture	Spasticity of the gastrocnemius muscles	A plantar flexion–knee extension couple can contribute to compensatory knee hyperextension ("recurvatum"). Rarely the soleus needs to be addressed except in hemiplegics. Over lengthening (especially the soleus) may weaken the muscle and contribute to other gait abnormalities, such as crouch
Crouch gait	Variable pelvis position, excessive hip and knee flexion and ankle dorsiflexion	Multifactorial: Hamstring, psoas, rectus femoris and contractures and weakness. Bony rotational deformities (LAD including foot deformity)	Most common diplegic gait pattern in older children Progressive and may lead to decline in functional independence May be iatrogenic—overlengthening of muscles
Stiff knee gait	Decreased knee flexion range of motion throughout the gait cycle	Overactive rectus femoris during swing phase	Commonly observed in hemiplegic CP

b. Angular—
 - Close wedge
 - Open wedge.
2. Arthodesis (joint fusion).

Q. What are the indications of surgery?
The indications of surgeries are as follows:
- Spastic deformity which cant be controlled by conservative measures
- Fixed deformity that interferes with function
- Secondary complication, such as bony deformity, dislocation of hip and joint instability.

Q. What is the age when surgery is done?
Brain development and gait patterns matures at 7–8 yrs . Generally surgery is deferred up to this age.
In some cases surgery is done even early, e.g. dislocation.

Q. IQ assesement in CP and grading of mental retardation?
The most common types of IQ tests are as follows:
- Stanford—Binet Intelligence Scale
- Universal Nonverbal Intelligence
- Differential Ability Scales
- Peabody Individual Achievement Test
- Wechsler Individual Achievement Test
- Wechsler Intelligence Scale for Children
- Woodcock Johnson III Tests of Cognitive Disabilities

Table 2.21: IQ assessment

IQ Range	*Classification*
50–69	Mild
35–49	Moderate
20–34	Severe
below 20	Profound

Q. Percentage of CP with normal IQ?
According to the National Institute of Neurological Disorders and Stroke, approximately two-thirds of patients with CP have some mental impairment. Mental retardation can range from mild to severe. People with the spastic quadriplegia are more likely to have mental disabilities than those with other forms of CP. CP patients with epilepsy are also more likely to have mental retardation.

Q. What is the prognosis of CP?
Good
1. Ability to sit independently by 2 years of age.
2. Less than 3 primitive reflexes present by 18–24 months.

Bad:
1. Inability to sit independently by 4 years of age.

N:B: GMFCS levels I and V tended to remain at these levels, but GMFCS levels II, III, and IV tended to need reclassification over time.

Q. How will you deal with adult CP and aging with CP?
- Preparing for transition begins early in the care of the individual with CP
- A child must be encouraged to become as independent as possible
- Therapy services for older individuals with CP are indicated for specific goals that will enhance functional independence or exercise capacity
- Children with significant cognitive and physical delays may require long-term support but may enjoy opportunities for socialization with peers other than their primary caregivers
- Transition of healthcare occurs in phases and requires preparation, readiness, and handoffs
- Patient counseling needs to include reminders about preventative health measures and screens
- There are some conditions that occur more frequently or earlier in the adult CP population because of aging and chronic alterations in biomechanics, such as cervical myelopathy and early development of degenerative joint disease
- Musculoskeletal conditions may worsen and energy consumption may increase for tasks previously accomplished easily
- Adults with CP may experience chronic pain and associated fatigue and depression.

SPONDYLOARTHROPATHY (ANKYLOSING SPONDYLITIS)

Summary

A 30-year-old right-handed literate male from a high socioeconomic status working as an IT professional presented with gradual onset chronic inflammatory LBP for last six months associated with bilateral knee pain, swelling and bilateral heel pain for last fifteen days. The episode was not proceeded by any loose motion, dysuria, hematuria or increased frequency. Pain responded partially to analgesics. He has a history of eye congestion and excessive lacrimation three months back which responded well to steroid eye drops. He is not suffering from any oral or urethral ulcer or any scarring of penis. His wife noticed that he is increasingly assuming a stooped posture slowly for last two months. He is having difficulty in assuming positions for coitus. He has taken more than two weeks leave in his office due to pain in the last three months. He does not have any constitutional symptoms.

On examination he is fully conscious but little bit depressed. Sacroiliac stress test is bilaterally positive along with decreased ROM of lumbar and cervical spine and decreased chest expansion <3cm. He has tender and swollen knee joints with bilateral hip adductor tightness but other joints are apparently normal. The tragus to wall distance is 18 cm, cervical rotation is 30 degree, inter malleolar distance is 80 cm, modified shoeber test is <10cm and lateral flexion is 5cm. He does not have any signs of uveitis, oral ulcer, skin lesion over palm or sole or any tophi over ears. His nails are normal. Cardiorespiratory findings are within normal limits. Current BASDAI score is 6.5.

Provisional diagnosis: A case of ankylosing spondylitis with peripheral arthritis and enthesitis with BASDAI 6.5 without any extra articular features.

Differential Diagnosis

- Reactive arthritis
- Crystal disease
- Tubercular arthritis.

Q. What are the features of inflammatory LBP?

Inflammatory low back pain according to ASAS criteria (four out of five of the following parameters present):

1. Age at onset 40 years.
2. Insidious onset.
3. Improvement with exercise.
4. No improvement with rest.
5. Pain at night (with improvement upon getting up).

According to ESSG (European Spondyloarthropathy Study Group) criteria:History or present symptoms of spinal pain in back, dorsal, or cervical region, with at least four of the following:

a. Onset before age 45.
b. Insidious onset.
c. Improved by exercise.
d. Associated with morning stiffness.
e. At least 3 months duration.

Q. What is spondyloarthropathy?

Spondyloarthropathies are a family of chronic diseases of joints including

- Ankylosing spondylitis
- Reiter's syndrome (reactive arthritis)
- Psoriatic arthritis
- Inflammatory bowel disease
- Undifferentiated SPA
- Juvenile Inflammatory arthritis.

Spondyloarthropathies are sometimes called spondyloarthritis.

Q. What are the different types of SPA?

See above.

Q. What is the diagnostic criteria of AS?

According to Modified New York Criteria

Clinical criteria:

- Low back pain and stiffness for more than 3 months that improves with exercise, but is not relieved by rest
- Limitation of motion of the lumbar spine in the sagittal and frontal planes
- Limitation of chest expansion relative to normal values correlated for age and sex

Radiological criterion:

- Sacroiliitis grade >2 bilaterally or grade 3–4 unilaterally.

Definite AS if the radiological criterion is associated with at least one clinical criterion

ASAS classification criteria for axial SPA in patients with ≥3 months back pain and age at onset <45 years.

- Sacroilitis on imaging plus ≥1 SPA features, or
- HLA-B27 plus ≥2 other SPA features.

SpA features:

- Inflammatory BP
- Arthritis
- Enthesitis (heel)
- Uveitis
- Dactylitis
- Psoriasis
- Crohn's/ colitis
- Family h/o SpA
- Good response to NSAIDS
- HLA B27
- Elevated CRP.

Sacroilitis on imaging:

- Active (acute) inflammation on MRI highly suggestive of sacroiliitis associated with SpA
- Definite radiographic sacroiliitis as per Modified New York Criteria.

Q. What are the points against reactive arthritis in this patient?

- No preceding history of urinary infection
- No preceding history of GI infection
- Long duration
- No skin lesion.

Q. Could it be a case of rheumatoid arthritis?

No because

- No symmetrical polyarthritis
- Axial back pain
- No small joint involvement
- Sacroilitis: Clinical.

Q. What are the hindrances of management of this patient?

- Iridocyclitis
- Decreased cervical ROM
- Decreased lumbar ROM
- Decreased ROM of involved joints
- Abnormal posture
- Decreased endurance
- Pain
- Fatigue.

Q. What are the different SI stress tests?

- **Patrick (Fabere) test:** The test is performed by having the tested leg flexed and the thigh abducted and externally rotated
- **Lateral compression test:** Patient is kept in lateral position and SI joints are given pressure
- **Gapping test (distraction test):** The patient lies supine and the examiner applies a vertically orientated, posteriorly directed force to both the anterior superior ilac spines
- **Gaenslen's test:** The hip joint is flexed maximally on one side and the opposite hip joint is extended, stressing both sacroiliac joints simultaneously
- **Direct pressure over the sacroiliac joint may elicit pain.**

Q. What are the different special tests of AS?

- Lateral spinal flexion
- Modified Schober test
- Tragus to wall distance
- Occiput to wall distance
- Cervical rotation
- Intermalleolar distance
- Chest expansion
- SI stress tests.

Q. What are the extra articular manifestations of AS?

- **Eye manifestations:** Anterior uveitis, hypopion, synechia, cataract, glaucoma
- **GI Tract involvement:** Crohn's disease, ulcerative colitis
- **CVS:** Aortic valve incompetence, conduction abnormality, ascending aortitis, cardiomegaly, pericarditis
- **Pulmonary:** Fibrosis of upper lobe of lung, interstitial lung disease, emphysema, bronchiectasis
- **Renal:** IgA nephropathy, amyloidosis
- **Bone:** Osteoporosis, osteopenia
- **Prostatism.**

Easy way to remember 10 A's in AS

- *Anterior uveitis*
- *Atlanto-axial subluxation*
- *Apical fibrosis*
- *Aortic regurgitation*
- *AV nodal delay*
- *IgA nephropathy*
- *Amyloidosis*
- *Adductor tightness*
- *HLA-B27*
- *(A)Ulcerative colitis.*

Q. What is the management?

1. **Investigations:**
   - Blood: CBC, ESR, CRP, LFT, urea, creatinine HLA-B27, RF, Anti CCP (to rule out RA)
   - Pulmonary function test (apical fibrosis)
   - ECHO (aortic regurgitation)
   - Slit lamp examination (for anterior uveitis)
   - USG—KUB
   - X RAY—SI joint, LS spine, peripheral joints involved
   - MRI—SI joints (if X-ray is not confirmatory).
2. **Patient education and counselling.**
3. **Goal setting after consultation with patient and family members.**
4. **Pharmacological management.**
   a. Topical—Very limited role, eye drops for uveitis
   b. Oral—Symptomatic (COX-2 inhibitors, indomethacin, naproxen, PPI)
   Disease modifiers (sulfasalazine, methotrexate)
   Biologics.
   c. Local intervention—SI joints, peripheral joints.
   d. Medicines for cardiovascular and pulmonary complication.
5. **Nonpharmacological management.**
   a. Physiotherapy—i. Exercise therapy
      - Exercise to start after hot shower
      - Postural care
      - Prone lying twice daily for half hour
      - Deep breathing exercise
      - Spinal extension exercise
      - SI joint mobilization
      - Squatting
      - AROM of all 4 limbs
      - Stretching of hip flexors, hamstrings, pectoralis and paraspinals
      - Swimming in shallow water.

ii. Modalities:
- UST: SI joint, L/S spine, enthesopathies.

b. Occupational therapy:
- Work station modification
- Assistive and adaptive devices
- Joint protection technique
- Energy conservation technique
- Endurance training

c. Orthotic Support:
- CASH brace (for compression fractures)
- Jewett brace (same).

Q. What are the NSAIDs most commonly prescribed?

Table 2.22: Commonly prescribed NSAIDs

Name	*Dosage*	*Adverse Effects*
Etoricoxib	Up to 120 mg OD	GI ulcer (less with COX-2 inhibitors)
Indometh-acin	75 mg ODHS, 25 mg OD morning	Exacerbation of inflammatory bowel disease
Naproxen	500 mg BD	Cardiovascular complications
Ibuprofen	400 mg BD	Renal impairment, raised hepatic enzyme
Diclofenac	50 mg BD	Chance of anaphylaxis, skin rashes, urticaria

Q. What are the disease modifiers commonly used?

Table 2.23: Commonly prescribed disease modifiers

Name	*Dosage*	*Uses*	*Adverse effects*
Sulfasalazine	2–3g/ DAY in divided doses	Reduces – spinal stiffness, – peripheral arthritis, – ESR	Rash, nausea diarrhea hepatic derangement Agranulocytosis Steven Johnson syndrome
Methotrexate	10 – 15 mg/week	Ameliorates symptoms (pain, swelling, stiffness) (no role in axial SpA)	Rash, nausea, oral ulcer, pancytopenia, hepatic derangement, renal impairment
Thalidomide		Enhances deg-radation of TNF messenger RNA	Drowsiness, constipation and dizziness
Pamindronate	i.v. monthly for 6 month	Evidence of symptomatic efficacy More effective in axial disease	

Q. What biologics will you refer?

See Page number 49

Q. What is HLA B27?

Human leukocyte antigen (HLA) B27 is a class I surface antigen encoded by the B locus in the major histocompatibility complex (MHC) on chromosome 6 and presents antigenic peptides (derived from self and nonself antigens) to T cells.

Q. Diseases that are associated with the HLA-B27 subtype ?

(mnemonic PAIR)
- Psoriasis
- Ankylosing spondylitis
- Inflammatory bowel disease
- Reactive arthritis.

Q. What is the sensitivity of HLA B27 in AS?
- Clinical sensitivity—90%.

Q. What is the specificity in AS?
- Clinical specificity in an unaffected individual without a family history—<1%.

Q. Positivity in normal population?

8% of Caucasians, 4% of North Africans, 2–9% of Chinese, and 0.1–0.5% of persons of Japanese descent possess this gene.

Q. What are the other blood investigations required for follow up?
- ESR
- CRP
- LFT, urea, creatinine
- CBC.

Q. What is the radiological grading of Sacroilitis?

Grade 0: Normal.

Grade 1: Suspicious changes.

Grade 2: Minimal abnormality—small localized areas with erosion or sclerosis, without alteration in the joint width.

Grade 3: Unequivocal abnormality—moderate or advanced sacroiliitis with one or more of: erosions, evidence of sclerosis, widening, narrowing, or partial ankylosis.

Grade 4: Severe abnormality—total ankylosis.

Q. How would you differentiate tubercular sacroilitis from AS?

Table 2.24: Difference between tubercular sacroilitis and AS

	Ankylosing spondylitis	*Tubercular sacroilitis*
Site	Usually bilateral	Unilateral
Involved side	Ilial side	Sacral side
Part of SI joint	Lower part	Upper part
SI joint pathology	Sclerosis	Erosion
Bamboo spine	Present	Negative

Q. Difference between ankylosing spondylitis and bilateral condensa ilei?

Table 2.25: Difference between AS and bilateral condensansa ilei

	Ankylosing spondylitis	*B/L Condensa ilei*
Erosion	Positive	Negative
Irregularities	Positive	Negative
Space reduction	Positive	Negative
HLA B27	Positive	Negative
Peripheral arthritis	Present	Absent
Extraarticular features	Present	Absent
Gender	Male	Female (multiparity)

Q. What are the vertebral changes in X-ray?

- Early spondylitis is characterized by small erosions at the corners of vertebral bodies with reactive sclerosis (Romanus lesions of the spine: Shiny corner sign)
- Vertebral body squaring
- Diffuse syndesmophyiticankylosis can give a "Bamboo spine" appearance
- Interspinous ligament calcification can give a "Dagger spine" appearance
- Ossification of spinal ligaments, joints and discs
- Apophyseal and costovertebral arthritis and ankylosis
- Pseudoarthroses may form at fracture sites
- Enthesophyte formation from enthesopathy
- Noninfectious spondylodiscitis: Andersson lesion.

Q. What is Bamboo spine?

Bamboo spine is a radiographic feature seen in ankylosing spondylitis that occurs as a result of vertebral body fusion by marginal syndesmophytes. It is often accompanied by fusion of the posterior vertebral elements as well.

Q. How do you differentiate between DISH and AS?

Table 2.26: Difference between DISH and AS

	AS	*DISH*
Patient group	Males	Males
Age	Young	Middle
Clinical	Inflammatory back pain SI joint tender Synovitis of joints	Mechanical back pain Nontender SI joint No synovitis
Associations	Uveitis, dactylitis, urethritis	Diabetis mellitus
Radiological	Syndesmophytes Sacroilitis	Osteophytes No sacroilitis
Investigation	HLA-B27 + CRP raised	No

Q. What are the things to see in chest X-ray of AS patient?

- Fibrosis
- Reticulonodular pattern.

Q. If you get changes in X-ray, what is the next investigation?

- PFT (to check restrictive lung disease)
- HRCT (to confirm ILD).

Q. What is the role of MRI in AS?

Detect early changes of S/I joints.

Q. What are the changes in MRI?

Active inflammatory lesions (STIR/post-gadolinium T1):

- Bone marrow edema (osteitis)
- Capsulitis
- Synovitis
- Enthesitis.

Chronic inflammatory lesions (normally T1):

- Sclerosis
- Erosions
- Fat deposition
- Bony bridges/ankylosis.

Q. Is there any role of DEXA scan?

Evaluation of osteoporosis and osteopenia in advanced AS.

Q. What are the common drugs prescribed for AS?

See Page number 48.

Q. What are the prerequisite and contraindication to start biologics?

Given earlier.

Q. What is the difference between biologics and biosimilars?

Because biologic medicines are made in living things like yeasts, bacteria or animal cells which are naturally variable that is why exact copies of biologic medicines cannot be made.

A biosimilar is a highly similar, comparable, version of an approved biologic medicine. Biosimilar medicines undergo clinical trials to demonstrate that they have comparable safety, quality and efficacy to an approved biologic medicine.

Q. What sports should be avoided in AS?

- Heavy contact sports
- Spinal flexion encouraging sports
- Golf, football, bowling.

Q. What are the assistive and adaptive devices?

- Bathing/grooming—Using long handled sponge to wash legs/feet/back to avoid bending

- Dresing—Wear loose clothing and slip on shoes, gather all clothes before dressing, using long handled shoe horn, sock aid, or reacher for donning shoes, socks, and pants
- Cooking—Use dishwasher, prepare recipes in large amount,all items should have easy access to prevent bending or reaching
- Housekeeping—Eliminate the need to iron by buying fabric that have wrinkle protection, avoid carring heavy packages during shopping.
- Driving—Wide angled panoramic mirrors for rear view.

  Prism glasses to accommodate decreased spinal motion.

Q. Why shallow water swimming is advised?

To prevent drowning in case the patient gets exhausted due to associated AR.

Q. What are the additive benefits of hydrotherapy?

- Decreases load on joints
- Strengthening exercise
- ROM exercise
- Warm water helps in circulation.

Q. What is joint protection technique?

- Avoid positions that foster deformity
- Avoid tight gripping
- Avoid placing excessive or constant pressure on joints
- Avoid prolonged static positions
- Using proper body mechanics
- Using the largest most stable joint for the task
- Respect pain and fatigue
- Prioritize and organize activities.

Q. What is question mark sign?

- Obliterated lumbar lordosis
- Buttock atrophy
- Accentuated thoracic kyphosis
- Forward stoop of the neck
- Flexion contractures at the hips compensated by flexion at the knees.

  That is why he looks like ? on standing.

Q. What are the sexual problems in AS?

- Fertility, pregnancy or childbirth are usually not a problem in AS
- Loss of libido may be present due to pain, joint stiffness or fatigue.

Q. What should be advised?

- Warm baths before intercourse may help
- Specific postures like lateral position for both the man and the woman is preferable
- In very advanced disease hip replacement may be a prerequisite to maintain sexual relationship
- Adverse effects of drugs on libido must be taken care of
- And finally understanding and counselling is needed.

Q. What are the surgeries done in AS?

- Joint replacement
- Vertebral stabilization.

Q. What are the salient features of psoriatic arthritis?

Types:

- DIP joint arthritis
- Symmetrical polyarthritis
- Asymmetrical oligoarthritis
- Arthritis mutilans
- Spondylitis.

Skin lesions

- Plaque
- Guttate
- Inverse
- Pustular
- Erythrodermic.

Nail changes

- Pitting
- Horizontal ridging
- Onycholysis
- Yellowish discoloration of the nail margins
- Dystrophic hyperkeratosis
- Combinations of these findings.

Q. What is the classification criteria of psoriatic athropathy?

CASPAR criteria

(As per the above criteria a patient must have inflammatory articular disease (joint, spine, or entheseal) with 3 points from any of the following five categories:

1. Evidence of current psoriasis, a personal history of psoriasis, or a family history of psoriasis.
2. Typical psoriatic nail dystrophy observed on current physical examination.
3. A negative test result for rheumatoid factor.

4. Either current dactylitis or a history of dactylitis recorded by a rheumatologist.
5. Radiographic evidence of juxtaarticular new bone formation in the hand or foot.

Q. What are the drugs to be avoided in psoriasis?

- Lead
- Beta blockers
- Chloroquines
- Lithium
- Intramuscular steroid.

Q. What are the treatment of PsA?

- Methotrexate to reduce disease activity
- Analgesics
- Infliximab if disease activity is not controlled.

Q. What is SAPHO?

- Serositis
- Acne
- Pustulosis
- Hyperostosis
- Osteitis.

Q. What are the salient features of reactive arthritis?

Triad of reactive arthritis

1. Conjunctivitis.
2. Arthritis.
3. Nongonococcal urethritis.
   - *Males >> females*
   - *Typically follows GI or GU infection*
   - *Organisms (2 main groups)*
     STDs: Chlamydia
     GI infection: Campylobacter, Yersinia, Shigella, Salmonella.
     3–10% of patients with reactive arthritis progress to AS.

- Clinical manifestations
  - Arthritis
    - Arthritis appears 2–4 weeks after initiating infectious event—GU or GI.
    - Asymmetric
    - Oligoarticular—average of 4 or fewer joints
      - LE involvement >> UE
      - More common in the knees, ankles, and small joints of the feet.
    - Sausage digits (dactylitis)
      - Swollen, tender digits with a dusk-like blue discoloration.
    - Enthesopathies—Achilles tendon
    - Low back pain—Sacroiliitis
  - Ocular
    - Conjunctivitis, iritis, uveitis, episcleritis, corneal ulceration.
  - Genitourinary
    - Urethritis, meatal erythema, edema
    - Balanitis circinata—small painless ulcers on the glans penis, urethritis.
  - Skin and nails
    - Keratoderma blennorrhagica—hypertrophic skin lesions on palms and soles of feet
    - Reiter's nails—thickened and opacified, crumbling, non-pitting.
  - Cardiac
    - Conduction defects.
  - General
    - Weight loss, fever
    - Amyloidosis.
  - Radiographic Findings
    - "Lover's heel"—erosion and periosteal changes at the insertion of the plantar fascia and Achilles tendons
    - Ischial tuberosities and greater trochanter
    - Asymmetric sacroiliac joint involvement
    - Syndesmophytes
    - Pencil-in-cup deformities of the hands and feet—more common in psoriatic arthritis.
  - Treatment
    - NSAIDs, such as indomethacin
    - Corticosteroids
    - DMARD: Sulphasalazine.

Q. What are the salient features of IBD?

- Arthritis secondary to inflammatory bowel disease (Crohn's disease and ulcerative colitis)
  - Males >> female
  - Peripheral arthritis occurs in ~ 10-20% of the patients with Crohn's disease and ulcerative coliti.

Clinical Manifestations

- Asymmetric joint involvement
- Synovitis affecting the peripheral joints
- Monoarticular or polyarticular
- Large joints—Knees, ankles, feet
- Two types of arthropathies can occur
  - Enteropathic arthritis
  - AS.
- Sacroiliitis
- Peripheral arthritis will subside with remission of bowel disease.

Extra-articular Manifestations

- Erythema nodosa—Crohn's
- Pyoderma gangrenosa—ulcerative colitis
- Painful deep oral ulcers
- Uveitis
- Fever and weight loss during bowel episodes.

Investigations

- Anti-neutrophil cytoplasmic antibodies (ANCA)~60% (antimyeloperoxidase)
- Increased incidence of HLA-B27.

Q. What are the salient features of USPA?

Diagnosed by ***modified AMOR criteria***

Box 2.1: Modified AMOR criteria

Inclusion Criteria Score			
Inflammatory back pain	1	Dactylitis (sausage digit)	2
Unilateral buttock pain	1	Acute anterior uveitis	2
Alternate buttock pain	2	HLA B27 positive or family history of SpA	2
Ethesitis	2	Good response to NSAID	2
Asymmetric peripheral arthritis	2		
Exclusion criteria			
Diagnosis of specific spondyloarthropathy		Keratoderma blenorrhagicum	
Sacroiliitis on radiograph ≥grade 2		IBD (crohn disease or ulcerative colitis)	
Precipitating genitourinary or GI infection		Positive antinuclear antibody titre >1; 80	
Psoriasis			
Diagnosis of USpA with 6 or more points			

Many patients present with features of two or more SpA or does not fall in any one category.

May present with dactylitis, synovitis and enthesitis.

Q. What are the difference between AS and Unclassified SPA?

2nd most common after AS

AS	USPA
Young age	Middle age
Males	Females
HLA-B27 +	HLA-B27 -ve

Q. Approach to SPA?

Approach to SPA has been shown in Flowchart 2.1.

Flowchart 2.1: Approach to SPA

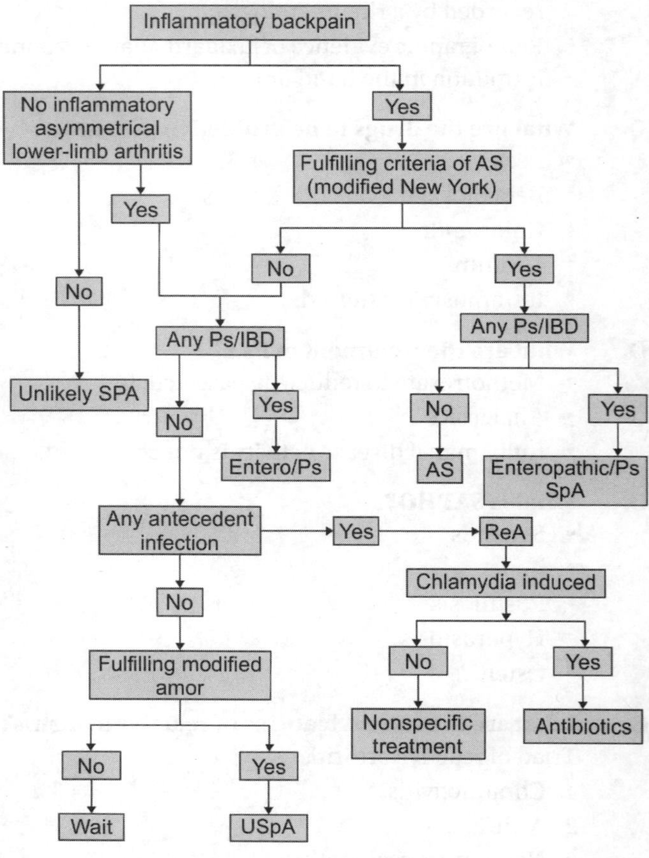

Q. How will you do Shoeber test?

- While standing erect, place a landmark midline at a point 5-cm below the iliac crest line and 10-cm above on the spinous processes
- On forward flexion, the line should increase by greater than 5 cm to a total of 20 cm
- Any increase less than 5 cm is considered negative.

Q. Difference from modified Shoeber test?

- Only the mark 10 cm above iliac crest is taken
- On forward flexion a rise by 5 cm to a total of 15 or more is normal.

Q. What is position of goniometer?

- **Cervical rotation:** Goniometer at the top of the head in line with the nose.

Q. How will you assess disease severity and impairment level of AS?

- Bath ankylosing spondylitis metrology index (BASMI)

- Bath ankylosing spondylitis disease activity index (BASDAI)
- Bath ankylosing spondylitis functional index (BASFI)
- Bath ankylosing spondylitis radiology index (BASRI)

See scales for details.

POLYARTHRITIS (RHEUMATOID ARTHRITIS)

Summary

A 32-years-old housewife from middle class family, mother of one baby presented with symmetrical inflammatory polyarthritis for last two years with small joint pain and early morning stiffness. She has taken pain killers intermittently for last few months. She had two episodes of eye congestion during this period. She also had few episodes of cough and shortness of breath in last one year. Her bladder and bowel habit is normal but she is struggling to do her household activities due to pain and restricted joint movement for last six months.

On examination she is anemic with few erythematous nodules on her shin bones. Her tender joint score is 16 and swollen joint count is 6. She also has swan neck deformity and Z deformity of hand and hallux valgus deformity of foot. There are bilateral basal end inspiratory crepitations on respiratory examinations without any organomegaly. Her FIM score is 116/126.

P/D: Rheumatoid arthritis complicated with anemia, erythyma nodusum joint deformity and probably interstitial lung disease with FIM score of 116/126.

D/D: 1. SLE.
2. Overlap syndrome.

Q. What is arthralgia and arthritis?

Table 2.27: Difference between athralgia and arthritis

	Athralgia	*Arthritis*
Pain	+	++
Swelling	-	++
Effusion	-	++
Tenderness	+	++
Synovitis	-	+

Q. What is mono arthritis,oligo arthritis and poly arthritis ?

- Mono arthritis is when only one joint is involved
- Oligo arthritis is when 2 to 4 joints are involved
- Poly arthritis is when greater than 4 joints are involved

Q. Give examples of each?

The most common causes of acute monarthritis are infection, crystal-induced arthritis, or the onset of a chronic inflammatory arthropathy

Other causes

- Traumatic
- Inflammatory:

Table 2.28: Inflammatory causes of acute mono arthritis

Infectious	*Noninfectious*
Septic arthritis	Psoriatic arthritis
Tuberculosis arthritis	Ankylosing spondylitis
Reactive arthritis (indirectly)	Rheumatoid arthritis:
	Juvenile idiopathic arthritis
	Adult-onset Still's disease
	Felty's syndrome
	Crystal arthropathy: Gout chondrocalcinosis

- Noninflammatory
  - Osteoarthritis
- Others
  - Hemarthrosis
  - Vilo nodular synovitis

Box 2.2: Causes of poly-arthritis

Inflammatory
- Peripheral polyarticular
  - Rheumatoid arthritis
  - Systemic lupus erythematosus
  - Viral arthritis
  - Psoriatic arthritis (occasionally)
- Peripheral pauciarticular
  - Psoriatic arthritis
  - Reiter's syndrome
  - Rheumatic fever
  - Polyarticular gout
  - Enteropathic arthritis
  - Behçet's disease
  - Bacterial endocarditis
- Peripheral with axial involvement
  - Ankylosing spondylitis (especially juvenile onset)
  - Reiter's syndrome
  - Enteropathic arthritis
  - Psoriatic arthritis

Noninflammatory (osteoarthritis)
- Hereditary
  - Osteoarthritis of the hands
  - Primary generalized osteoarthritis
- Traumatic osteoarthritis
  - Osteoarthritis after local injury
  - Osteoarthritis of the knees in obese individuals
  - Chondromalacia after aggressive exercise programs
  - Osteoarthritis in the elderly
- Metabolic diseases (may have an unusual pattern)
  - Hemochromatosis
  - Ochronosis
  - Acromegaly
  - Idiopathic

Oligoarthritis

- Evolving RA
- Palindromic RA
- Degenerative joint disease
- Reactive arthritis
- Crystal disease
- Enteropathic SpA
- Psoriatic SpA.

Q. What is the diagnostic criteria of RA?

1987 ACR criteria

1. *Morning stiffness*—Lasting ≥1 hour before maximum improvement.
2. *Arthritis of ≥3 joint areas*—Simultaneous soft tissue swelling or effusion (not bony overgrowth alone) of atleast 3 joint areas.
   (Note: The 14 possible joint areas involved are right or left PIP, MCP, Wrist, Elbow, Knee, Ankle, MTP)
3. *Arthritis of hand joints*—At least 1 joint area swollen in wrist,MCP,PIP.
4. *Symmetric arthritis*—Simultaneous involvement of the same joint area on both side.
   (absolute symmetry is not needed)
5. *Rheumatoid nodules*—Subcutaneous nodules over bony prominences or extensor surfaces or juxta articular regions.
6. *Serum RF*—Demonstration of abnormal amount of RF by any method that has been positive.
7. *Radiographic changes*—Typical changes on posteroanterior hand and wrist include erosions or unequivocal bony decalcification.
   (*Note*: In 1987 criteria to diagnose RA, 4 out of 7 criteria required.
   Criteria 1–4 must be present for at least six weeks.)

Q. What is the screening criteria of RA?

The 2010 American College of Rheumatology/ European League Against Rheumatism classification criteria for rheumatoid arthritis

Score Target Population (Who Should be Tested?) Patients who

1. Have at least 1 joint with definite clinical synovitis (swelling).
2. With the synovitis not better explained by another disease.

Classification criteria for RA (score-based algorithm: Add score of categories A–D; a score of 6/10 is needed for classification of a patient as having definite RA)‡

A. Joint involvement
   1 large joint 0
   2–10 large joints 1
   1–3 small joints (with or without involvement of large joints) 2
   4–10 small joints (with or without involvement of large joints) 3
   10 joints (at least 1 small joint) 5

B. Serology (at least 1 test result is needed for classification)
   Negative RF and negative ACPA 0
   Low-positive RF or low-positive ACPA 2
   High-positive RF or high-positive ACPA 3

C. Acute-phase reactants (at least 1 test result is needed for classification)
   Normal CRP and normal ESR 0
   Abnormal CRP or abnormal ESR 1

D. Duration of symptoms
   Less than 6 weeks 0
   Greater than 6 weeks 1

Q. What is the diagnostic criteria of SLE?

Mneumonic: MD SOAP NIHAR (Box 2.3)

Box 2.3: Mneumonics for diagnostic criteria of SLE

Malar rash
Discoid rash
Serositis
Oral ulcers
Arthritis
Photosensitivity
Neurologic disorder
Immunologic disorder
Hematologic disorder
ANA
Renal disorder

Q. What are the causes of anemia in RA?

The causes of anemia in RA in are:

1. Anemia of chronic disease.
2. Iron deficiency anemia.
3. Folate plus Vit B12 deficiency.
4. NSAIDS induced chronic GI blood loss.
5. Felty's syndrome.
6. Marrow suppression due to DMARDS.

Q. What are the common hand deformities in RA?

- Spindle-shaped swelling of PIP
- Grasshopper deflection

- Swan neck deformity
- Boutonniers deformity
- Z deformity
- Game keepers thumb
- Ulnar deviation of hand.

Q. What are the causes of foot drop in RA?

- Vasculitis
- Extensor tendons rupture.

Q. What are the lung complications in RA?

- Pleura: Pleuritis, pleural effusion
- Interstitial pneumonitis and fibrosis
- Nodular lung disease
- Bronchiolitis
- Pulmonary hypertension
- Small airway diseases.

Q. Name the eye complications of RA?

- Keratoconjuctivitis sicca
- Scleritis
- Episcleritis.

Q. What are the other extra-articular complications seen in RA?

1. Bone: Osteopenia, osteoporosis.
2. Rheumatoid nodule.
3. Muscles: Decreased bulk, peripheral neuro-myopathy, steroid myopathy, active myositis, myopathy.
4. Skin: Senile purpura, vasculitis changes, livedo reticularis.
5. Vasculitis.
6. Renal: Amyloidosis (rare) due to NSAIDS and gold.
7. Heart: Pericarditis, myocarditis, conduction defect, atherosclerosis.

Q. What is the role of tender joint count, swollen joint count and DAS score?

- To monitor severity of disease
- For initiation of drugs
- To assess remission.

Q. Formula of DAS (ESR)?

- DAS28 = 0.56 * sqrt(tender28) + 0.28 * sqrt (swollen28) + 0.70 * ln(ESR) + 0.014 * GH

Q. What is DAS (CRP) and when is it used?

- Sometimes ESR may be raised due to severe anemia (measurement if taken in Western green method)
- There are many physiological causes of raised ESR.

Q. What are the hindrances in RA?

- Pain
- Deformity
- Extra articular complications.

Q. What is overlap syndrome?

When the disease process does not fall into anyone of the disease processes or has features of two or more of the following diseases:

- RA
- Dermatomyositis
- Polymyositis
- SLE
- Sjogrens syndrome
- Scleroderma.

Q. What is MTCD?

It stands for mixed tissue connective disorder.

Q. What is the diagnostic criteria?

Diagnostic criteria of MTCD have been discussed in Table 2.29.

Table 2.29: Diagnostic criteria of MTCD

	Alarcon-Segovia Criteria	*Kahn Criteria*
Serologic criteria	Anti-RNP at hemagglutination titer of ≥1:1600	High-titer anti-RNP corresponding to a speckled ANA of ≥1:1200 titer
Clinical criteria	1. Swollen hands	1. Swollen fingers
	2. Synovitis	2. Synovitis
	3. Myositis (biologically proven)	3. Myositis
	4. Raynaud's phenomenon	4. Raynaud's phenomenon
	5. Acrosclerosis	
MTCD present if	Serologic criterion accompanied by 3 or more clinical criteria, one of which must be synovitis or myositis	Serologic criterion accompanied by Raynaud's phenomenon and at least 2 of the 3 remaining clinical criteria

Q. How will you manage this case of RA?

- Councelling of patient and family
- Patient education about the disease process and progression
- Goal setting: After discussing with patient and family
- Rest: Local rest
- Investigations:

- Blood: ESR, CRP, Hb%, RF, ANTI CCP, ANF, SGPT, SGOT, urea, creatinine
- X-ray of hands, foot, chest
- Doppler USG of hand
- Urine RE/ME/CS
- ECG
- PFT to rule out restrictive lung disease
- HRCT to confirm ILD.
- Pharmacological management:
  - Supportive analgesics.
- Etoricoxib
- Naproxen
  - Specials: DMARDS
    - Methotrexate, sulphasalazine (SSZ), hydroxy choloroquine (HCQ)
    - If nonresponsive: Lefunomide in place of SSZ and HCQ
    - If nonresponsive >3 weeks: Biologics can be started
  - Steroids: Mainly methylprednisolone
  - (if ILD and EN).
- Nonpharmacological management:
  - PT: Exercise:
    - Deep breathing exercise
    - Range-of-motion exercise
    - Intrinsic hand muscle strengthening exercise
    - Stretching and strengthening exercises.

Modalities:
Contrast bath
Hydrotherapy
Paraffin wax bath
  - OT: Joint protection and energy conservation techniques
  - PO: Splints as described on Page number 50
  - Home modifications
  - Vocational rehabilitation.

Q What are the NSAIDS given to reduce pain in symptomatic patients?

NSAIDs that can be given in symptomatic patients have been given in Table 2.30.

Table 2.30: Various NSAIDs

Name	*T1/2*	*Max dose*	*S/E*
Indo-methacin	4.5 hours	Maximum single dose: 100 mg Maximum daily dose: 200 mg	Upset stomach, nausea, vomiting; Diarrhea, constipation; Headache, dizziness, drowsiness; Feeling tired or depressed; or Ringing in ears
Etoricoxib	22 hours	Maximum single dose: 120 mg Maximum daily dose: 120 mg	Stroke Edema Hepatic toxicity GI effects Renal toxicity Skin rashes
Naproxen	12–17 hours	Maximum single dose: 750 mg Maximum daily dose: 1500 mg	Myocardial infarctions Strokes Gastrointestinal problems

Q. What are the different types of steroid with potency and half life?

Potency and half life of different steroids have been discussed in Table 2.31.

Table 2.31: Potency and half life of different steroids

Glucocorticoid	*Approximate equivalent dose (mg)*	*Half-life (hr)*
	Short-acting	
Cortisone	25	8–12
Hydrocortisone	20	8–12
	Intermediate-acting	
Methylprednisolone	4	18–36
Prednisolone	5	18–36
Prednisone	5	18–36
Triamcinolone	4	18–36
	Long-acting	
Betamethasone	0.6–0.75	36–54
Dexamethasone	0.75	36–54

Q. What are the disease modifying drugs (DMARDS) given in RA?

- First line—Methotrexate (MTX), hydroxychloroquine (HCQ), sulfasalazine (SSZ)
- Less commonly used—Leflunomide, mino and doxycycline
- Others—Gold salts, penicillamine, azathioprine, cyclosporine and tacrolimus.

Q. What are the occupational therapy advices given in RA?

- Correction of deformity
- Maintainence of range of motion
- Energy conservation technique
- Joint protection technique
- Work place modification
- Work simplification
- Adaptive devices

- Hand function activity: Peg board training, ADL board, dexterity board.

Q. What is RF ?

It stands for rheumatoid factor (RF).

It is the autoantibody that was first found in rheumatoid arthritis. It is defined as an antibody against the Fc portion of IgG (an antibody against an antibody). RF and IgG join to form immune complexes that contribute to the disease process.

Q. What are the types of RF?

Although predominantly encountered as IgM, rheumatoid factor can be any isotype of immunoglobulins, i.e. IgA, IgG, IgM, IgE, IgD.

Q. What is the role of RF?

1. Diagnosis of RA.
2. Prognostic factor (Higher the titre more the joint destruction).

Q. What is the sensitivity and specificity of RF?

Sensitivity is 60–70%

Specificity is 78%.

[High levels of RF (in general, above 20 IU/mL, 1:40, or over the 95th percentile) occur in rheumatoid arthritis (present in 80%) and Sjögren's syndrome (present in 70%).]

Q. What is the normal population with RF positivity?

5–10% of healthy persons, especially the elderly.

It is also found in Epstein-Barr virus or Parvovirus infection.

Q. Mention the false positive causes of RF?

Other than in rheumatoid arthritis, rheumatoid factor may also be elevated in:

- Systemic lupus erythematosus (SLE)
- Sjögren's syndrome
- Interstitial pulmonary fibrosis
- Hepatitis B, chronic liver disease and chronic hepatitis
- Essential mixed cryoglobulinemia
- Primary biliary cirrhosis
- Infectious mononucleosis and any chronic viral infection
- Bacterial endocarditis
- Leprosy
- Sarcoidosis
- Tuberculosis
- Syphilis
- Visceral leishmaniasis
- Malaria
- Leukemia
- Dermatomyositis
- Systemic sclerosis
- After vaccination/transfusion in normal individuals.

Q. What is anti CCP?

Antibodies to citrullinated protein antigens (ACPAs) are autoantibodies that are directed against peptides and proteins that are citrullinated. They are present in the majority of patients with rheumatoid arthritis (RA).

ACPAs have proved to be powerful biomarkers that allow the diagnosis of RA to be made at a very early stage.

N.B.: *In July 2010, the 2010 ACR/EULAR Rheumatoid Arthritis Classification Criteria* were introduced. These new classification criteria include ACPA testing, and overruled the "old" *ACR criteria of 1987* and are adapted for early RA diagnosis.

Q. What is the sensitivity and specificity of anti CCP?

Sensitivity between 69.6% and 77.5% and a specificity between 87.8% and 96.4%.

(ACPA are more specific than rheumatoid factor)

Q. What are the range of anti CCP?

The reference ranges for blood tests of anti-citrullinated protein antibodies are shown in Table 2.32.

Table 2.32: Range of anti CCP

Negative	*Low/weak positive*	*Moderate positive*	*High/strong positive*	*Unit*
< 20	20–39	40–59	> 60	EU

Q. What is Felty's syndrome?

It's a triad of chronic arthritis, splenomegaly, and granulocytopenia. It occurs in patients with unusually severe extra-articular disease and immunologic abnormalities. Persistent granulocytopenia (<2000/mm) must be present, but the complete triad is not required for a diagnosis of Felty's syndrome as patients without splenomegaly resemble patients with full-blown Felty's syndrome in terms of most clinical, serologic, and immunogenetic features.

Q. Comparative notes on DMARDS.

Various DMARDS have been described in Table 2.33.

Table 2.33: Various DMARDS

Name	*Mechanism of action*	*Dose*	*Side effects*	*Contraindication*
Methotrexate	Inhibits dihydrofolate reductase enzyme	7.5–25mg weekly, can be escalated at 2.5 mg weekly basis in 8wks	Nausea and mucosal ulcers most common Diarrhea Heptotoxicity Severe myelosuppression Interstitial pnuemonitis	Pregnancy Breast feeding Liver disease Severe renal failure
Sulphosalazine	Multiple anti-inflammatory properties Multiple immuno modulatory properties	Starting dose is 500mg/day for the 1st week which is increased by 500mg/day on a weekly basis until a max of 2–3 g/day is attained	Nausea,vomiting, headache and rash Hemolytic anemia Hypersensitivity reactions SJS	
Hydroxychloro-quine	i. Inhibit antigen processing and presentation leading to down regulation of CD4+ response in sites of immune damage ii. Leads to decreased production of cytokines and other inflammatory mediators	200–400 mg per day orally	GI disturbances Pruritic maculopapular rash Headaches and light headedness Rarely psychosis and convulsions Ocular toxicity i. Corneal deposits ii. Retinopathy	
Leflunomide	Inhibition of pyrimidine (rUMP) through inhibition mitochondrial enzyme dihydroorotate dehydrogenase (DHODH)	10–20mg daily	Diarrhea Headache Nausea Rash Hepatotoxicity alopecia	Pregnancy

Q. What special advices will you give regarding contraceptions?

- To avoid estrogen based contraception
- Avoid pregnancy during DMARDS therapy
- Atleast 3 months discontinuation of DMARDS before conception
- Proper monitoring of fetus for congenital anomalies if already became pregnant.

Q. What is the best contraception possible?

Barrier methods are the best methods in RA.

Q. Mention the target DAS 28?

Target DAS 28 have been mentioned in Table 2.34.

Table 2.34: Target DAS 28

Instrument	*Score range*	*Remission*	*Low*	*Moderate*	*High*
Das 28	0–9.4	<=2.6	<=3.2	>3.2 and <=5.1	>5.1

Q. What is the role of steroid in RA?

- Vasculitis
- Flare up
- To cover up window period
- Critically ill
- Serositis
- Low dose may be used as disease modifier.

Q. Classify the biologics used in RA?

- TNFα inhibitors—Infliximab, etanercept, adalimumab, golimumab, certolizumab
- Interleukin-1 receptor antagonist—Anakinra
- Selective costimulatory modulator—Abatacept
- Anti CD20—Rituximab
- Interleukin 6 antagonist—tocilizumab.

Q. What are the prerequisites before starting biologics?

- Infection of any kind should be ruled out
- Low ejection fraction and heart failure are to be excluded
- Hyperlipidemia should be ruled out before initiation of tocilizumumab
- Standard investigations: HbsAg, anti HCV, HIV,
  CXR
  Mantaux test
  - Vaccination for pneumoccocus.

Q. What is the role of rest in RA?

There are three types of rest in RA:

- Systemic rest: Severe disease or new-onset RA
- Local rest: Affected joints in acute or subacute stages with static orthosis. (one ROM exercise per day is needed to prevent contracture)
- Short rest: A brief 20–30 mins of rest throughout day to avoid fatigue.

Q. Biologics in brief?

Various biologies have been described in Table 2.35.

Table 2.35: Biologics

Name	*Route of administration*	*Half life*	*Dose*	*Side effects*
Infliximab	i.v.	8–10 days	3mg/kg i.v. infusions at 0, 2 and 6 wks then every 8wks If pts fail to respond then up to 10 mg/kg or it can be given every 4 weeks	Reactivation of TB Infusion site reactions Demyelinating syndromes can occur
Etanercept	s.c.	3–5 days	25mg twice weekly or 50mg once weekly	Effects—Increased incidence of bacterial infections, reactivation of latent tuberculosis (less than others), lymphomas, injection site hypersensitivity
Adalimumab	S.C.	6–14 days	40mg every alternate week	
Rituximab	Slow i.v.	40–400hrs	Two 1g i.v. infusions separated by 2wks to be repeated every 6 months	Infusion reactions, interference with vaccinations
Abatacept	Slow i.v.	2 weeks	12 mg/kg. 2nd dose after 2 wks followed by subsequent doses at monthly intervals	Infection

Q. Compare the efficacies of DMARDS and Biologics?

Comparison of the efficacies of DMARDS and biologics have been given in Table 2.36.

Table 2.36: Differences in efficacies of DMARDS and biologics

	DMARDS	*Biologics*
Chances of remission	High	Very high
Control of extra articular disease	To some extent	High
Prevention of radiographic damage	To some extent	Highly effective
Adverse drug reaction	Acceptable	Acceptable
Control of associated co- morbidities	Only to limited extent	Very effectively
Cost of treatment	Cheaper	Expensive but if given early then lifetime treatment cost will be cost effective

Q. What are types of DAS?

DAS 28

DAS 68.

Q. What are the modalities used in RA?

- Heat: Superficial heat with hot packs, paraffin bath
- Cold therapy
- TENS: In neuropathy
- Galvanic stimulations
- Faradic stimulations
- Faradic foot bath
- Iontophoresis: For pain release
- Interferential current
- Low-level laser therapy.

Q. Mention the complications of deep heat?

- When joint temperature is increased from 30.5–36 degree C cartilage or joint destruction occurs due to increased activity of collagenase released from inflamed joint.

Q. Describe the joint protection technique in RA?

The main idea in joint protection is to minimize the strain on joints in daily activities by

- Respect pain
- Avoid positions of deformity
- Avoid awkward positions
- Use strongest joints or several joints (distribute force)
- Interrupt sustained activity with rest
- Exercise in pain-free range
- Reduce effort
- Use larger joints
- Use adaptive equipments.

Q. Describe the energy conservation technique in RA?

It is not so much what, but how that can help control fatigue.

- Plan the task.
- Eliminate extra trips.

- Use good posture and body mechanics.
- Don't fight gravity.
- Proper rest
- Use energy-saving devices.

Q. Describe the biomechanics of hand deformity?

Biomechanics of hand deformity have been given in Table 2.37.

Table 2.37: Biomechanics of hand deformity

Deformity	*Mechanism of action*
Swan-neck deformity	Rupture of lateral retinaculum of extensor tendon at proximal interpharangeal joint
Boutonniere deformity	Rupture of central slip of extensor tendon allows migration of proximal interphalangeal joint between lateral slips
Ulnar deviation of fingers	Rupture of radial retinaculum produces ulnar subluxation of metacarpal phalangeal joints
Game keepers thumb	Torn ulnar collateral ligament

Q. Mention the other hand problems in RA?

- CTS
- Vasculitis
- Muscle wasting
- Peripheral neuropathy.

Q. What is spiral hand orthosis?

It's wrapped spirally around the arm, providing constant but gentle pulling force to stabilize, mobilize and position the arm in correct possible posture.

Q. What are the advantages of spiral hand orthosis?

- Allows wrist and hand to move freely
- Helps in decreasing abnormal tone
- Increases forearm range of motion.

In case of severe deformity or contracture or open wound it should not be used.

Q. What are the static and dynamic orthosis?

Static orthosis:

- Used for immobilization or support
- Help prevent deformity
- Prevent soft-tissue contracture
- Allow attachment of assistive devices

Dynamic orthosis:

- Used to substitute for loss of motor function
- To correct an existing deformity
- Aid in fracture alignment and wound healing

Q. What are the common orthosis and there mechanism of action?

Common orthosis and their mechanism of action have been discussed in Table 2.38.

Table 2.38: Common orthosis

Name	*Deformity*	*Orthosis*	*Mechanism of action*
Ring orthosis	Swan-neck deformity		Prevents PIP joint hyperextension through a 3-point pressure system but allows full IP flexion
Ring orthosis	Boutonniere deformity		Immobilizes the PIP in extension and prevents flexion through a 3-point pressure system
Ulnar deviation orthosis	Ulnar deviation of fingers		The ulnar deviation orthosis provides support to the MCP joints, which restricts flexion and may assist in proper alignment by pulling the fingers radially out of ulnar deviation. The IP joints are left free to encourage proximal IP flexion during activities

Contd...

Contd...

Name	*Deformity*	*Orthosis*	*Mechanism of action*
Ring orthosis	Z deformity thumb	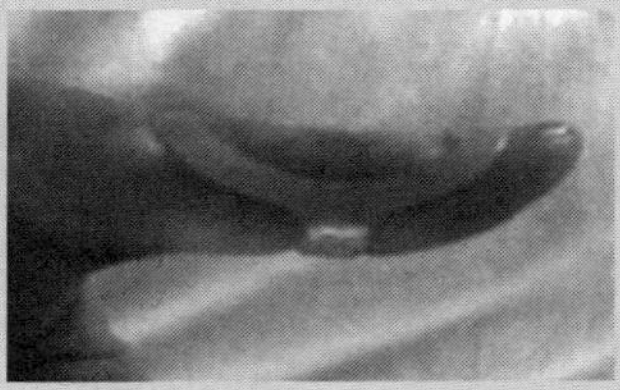	3 point pressure system
Thumb abduction splint	Game keepers thumb	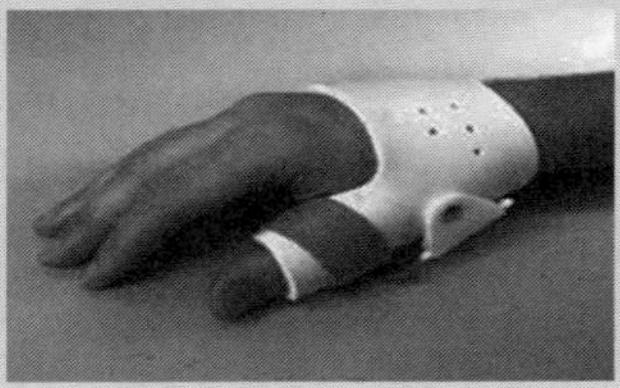	Immobilize the thumb to promote tissue healing and/or protection or for positioning of the weak thumb in opposition to other fingers to facilitate 3-jaw-chuck pinch
Abduction splint	Halux valgus	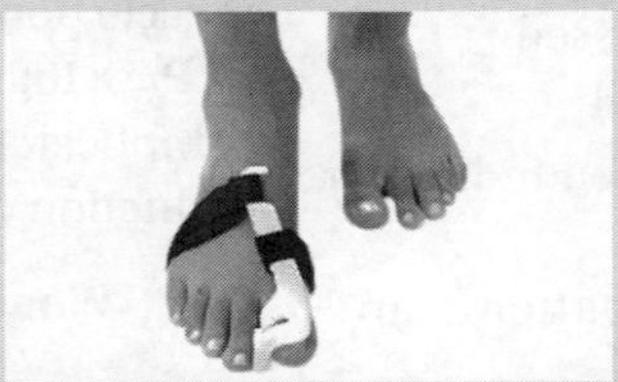	
Toe crest	Hammer toe	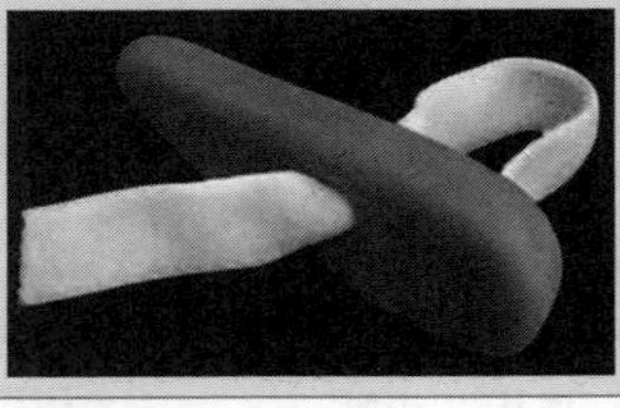	

PIP: Proximal interphalangeal
MCP: Meta carpophalangeal

Q. What home modifications will you suggest in RA?

Access routes—At least two for entrance/exits and emergency evacuation plans.

Staircase—4-7 inch height x 11 inch depth with non-skid surface with continuous handrails with height of 34-38 inch, 1.5 inch from wall and 1.25-2 inch cross sectional area.

Wide doorways (at least 32 inch) with level threshold and easy grab doorknobs

Ramp—Slope of 12 inch of ramp length for every inch of vertical rise with 3-4 feet width for walker/ wheelchair with continuous hand rails, rest platforms at 10 foot interval.

In kitchen, spice rack and milk box at wheelchair level, push button controls on stove.

Patient has two special sticks to operate stove. Front loading dishwasher.

In bathroom, Floor—stable, firm, skid resistant and unobstructed.

It should have grab bars, elevated toilet seats/ basin, non-skid strips in bath tubs, angled lever type handles in shower spray, flush controls and toilet paper dispenser within reach.

Cabinets—not very high up in the wall (between 36 and 44 inch).

Q. What are the goals of surgery in RA?

- Relieve pain
- Prevent destruction of cartilage or tendon
- Improve function of joints
- Correcting deformity
- Increasing stability
- Improving effective muscle forces.

Q. What are the surgeries done in RA?

- PROPHYLACTIC : Synovectomy
  THERAPEUTIC : Tendon repair and realingment

Osteotomy
Arthrodesis
Arthroplasty.

Q. What are the poor prognostic factors associated with RA?

- Presence of rhematoid factor and titer
- Presence of antibodies to anti ccp and titer
- Erosive disease at presentation
- Magnitude of acute phase reactants
- Presence of nodules or other extra articular features
- Disease activity at presentation
- Presence of shared epitope (HLA-DR alleles) and no of copies
- Female gender
- Current or past smoking
- Obesity.

Q. Describe the councelling in RA.

To patient and next of kin

- Disease and its course is to be discussed
- Possible complications is mentioned
- Treatment plan should be mentioned in his/her own language
- Rehab goals are set along with patients and families expectations are noted.

Q. What is the advantages of aqua therapy in RA?

- Elimination of gravity
- Positive effect of water buoyancy
- Decreased joint compression and pain
- Increased muscle relaxation
- Greater level of aerobic exercise may be tolerated in the water than on land.

Q. What are the safe DMARDS in Pregnancy?

- Safe with high-level evidence: Azathioprine
- Safe with low-level evidence: HCQ, rituximab, sulfasalazine
- Contraindicated: Methotrexate, leflunomide
- Inadequate data: Abatacept, toclizumab, anakinra.

Q. What DMARDS safe during lactations?

Safe to continue during lactation: NSAIDs, corticosteroid, HCQ, sulphasalazine.

Inadequate data regarding lactation: TNF alpha inhibitors, anakinra, abatacept, rituximab, toclizumab, tofacitinab.

Contraindicated during lactation: Methotrexate, leflunomide, azathioprine.

AMPUTATION (ABOVE KNEE)

Summary: A 30-years-old male shopkeeper presented with loss of right lower limb after road traffic accident two months back. Initially he was treated in orthopedic ward by surgery followed by regular dressing and antibiotics. Thereby wound healed completely though he is complaining about pain from the residual limb. Not only that but also sometime he has feeling that something is touching on his right toes intermittently. He is severely depressed at this moment. Although he is managing his ADL independently, his mobility at this moment is mainly by two axillary crutches. His bladder bowel appetite is normal. After the incident he did not receive any active rehabilitation care or immediate prosthetic fitting. Now he has been referred to rehabilitation ward for further care.

On examination, he is fully oriented and conscious cooperative. He has right mid thigh amputation with cylindrical stump without any bony prominence. But there is a neuroma at the end of the stump. Stump length is 25 cm from the right greater trochanter. Hip range of motion is full apart from restricted range of motion of right side. Hip muscle power is 5/5 in both the limbs.

P/D: Right-sided above knee post-traumatic amputation complicated with phantom limb sensation, neuroma and abduction deformity with FIM score of 101.

Q. What are the different etiology of amputation?

- Vascular disease
- Trauma
- Infection
- Cancer
- Congenital deformities.

Q. What is the difference between disarticulation and amputation?

Amputation is a procedure where a part of limb is removed through one or more bones.

Disarticulation is the separation of two bones from their joint.

Q. What are the level of amputation in upper limb and lower limb?

- Upper Limb
  - Transphalangeal
  - Transmetacarpal
  - Transcarpal
  - Wrist disarticulation
  - Transradial (below elbow) amputation
  - Elbow disarticulation
  - Transhumeral (above elbow) amputation—6.5 cm or more proximal to the elbow joint
  - Shoulder disarticulation
  - Forequarter amputation
- Lower limb
  - Partial toe—Excision of any part of 1 or more toes
  - Toe disarticulation—Disarticulation at the MTP joint
  - Partial foot/Ray resection—Resection of a portion of up to 3 metatarsals and digits

- Transmetatarsal amputation—Amputation through the midsection of all metatarsals
- Lisfranc—Amputation at the tarso-metatarsal junction
- Chopart—Midtarsal amputation—only talus and calcaneus remain
- Syme's—Ankle disarticulation with attachment of heel pad to distal end of tibia. It may include removal of malleoli and distal tibial/fibular flares
- Long BKA (transtibial)—> 50% of tibial length (residual)
- Standard BKA—20–50% of tibial length (residual)
- Short BKA (transtibial)—< 20% of tibial length (residual)
- Knee disarticulation—Amputation through the knee joint, femur intact (residual)
- Long AKA (transfemoral)—>60% of femoral length (residual)
- AK (transfemoral)—35–60% of femoral length (residual)
- Short AKA (transfemoral)—<35% of femoral length (residual)
- Hip disarticulation—Amputation through hip joint, pelvis intact
- Hemipelvectomy—Resection of lower half of the pelvis
- Hemicorporectomy—Amputation of both lower limbs and pelvis below L4, 5 level

Q. What are the standard length of amputation in upper limb and lower limb ?

See above

AK—10–12 inches from tip of greater trochanter

BK—5.5 inches from medial edge of tibial plateau

AE—8 inches from tip of acromion

BE—7 inches from tip of olecranon.

Q. Do you think this length is ideal?

Yes.

Q. What do you mean by ideal stump ?

- Stump must be covered by healthy skin
- Must not have any joint contractures
- Stump should not be flabby
- No fixed deformity
- Should have adequate muscle power
- Must be free from pain
- Bone end well covered with muscles
- Should have end bearing
- Incision scar should not be adherent to bone
- Absence of neuroma
- Free from infection
- Must have proper skin and joint senses
- Should have a proper length to fit with a prosthesis.

Q. Why is it ideal in this patient?

Because of the length, covered with healthy skin without any contracture.

Q. What is myodesis and myoplasty?

Stable distal muscle padding can be accomplished through *myodesis,* in which the deep layers are sutured directly to the periosteum. It can also be accomplished by *myoplasty,* in which the superficial antagonistic muscles are sutured together and to the deeper muscle layers.

Q. What are the complications of amputee?

Early complications:

- Secondary hemorrhage
- Breakdown of the skin flaps (may be due to ischemia or excessive suture tension)
- Gas gangrene.

Late complications:

- Dermatological
  - Eczema
  - Purulent lumps
  - Fissuring and ulceration
  - Infected epidermoid cyst
  - Squamous cell carcinoma
  - Verrucous hyperplasia.
- Muscular
  - Weakness
  - Imbalance
  - Tightness.
- Vascular
  - Ischemia
  - Necrosis.
- Neurological
  - Phantom pain
  - Phantom limb
  - Reflex sympathetic dystrophy.
- Joints
  - Contracture.
- Bone
  - Heterotrophic ossification
  - Bone spur.

Q. What are the complications before and after prosthetic fitting?

Complications occuring before and after prothetic fitting are given in Table 2.39.

Table 2.39: Complications before and after prothetic fitting

Preprosthetic	*Postprosthetic*
Delayed healing	Painful residual limb
Skin adherence to bone of residual limb	Adherence of skin to bone
Problems in shaping of residual limb	Insensitive skin
Chronic wound sinus	Poor fit
Contractures	Bony overgrowth in children
	Fractures
	Degenerative arthritis

Q. What are the hindrances in management of this patient?

Stump complications:
- Phantom limb
- Neuroma
- Hip-abduction deformity.

Systemic complication:
- Depression
- Low endurance.

Q. What is the management?

1. Patient education and counselling.
2. Goal setting after discussion with the patient and party.
3. Proper positioning of the residual limb.
4. Investigations:
   - Routine blood
   - FBS, lipid profile, ECG, Doppler—if diabetic
   - Gait analysis with/without prosthesis.
5. Medical management:
   - Anti-depressant
   - Pain management (stump and neuropathic)
   - Wound dressing
   - Local and systemic steroids
   - Antioxidants.
6. Nonpharmacological:

- Stump care:
  - Wound care
  - Edema control
  - Desensitization technique
  - Sensory reeducation in healed stump
  - Keep the stump clean, dry, and free from infection at all times
  - If fitted with a prosthesis, it should be removed before going to sleep
  - Inspect and wash the stump with mild soap and warm water every night, then dry thoroughly and apply talcum powder
  - Do not use the prosthesis until the skin has healed
  - The stump sock should be changed daily, and the inside of the socket may be cleaned with mild soap.
- Physiotherapy:
  - Maintaining ROM of proximal joints
  - Crutch muscle strengthening
  - Strengthening of hip extensors, adductors, abductors
  - Stretching of hip abductors and flexors
  - Deep breathing exercise
  - Endurance training.
- Modalities:
  - TENS (neuropathic pain)
  - UST (for neuroma)
- Prosthetic management:
  - Preprosthetic counselling
  - Preprosthetic training
  - Measurement and fitting of right AK prosthesis
  - Prosthetic checkout.
- Occupational therapy:
  - Weight bearing with prosthesis
  - Weight shifting initiated with prosthesis
  - Gait training with axillary crutch
  - Gait training with prosthesis
  - Obstacle walking
  - Independent walking without crutch
  - Staircase climbing
  - Simulated task training.
- Psychological counselling
- Vocational rehabilitation
- Home modification
- Resettlement.

N.B.—As a shopkeeper he can maintain his current job by proper rehab program.

- Follow-up for further checkout and assessment of performance level and adjustment of rehab program accordingly.

Q. What are the don'ts in this patient?

- Rigid dressing must not be off for more than 20 minutes
- No pillow under affected leg when supine and between the legs
- No crossing leg in bed
- Avoid dangling right leg over the side of the bed

- Not to sit longer than 30 minutes
- Should not put pressure on the limb or drag it on the bed.

Q. What are the preoperation rehab plans?
- Patient education
- Psychological counselling
- Nutritional care
- Endurance training
- Maintaining ROM of proximal joints
- Maintaining muscle mass
- Transfer training
- Crutch gait training.

Q. What is the postoperative rehab management?
- Prevention of complications
- Promotion of wound healing
- Strength and mobility of the whole body
- To strengthen and mobilize unaffected leg
- To strengthen and co-ordinate the muscles controlling the stump
- To strengthen and mobilize the trunk and retrain balance
- Initiate remobilization and pre prosthetic training
- Prevention of joint contracture
- To teach the patient to regain independence in functional activities
- To control edema of the stump and commence early ambulation
- Re-education of sensation in healed stump
- Psychological support
- Successful discharge into community.

Q. Positioning of the residual limb?
- In supine lying:
  - Pillow should not be used below the residual limb
  - Limbs not to be kept abducted.
  - Place a pillow laterally along the residual limb to maintain neutral rotation with no abduction.
- In prone lying:
  - Should be encouraged keeping the pelvis flat on bed,
  - Legs close together
  - A pillow is placed anteriorly under the residual limb for 20–30 minutes, two to three times daily, to maintain hip extension.
- Side lying:
  - On the unaffected side
  - Flexing the hip on that side
  - The amputee limb should lie behind the normal limb and at level to the hip on same side.
- The patient should not put pressure on the limb or drag it on the bed
- Slightly raising the residual limb and moving it to the side while rolling to the unamputated side is the best way to come to sitting.
- Not to sit longer than 30 mins.

Q. What is the ambulatory level of this patient?
See Page number 258, Chapter 11.

Q. What are the prosthetic gait deviation of above knee amputee?
Prosthetic gait deviation is given in following Table 2.40.

Table 2.40: Prosthetic gait deviation

Problem	*Prosthetic causes*	*Amputee causes*
Lateral bending of trunk: Excessive bending occurs laterally from midline, generally to prosthetic side	Prosthesis may be too short Improperly shaped lateral wall High medial wall Prosthesis aligned in abduction	• May not have adequate balance • May have hip abduction contracture • Residual limb may be painful • Very short residual limb • Defect may be due to habit pattern
Abducted gait: Very wide-based gait with prosthesis held away from midline at all times	• Prosthesis may be too long • Too much adduction may have been built into prosthesis • High medial wall may cause amputee to hold prosthesis away to avoid ramus pressure • Improperly shaped lateral wall can fail to provide adequate support for femur • Pelvic band may be positioned too far away from patient's body	• Patient may have hip abduction contracture • Defect may be due to habit pattern

Contd...

Contd...

Problem	*Prosthetic causes*	*Amputee causes*
Circumducted gait: Prosthesis swings laterally in wide area during swing phase	• Prosthesis may be too long • Prosthesis may have too much alignment stability or friction in knee, making it difficult to bend knee in swing-through	• Inadequate suspension • Amputee may have abduction contracture of residual limb • Patient may lack confidence for flexing prosthetic knee because of muscle weakness or fear of stubbing toe and falling • Defect may be due to habit pattern
Vaulting: Rising on toe of sound foot permits amputee to swing prosthesis through with little knee flexion	• Prosthesis may be too long • Socket suspension may be inadequate • Excessive stability in alignment or some limitation of knee flexion, such as knee lock or strong extension aid, may cause this deficit	• Vaulting is fairly frequent habit pattern • Fear of stubbing toe may cause this defect • Residual limb discomfort may be a factor
Medial or lateral whips: Whips best observed when patient walks away from observer; a medial whip is present when heel travels medially on initial flexion at beginning of swing phase; a lateral whip exists when heel moves laterally	• Lateral whips may result from excessive internal rotation of prosthetic knee • Medial whips may result from excessive external rotation of knee • Socket may fit too tightly, thus reflecting residual limb rotation • Excessive valgus or "knock" in prosthetic knee may contribute to this defect • Badly aligned toe break in a conventional foot may cause twisting on toe-off	• Improper donning of socket or socket rotated on limb
Foot rotation at heel strike: As heel contacts the ground, the foot rotates laterally, sometimes with vibrating motion	• Too hard heel cushion or plantar flexion bumper	• Weakness at hip muscles
Foot slap: The foot plantar flexes too rapidly and strikes the floor with a slap	Plantar flexion bumper is too soft, offering insufficient resistance to foot motion as weight is transferred to the prosthesis	• None
Uneven heel rise: Prosthetic heel rises quite markedly and rapidly when knee is flexed at beginning of swing phase	• Knee joint may have insufficient friction • Extension aid may be inadequate	• Amputee may be using more power than necessary to force knee into flexion
Terminal swing impact: Rapid forward movement of shin piece allows knee to reach maximum extension with too much force before heel-strike	• Knee friction is insufficient • Knee extension aid may be too strong	Amputee may try to assure himself or herself that knee is in full extension by deliberately and forcibly extending the residual limb
Uneven step length: The length of the step taken with the prosthesis differs from that of the sound leg	• Insufficient socket flexion • Insufficient friction at the prosthetic knee or too loose an extension aid	• Pain or insecurity causing amputee to transfer weight quickly from the prosthesis to the sound leg • Hip flexion contracture
Exaggerated lordosis: The lumbar lordosis is exaggerated when the prosthesis is in stance phase, and the trunk may lean posteriorly	• Insufficient socket flexion • Insufficient support from the anterior socket brim	• Hip flexion contracture • Weak hip extensors • Weak abdominal muscles

Contd...

Contd...

Problem	*Prosthetic causes*	*Amputee causes*
Instability of the prosthetic knee creating a danger of falling	• Knee joint may be too far ahead of trochanter-knee ankle (TKA) line • Socket is mounted with excess flexion • Plantar flexion resistance may be too great, causing knee to buckle at heel-strike • Failure to limit dorsiflexion can lead to incomplete knee control	• Amputee may have hip extensor weakness • Severe hip flexion contracture may cause instability
Drop-off at end of stance phase; downward movement of trunk as body moves forward over prosthesis	• Limitation of dorsiflexion of prosthetic foot is inadequate • Heel of SACH-type foot may be too short, or toe break of a conventional foot may be too far posterior • Socket may have been placed too far anterior in relation to foot	• None

Q. What is IPOP cast?

It is immediate postoperative cast given in transtibial amputee for early ambulation. This rigid plaster casts result in accelerated rehabilitation times and significantly less edema compared with soft dressings; and were found to have significantly fewer postsurgical complications and fewer higher level revisions compared with soft gauze dressings. Only limited weight bearing can take place with an IPOP.

Q. What are the nature of different types of pain and management strategies ?

Nature of different types of pain and their management strategies have been given in Table 2.41.

Table 2.41: Different types of pain

Type of pain	*Cause*	*Features*	*Management*
Phantom pain	Due to loss of inhibitory influences normally inhibited through the afferent impulses from the limb and associated central connections	Cramping, crushing, burning, shooting Located in phantom	Desensitization technique Antidepressant Anticonvulsant TENS
Residual limb (intrinsic)	Neuroma	Local pain in the stump Increases with activity	Rubbing, tapping, massaging, TENS, nerve block. Proper fitting of the prosthesis
Residual limb (extrinsic)	Ill-fitting prosthesis		
Biomechanical	Muscular imbalance	Mechanical pain	Correction of biomechanical factors

Q. Why neuroma forms?

Formation of scar tissue around the distal end of the severed nerve. Every time a nerve is cut it forms a neuroma.

Q. How to prevent neuroma formation?

- Cutting the nerves sharply
- Gentle traction on nerves as being cut
- Avoiding nerve in the suture lines.

Q. What is definition, pathogenesis and management of phantom limb sensation?

- Phantom sensation is a normal occurrence after amputation of a limb. This is the sensation that the amputed part is present
- Almost all amputees except young children and those with brain damage have phantom sensation
- Pathogenesis: Arises from excessive, spontaneous firing of the spinal cord neurons that have lost their normal sensory input from missing body part
- Management: Does not need treatment, diminishes over time.

Q. What are the effects of abduction deformity in rehabilitation?

- Difficulty in prosthetic fitting
- Circumduction gait.

Q. How will you overcome this problem?

- Proper positioning of residual limb
- Stretching of hip abductors
- Strengthening of hip adductors
- Reattachment of adductor mechanism during surgery.

Q. What is the problem with too long or too short stump?

Too short a stump—slips out from the prosthesis

Too long a stump—painful, ulcerate, complicates the incorporation of the joint in the prosthesis (with current suspension and prosthetic design there is no such problem)

Q. Which stump shape is ideal for prosthetic fitting?

Cylindrical for above knee amputation

Conical for below knee amputation.

Q. How will you manage if further wound develops after prosthetic fittings?

- Wound care
- Avoid wearing prosthesis till wound is healed
- Relief areas on the corresponding portion of prosthesis.

Q. How will you do figure of 8 bandaging?

As per Figure 2.1.

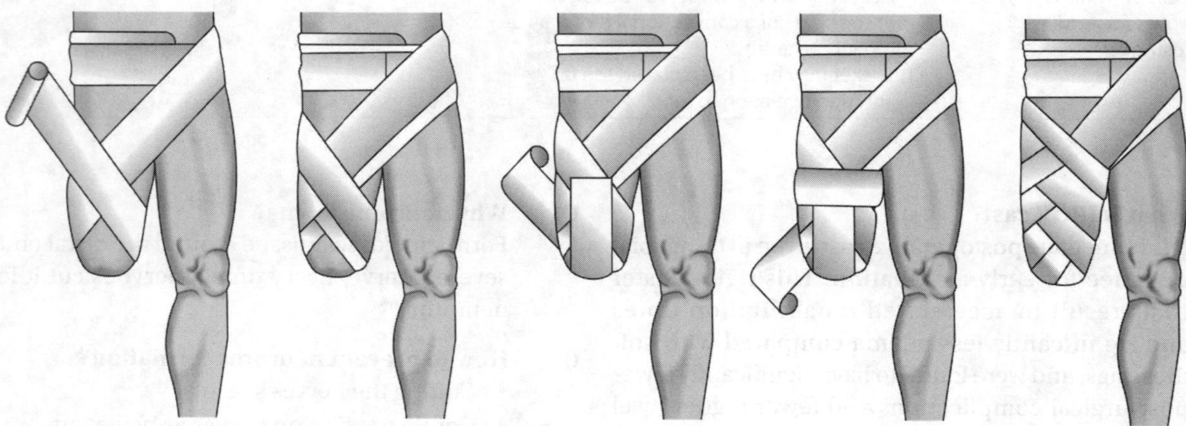

Figure 2.1: Figure of 8 bandaging

Q. What are the other bandage types?

- Soft
  - Shrinkers
  - Elastic wraps
- Semi rigid
- Rigid
  - Removable
  - Nonremovable.

Q. What are the causes of bony projection? How will you manage?

- The most common type of bony overgrowth is associated with production of bone spurs from remnants of periosteum left in the stump at surgery
- Managed by socket modifications, surgical removal of the spur and periosteum.

Q. What are the modifications for prosthesis in this patient?

No modification required.

Q. When will you consider the stump is ready for definite prosthesis?

- No discharge
- No pain
- No deformity
- No fluctuation in limb size.

Q. Other questions in AK prosthesis.

See Page number 139, Chapter 4.

Q. What are the occupational therapy needed in case of upper limb amputation?

- Postprosthetic stage
  - Prehension training
  - ADL training
  - Terminal device control training.
- Psychological counselling and social acceptance
- Simulated task/work training with the prosthesis
- Vocational rehabilitation.

Q. Classify congenital absence of limbs.

- *Amelia:* Absence of a limb
- *Meromelia:* Partial absence of a limb
- *Phocomelia:* Flipper-like appendage attached to the trunk
- *Adactyly:* Absent metacarpal or metatarsal
- *Hemimelia:* Absence of half a limb
- *Acheiria:* Missing hand or foot
- *Aphalangia:* Absent finger or toe.

Q. What is ISPO Classification System for congenital upper limb reductions?

- *Transverse deficiency:* (No remaining distal portions). (Transverse level is named after the segment beyond which there is no skeletal portion)
- *Longitudinal deficiency:* Some remaining distal portions. (Longitudinal deficiencies name the bones that are affected).

Q. What are the salient points to consider in this patients?

- The child with a congenital condition may be provided with a passive hand within 60-90 days after birth
- Maintenance of muscular development in residual limb
- Prevention of progressive deformity
- Retention of all long bone growth plates
- Preservation and stabilization of proximal joints
- Only one type of prosthesis should be used for the very young child
- Try to avoid hook in UL prosthesis
- Use myoelectric prosthesis if feasible
- The more cosmetic the prosthesis, the greater the chance of a positive reaction to the child.
- The rapid growth of their limbs requires replacement of all or part of the prosthesis annually
- The use of multilayered sockets or thick limb socks will delay the replacement
- The use of thermoplastics that are adjustable will also help
- The life-style of the child requires that the prostheses be functional, durable, and cosmetic.

Q. How will you assess the disability of amputation?

Basic guidelines

1. In case of multiple amputees, if the total sum of percentage permanent physical impairment is above 100%, it should be taken as 100%.
2. *Amputation at any level with uncorrectable inability to wear and use prosthesis, should be given 100% permanent physical impairment.*
3. In case of amputation in more than one limb percentage of each limb is counted and another 10% will be added, but when only toes or fingers are involved only another 5% will be added.
4. Any complication in form of stiffness, neuroma, infection, etc. has to be given a total of 10% additional weightage.
5. Dominant upper limb has been given 4% extra percentage.

Upper limb amputation percent permanent physical impairment and loss of physical function of each limb

- Fore-quarter amputation—100%
- Shoulder disarticulation—90%
- Above elbow up to upper 1/3 of arm—85%
- Above elbow up to lower 1/3 of arm—80%
- Elbow disarticulation—75%
- Below elbow up to upper 1/3 of forearm—70%
- Below elbow up to lower 1/3 of forearm—65%
- Wrist disarticulation—60%
- Hand through carpal bones—55%
- Thumb through CMC or through 1st MC joint—30%
- Thumb disarticulation through metacarpophalangeal joint or through proximal phalanx—25%
- Thumb disarticulation through interphalangeal joint or through distal phalanx—15%.

Table 2.42: PPI in amputation of digits

	Index finger	*Middle finger*	*Ring finger*	*Little finger*
Amputation through proximal phalanx or disarticulation through MP joint	15%	5%	3%	2%
Amputation through middle phalanx or disarticulation through PIP joint	10%	4%	2%	1%
Amputation through distal phalanx or disarticulation through DIP joint	5%	2%	1%	1%

Lower Limb Amputations

- Hind quarter—100%
- Hip disarticulation—90%
- Above knee up to upper 1/3 of thigh—85%
- Above knee up to lower 1/3 of thigh—80%
- Through knee—75%
- BK up to 8 cm—70%
- BK up to lower 1/3 of leg—60%
- Through ankle—55%
- Syme's—50%
- Up to mid-foot—40%
- Up to fore-foot—30%
- All toes—20%
- Loss of first toe—10%
- Loss of second toe—5%
- Loss of third toe—4%
- Loss of fourth toe—3%
- Loss of fifth toe—2%.

3

Chapter

Short Cases

ABNORMAL GAIT

Summary 1

The patient is having steppage gait with low cadence, absent heel strike without any heel-to-toe rhythm. He is also having high ground clearance.

1. Lateral peroneal nerve palsy.
2. HSMN/CMT.
3. Post-polio residual palsy (PPRP).

Summary 2

This patient is walking on wide base with increased lumbar lordosis, side-to-side trunk movement and dropping of pelvis on each side once leg is off the ground. His toes touches the ground before heel. So I think he is having waddling gait.

Etiology:

1. BMD/DMD (Becker's/ Duschene's muscular dystrophy).
2. Dermatomysosis.
3. Rickets/Osteomalacia.

Summary 3

This patient is walking with stiff right leg along with each step. He tilts the pelvis to the other side trying to keep his toe off the ground. His right leg is following semicircular motion to maintain the ground clearance and forefoot touches the ground before heel. At the same time right hand is flexed and trying to maintain the balance and keep center of gravity in near neutral position. So I think he is having circumduction gait.

Etiology: All cause of hemiplegia.

Summary 4

This patient is walking with low speed and cadence. At the same time his lower limb is crossing the midline every time. So I think he has scissoring gait.

Etiology:

1. Spastic paraplegia.
2. Cord compression.
3. Demylinating disease.
4. Hereditary spastic paraparesis.
5. Diplegic CP.

Summary 5

The patient walks with wide base and arm held wide with tremor of right hand. He has ataxia of trunk and tends to fall on right side specially during tandem walk. Romberg sign is negative.

I think he is having ataxic gait due to cerebellar origin.

Etiology:

1. Demylenation.
2. SOL (Cerebellar).
3. Vasculitis.
4. Alcoholic cerebellar degeneration.
5. Friedrich ataxia.

Summary 6

This patient is walking with a wide base and both heels and toes are slapping on the ground almost at the same time. He is continuously watching his feet and ground to compensate sensory feedback for muscles and joints. His heel-to-toe rhythm is broken and ataxia is becoming worse on eye closure. So I think he has sensory ataxia.

Etiology:

1. Subacute combined degeneration of cord (SCD).
2. Tabes dorsalis.
3. Friedrich ataxia.
4. Demylinating disease.
5. Diabetes pseudo tabes.

Summary 7

The elderly patient with expressionless, depressed facies is walking with initial hesitancy and is suffling continuously. Arm swing is quite low along with pen rolling movement of his hand. He is continuously about to fall as if he is trying to catch his own center of gravity.

I think he is having fastinating gait due to Parkinsonism.

Summary 8

This elderly patient walks on broad base, short steps, and places his foot flat cautiously as if is walking on ice, so called sticky feet. His turning and straight walking is not that fluid.

I think this is magnetic gait in gait apraxia.

Etiology:

1. Alzheimers disease.
2. Subdural hematoma.
3. Normal pressure hydrocephalus.

Q. What is gait?

A translatory progression of the body as a whole, produced by coordinated, rotatory movement of body segments.

Q. What is normal gait cycle?

It is the activity that occurs between the time one foot touches the floor and same foot touches the floor again.

It is also called stride.

Q. What are the phases of gait cycle?

There are two types of gait phase.

- **STANCE PHASE:** Activity that occurs when the foot is in contact with the ground.

This is 60% of gait cycle

- **SWING PHASE**: Activity that occurs when the foot is not in contact with the ground.

This is 40% of gait cycle.

Further classified into (Table 3.1):

Table 3.1: Phase of gait cycle

Stance phase		*Swing phase*	
Traditional	*Rancho Los amigos*	*Traditional*	*Rancho Los amigos*
Heel strike	Initial contact	Acceleration	Initial swing
Foot flat	Loading response	Midswing	Midswing
Midstance	Midstance	Deceleration	Terminal swing
Heel off	Terminal stance		
Toe off	Preswing		

Q. What are the determinants of gait?

It is applied in normal human gait to minimize the excursion of the body's center of gravity and help for forward progression with the least expenditure of energy. The six determinants of gait are as follows:

1. Pelvic rotation.
2. Pelvic tilt.
3. Knee flexion in stance phase.
4. Foot mechanisms.
5. Knee mechanisms.
6. Lateral displacement of the pelvis.

Q. How will you assess gait?

Components of gait analysis:

- Observational gait analysis
  - Clinic-based approach
  - Relevant history
  - Physical examination of the patient
  - Gait cycle observation and documentation
  - Videotaping if required for slow-motion analysis.
- Functional community analysis
  - Observation in outdoor setting
  - Maneuvering at different surface
  - Feasibility of community ambulation.
- Quantitative gait analysis
  - Kinetics
  - Kinematics
  - Poly-EMG or dynamic EMG
  - Energetics.

Q. How gait training is done?

See Chapter 10, Page number 253.

ACHONDROPLASIA

Summary

This 13-year-old right-handed school kid studying in class eight presented with short stature and associated mechanical low-back pain. His father along with his elder sister also has similar stature. There is associated frontal bossing and facial hypoplasia on examination along with disproportionate shortening of the proximal parts of limb and lengthening of the axial skeleton. There is radicular pain and SLR is forty degrees bilaterally.

So this is a case of achondroplasia with discogenic low-back pain.

Q. What is achondroplasia?

It is a clinical condition caused by the failure of normal ossification of bones primarily affecting the long bones which results in dwarfism.

Q. What is the pathogenesis?

It is essentially an abnormality of endochondral longitudinal growth resulting in diminished length of the tubular bones. Membrane bone formation is unaffected, hence the normal growth of the skull vault and the periosteal contribution to bone width.

Q. What are the other causes of dwarfism?

- Dyschondroplasia
- Diaphysialaclasis
- Multiple epiphyseal dysplasia
- Spondylo epiphyseal dysplasia
- Cretinism
- Malnutrition
- Metabolic storage disorders.

Q. What is the hereditary pattern of acho ndroplasia?

Autosomal dominant.

Q. What are the clinical features?

- Severely stunted growth
- Short limbs—Particularly the proximal segments are disproportionately short (rhizomelic shortening)
- Large skull with prominent forehead
- Saddle-shaped nose
- Stubby fingers and somewhat splayed *(trident hands)*
- Increased lumbar lordosis
- Joint laxity.

Q. What are the other types of epiphyseal dysplasias?

- Dysplasias with predominantly physeal and metaphyseal changes
  - Hereditary multiple exostosis
  - Achondroplasia
  - Hypochondroplasia
  - Metaphyseal chondrodysplasia
  - Dyschondroplasia (enchodromatosis, Ollier's disease).
- Dysplasias with predominantly epiphyseal changes
  - Multiple epiphyseal dysplasia
  - Spondyloepiphyseal dysplasia
  - Dysplasia epiphysealishemimlica (Trevor's disease)
  - Chondrodysplasia punctata (stippled epiphysis).
- Dysplasias with predominantly metaphyseal anddiaphyseal changes
  - Metaphyseal dysplasia (Pyle's disease)
  - Craniometaphyseal dysplasia
  - Diaphyseal dysplasia (Engelmann's disease, Cumurati's disease)
  - Craniodiaphyseal dysplasia
  - Osteopetrosis (marble bones, Albers-Shönbert disease)
  - Pyknodysostosis
  - Candle bones, spotted bones and striped bones.
- Combined and mixed dysplasias
  - Spondylometaphyseal
  - Pseudoachondroplasia
  - Diastrophic dysplasia
  - Cleidocranial dysplasia
  - Nail-patella syndrome
  - Craniofacial dysplasia.

Q. How will you manage this case?

- Reassurance
- Counselling
- Pharmacological:
  - NSAIDS
  - Gabapentin or Pregabalin
  - Methylcobalamin.
- Nonpharmacological:
  - ROM exercises
  - Postural care
  - Management of PIVD.

Q. Why low-back pain in this patient?

Due to prolapsed intervertebral disc.

Q. What are the major causes of LBP in these patients? Why?

- PIVD
- Spinal canal stenosis.

Since there is shortening of the vertebral pedicles.

Q. What are the secondary complications of achondroplasia?

- Lower-limb deformity
- Cervical stenosis
- Thoracolumbar kyphosis
- Foramen magnum stenosis
- PIVD
- Lumbar canal stenosis.

ADHESIVE CAPSULITIS

Summary

A 45-year-old diabetic office worker presented with restricted ROM of right shoulder along with mechanical shoulder pain for last three months. Initially only pain was there but was followed by progressive restriction of right shoulder. The pain is intense enough to disturb his sleep while trying to change sleeping positions. He also has difficulty in wearing T-shirts and in reaching his back while bathing. There is no neurodeficit or any vascular compromise. His ROM is restricted in all direction and in both active and passive movements.

So, this is a case of right-sided Stage II adhesive capsulitis of shoulder.

Q. What is adhesive capsulitis?

Adhesive capsulitis, or "frozen shoulder," is characterized by painful, restricted shoulder ROM in patients with normal radiographs.

Q. What are its stages?

Stage I to IV (See chapter 11, Page number 263)

Q. What are the risk factors?

- Intracranial lesions: CVA, hemorrhage, and brain tumor
- Depression
- Parkinson's disease
- Iatrogenic disorders (prolonged immobilization)
- Post CABG/Myocardial infarction
- Diabetes mellitus
- Hypothyroidism
- Rheumatoid arthritis
- Crystal diseas.

Q. What are the clinical signs related to examination of rotator cuff muscles?

Clinical signs related to examination of rotator cuff muscles are given in the Table 3.2.

Table 3.2: Examination of rotator cuff muscles

Test	*Description*	*Positive test*
Subscapularis		
Lift off test	Dorsum of hand on back and raise off the back	Patient is unable to lift dorsum of hand off the back
Belly press test	Press abdomen with hand flat and elbow forward	Elbow drops back behind the trunk
Supraspinatus and Infraspinatus		
External rotation lag sign at 0 degree	Elbow flexed at 90 degree, shoulder in 20 degree of elevation and near maximal external rotation and release examiners hand off the wrist	Lag or angular drop occurs
External rotation lag sign at 90 degree	Same as above except done with arm in 90 degree elevation	Lag or angular drop occurs
Empty can sign	First arm at 90 degree of abduction and neutral rotation then shoulder internally rotated and angulated at 30 degree	Weakness to resistance with second maneuver as compared with first
Bicep tendon		
Speed test	Flex shoulder against resistance while elbow extended and forearm supinated	Pain localized to bicepital groove
Impingement sign		
Neer sign	One hand of examiner is on top of shoulder and examiner raises the arm in forced forward elevation	Pain
Hawkin sign	Forward flex humerus to 90 degree and internally rotate	Pain

Q. How will you manage?

- **Investigations:**
  - Routine blood, FBS, PPBS, TSH, Free T4, T3,
  - X ray shoulder, AP view
  - USG of shoulder
  - MRI.

Q. What are the intra-articular approaches for shoulder joint?

- Anterior approach
- Posterior approach.

Q. Contraindications of intra-articular steroid?

- Uncontrolled hypertension
- Uncontrolled diabetes
- Infection
- Partial tear of supraspinatus
- Bleeding diathesis/coagulopathy.

Q. What is the supply of suprascapular nerve?

Motor innervation

- Supraspinatus muscle
- Infraspinatus muscle (through the spinoglenoid notch).

Sensory innervation

- Acromioclavicular joint
- Glenohumeral joint.

Q. What is the procedure of suprascapular nerve block?

In sitting position: The spine of the scapula is divided by line formed by the bisection of the scapular angle. The upper outer quadrant formed from the spine of the scapula and the vertical line bisecting the angle of the scapula is marked and a point is marked 2 cm anteriorly along this line for needle insertion. A 3-inch (8-cm), 23- to 25-gauge needle is inserted perpendicular to the skin and, using a nerve stimulator, advanced until needle placement is confirmed by movements of the supraspinatus and infraspinatus muscles. After negative aspiration, 5 mL of local anesthetic is injected.

It can be given by USG-guided method also.

Q. What are the complications?

- Intraneural injection
- Intravascular injection
- Hematoma
- Pneumothorax.

Q. How to assess impairment?

See Chapter 11, Page number 264.

Q. What is the prognosis?

Most patients will have restoration of normal function over a 12- to 14-month period. In patients who do not improve after 6 months of nonoperative treatment, more aggressive treatments, such as capsular hydrodilatation, manipulation under anaesthesia, and arthroscopic lysis of adhesions can be considered.

Q. What is impingement syndrome?

It is a clinical syndrome which occurs when the tendons of the rotator cuff muscles become irritated and inflamed as they pass through the subacromial space, the passage beneath the acromion. This can result in pain, weakness and loss of movement at the shoulder.

Q. What are the causes of impingement syndrome?

- Subacromial spurs (bony projections from the acromion)
- Osteoarthritic spurs on the acromioclavicular joint
- Variations in the shape of the acromion
- Thickening or calcification of the coracoacromial ligament.

Q. What is painful arc syndrome?

Same as Impingement syndrome.

Q. What is bicipital tendinitis?

Bicipital tendinitis, or biceps tendinitis, is an inflammatory process of the long head of the biceps tendon and is a common cause of shoulder pain due to its position and function.

Q. What is scapula thoracic rhythm?

Every 2 degree of shoulder abduction is accompanied by 1 degree of scapular motion, except for initial 30 degree. This is called scapula thoracic rhythm.

BELL'S PALSY (LMN VII CRANIAL NERVE PALSY)

Summary

A young female patient presented with sudden-onset right-sided weakness of upper and lower face so that the eyes cannot be closed. The eyeball rolled upward in an attempt to close the eyes with deviation of angle of mouth to the opposite side. This was preceded by a febrile illness and cough, coryza. Her nasolabial fold has smoothened out. She does not have any other weakness or tinnitus on examination. There is no parotid swelling, scar mark, ear surgery or vesicular eruption.

So this is a case of right LMN VII nerve palsy also called Bell's palsy.

Q. Why is it Bell's palsy?

- Bell's phenomenon (upward rolling of eye ball during attempted closure of eyelid)
- Preceding viral infection
- No other cause apparently found.

Q. What is Ramsay-Hunt Syndrome?

It is the reactivation of herpes zoster in the geniculate ganglion. It is sometimes called herpes zoster oticus. A triad of ipsilateral LMN facial paralysis, ear pain, and vesicles on the face, on the ear, or in the ear is the typical presentation and loss of taste sensation in anterior two third of tongue.

Q. What are the other etiologies of LMN facial nerve palsy?

- CP angle tumor—V, VI, VII, VIII nerve involved plus cerebellar signs plus loss of unilateral corneal reflex
- Parotid tumor
- Trauma
- Mononeuritis multiplex (other causes)
- Middle ear disease.

Q. Is there only motor and no sensory features in LMN VII nerve palsy?

Sensory loss in the anterior 2/3rd of tongue of the involved side is also present.

Q. What is the motor supply of face?

All muscles of face are supplied by the facial nerve except masseter and temporalis.

Q. What are the branches of the facial nerve?

Intracranial branches

- Greater petrosal nerve— It arises at the geniculate ganglion and provides parasympathetic innervation to several glands, including the nasal gland,palatine gland, lacrimal gland, and pharyngeal gland. It also provides parasympathetic innervation to the sphenoid sinus, frontal sinus, maxillary sinus, ethmoid sinus and nasal cavity.
- Communicating branch to the otic ganglion— It arises at the geniculate ganglion and joins the lesser petrosal nerve to reach the otic ganglion.
- Nerve to stapedius—provides motor innervation for stapedius muscle in middle ear
- Chorda tympani
  - Submandibular gland
  - Sublingual gland
  - Special sensory taste fibers for the anterior 2/3 of the tongue.

Extracranial branches

Distal to stylomastoid foramen, the following nerves branch off the facial nerve:

- Posterior auricular nerve—controls movements of some of the scalp muscles around the ear
- Branch to posterior belly of digastric muscle as well as the stylohyoid muscle
- Five major facial branches (in parotid gland)—from top to bottom:
  - Temporal branch
  - Zygomatic branch
  - Buccal branch
  - Marginal mandibular branch
  - Cervical branch.

Q. What are the cause of bilateral LMN facial palsy?

- GB Syndrome
- Sarcoidosis
- Bilateral Bells palsy
- Myasthenia gravis
- MND (rarely).

Q. What is the difference between LMN and UMN facial palsy?

Difference between LMN and UMN facial palsy have been given in Table 3.3.

Table 3.3: Different between LMN and UMN facial palsy

Features	*LMN*	*UMN*
Upper face	Involved	Escapes
Bell's phenomenon	Present	Ansent
Atrophy	Present	Absent
Taste sensation	Lost	Preserved
Other UMN features	Absent	Present
Hemiplegia	Always crossed	Always same sided
Investigation	NCS of facial nerve	CT/MRI of brain
Role of electric stimulation	Present	Absent

Q. What is the management?

- Investigation: FBS (DM), CBC, ESR, CRP (vasculitis)
- NCS of facial nerve
- Medicine:
  - Eye drops/ cream/ eye protection
  - Short course of steroid: Tapering dose
  - Vitamin B_{12} and pregabalin
  - Acyclovir 800 mg 5 times a day for 5–7 days
- Nonpharmacological
- Exercise:
  - Facial muscles strengthening
  - Maintaining ROM
  - Modalities Galvanic stimulation after 2 weeks followed by faradic

- Splint: To prevent or correct facial deviation
- Surgical decompression.

NB

1. Most common cranial nerve palsy of diabetes patients—VII nerve
2. Most common cause of III cranial nerve palsy—Diabetes mellitus

Q. What is crocodile tear syndrome or Bogard's syndrome?

It is due to faulty connection between regenerating facial nerve with lacrimal gland. There is excessive tearing while chewing foods due to wrong connection.

Q. What is Frey's syndrome?

It is is a rare neurological disorder resulting from damage to or near the parotid glands responsible for making saliva, and from damage to the auriculotemporal nerve often from surgery.

The symptoms of Frey's syndrome are redness and sweating on the cheek area adjacent to the ear. They can appear when the affected person eats, sees, dreams, thinks about or talks about certain kinds of food which produce strong salivation due to faulty reinnervations of auriculotemporal nerve to sweat glands during regeneration stage.

BELOW ELBOW AMPUTATION

Summary

A 23-year-old male industrial worker presented with loss of his part of right fore arm and hand after a machine injury two months back. Initially, he was treated with surgery followed by regular dressing and antibiotics. Now his wound has healed completely with a pain sensation over stump area. He is quite depressed because he has lost his job.

On examination, his stump length is 7 cm from epicondyle, conical in shape with a painful neuroma on stump. His FIM Score is 100/126.

P/D: Below elbow amputation with painful neuroma.

Q. What are types of upper limb amputation?

1. Transphalangeal.
2. Transmetacarpal.
3. Transcarpal.
4. Wrist disarticulation.
5. Transradial (below elbow) amputation.
6. Elbow disarticulation.
7. Transhumeral (above elbow) amputation—6.5 cm or more proximal to the elbow joint.
8. Shoulder disarticulation
9. Forequarter amputation.

Q. What are the hindrances in management of this case?

- Stump hindrance
  - Stump pain
  - Neuroma
- Depression
- Economic condition.

Q. How will you manage this case?

- Counceling
- Patient education
- Goal setting
- Investigations:
  - Routine blood
  - X-ray of the residual limbs.

Treatment:

- Pharmacological:
  - Wound care
  - Anti depressents
- Nonpharmacological:
  - Stump care
  - Range of motion exercise of elbow and shoulder joint.

Modalities: UST over Stump area for neuroma

Orthosis: Below elbow prosthesis: See prosthesis section.

Q. What are the Do's and Don't's ?

See Chapter 2, Long cases.

Q. What is the ideal stump?

See Chapter 2, Long cases.

Q. What are the different types of grips?

1. *Precision grip (i.e., pincher grip):* The pad of the thumb and index finger are in opposition to pick up or pinch a small object (e.g., a small bead, pencil, grain of rice).
2. *Tripod grip (i.e., palmar grip, three-jaw chuck pinch):* The pad of the thumb is against the pads of the index and middle finger.
3. *Lateral grip (i.e., key pinch):* Tips of the fingers and thumb are flexed (e.g., when screwing in a light bulb or turning a doorknob).
4. *Hook power grip:* The distal interphalangeal joint and proximal interphalangeal joint are flexed with

the thumb extended (as when carrying a briefcase by the handle).

5. *Spherical grip*: Tips of the fingers and thumb are flexed (e.g., when screwing in a light bulb or opening a doorknob).

Q.48 What are the different Grasps ?

Ans.
- Cylindrical grasp
- Tip grasp
- Hook grasp
- Palmar grasp
- Spherical grasp
- Lateral grasp.

Q. What is the difference between grip and grasp?

It is more or less similar: holding the object

Grasp: To take hold of something

Grip : To have hold of something

Q. Which functions are achieved by conventional BE prosthesis?

- Active lateral pinch grip
- Hook grip

Q. What is cosmetic BE prosthesis?

It is a passive terminal device with no active function.

Q. What are the advantages of myoelectric prosthesis?

- Do not require a harness or cable
- Looks like natural-appearing arm
- Battery powered, so motor strength and coordinated mobility are not as important as other prosthesis
- Newer batteries have reduced weight.
- Provides strong grip force
- Greater ROM.

Q. What are the advantage of neuronal prosthesis?

See Chapter 4.

Q. What is robotics?

Rehabilitation robotics is the field of science and engineering concerned with powered devices for improving function or mobility in individuals with disabilities. It includes powered devices for movement therapy (e.g., after a stroke or spinal cord injury) and of robotic devices for the chronic assistance of human function (e.g., powered prosthetics and orthotics).

Q. What are the basic differences in amputation care of UL and LL?

Basic differences in amputation care of Upper limb (UL) and Lower limb (LL) has been given Table 3.4.

Table 3.4: Differences in amputation care of UL and LL

Rehabilitation concern	*Upper limb*	*Lower limb*
Range of motion	More required	Lesser
Stability	Less important	More important
iADL and ADL	More	Less
Weight bearing	Not done	Done
Endurance in training	Normal	Increased training
Work-station modification	Required	Less required
Home modification	Same	Same

Q. What are the specific hindrances of bilateral UL amputation?

- No "sound limb"for the prosthetic limb to assist
- The ability to handle complex sensory feedback and fine manipulation is lost
- The sockets need to be easily donned and doffed for independence to occur.

Q. What is Caryle formula

It is the formula for measurement of prosthesis requirement in bilateral amputee.

- *Bilateral transradial amputee:* The formula for the distance from the apex of the lateral epicondyle to thumb tip (forearm) is the patient's body height × 0.21 (in either English or metric units).
- *Bilateral transhumeral amputee:* The formula for the distance from the acromion to the lateral epicondyle (arm) is the patient's body height × 0.19.

Q. How will you manage the case?

- Bilateral wrist flexion units are mandatory to obtain the positioning necessary to master basic hygiene
- The socket is aligned in such a way that it brings the terminal device closer to the center of the body.

BENIGN HYPERMOBILE JOINT SYNDROME

Summary

A 17-year-old male patient presented with polyarthralgia in mainly the large joints which is worsening after working and playing contact sports. His joints are hyperextensible with genu recurrvatum and pes planus deformity of both lower limbs.

His palate is not high arched and there is no skin laxity or changes. His intelligence level is absolutely

normal. He did not suffer from any lens subluxation. His CVS examinations did not reveal any murmur in auscultation he did not have any pneumothorax or DVT in his life

P/D: Benign hyper mobile joint syndrome (BHJS)

Q. What are the causes of hypermobile joint syndrome?

- BHJS
- Marfans syndrome
- Osteogenesis imperfacta
- Noonans syndrome
- Pseudo xanthoma elastic
- Downs syndrome
- Familial.

Q. What is the diagnostic criteria of BHJS?

By Beightons Critria

Major criteria

- Beighton score of 4 or more
- Joint pain affecting 4 or more joints and lasting more than 3 months.

Minor criteria

- Beighton score of 1, 2, or 3
- Back pain or pain in one to three joints lasting more than 3 months, or spinal spondylosis, spondylolysis, or spondylolisthesis joint hypermobility
- Dislocation of more than one joint, or of one joint more than once
- 3 or more soft-tissue problems (e.g., tendonitis, bursitis)
- Tall, thin body shape
- Skin hyperextensibility, stretch marks, thin skin, or abnormal scarring
- Drooping eyelids, near sightedness
- Varicose veins, hernia or uterine or rectal prolapse
- Mitral valve prolapse

(Any of the following required for diagnosis)

- 2 major criteria
- 1 major and two minor criteria
- 4 minor criteria
- 2 minor criteria and a clearly affected first-degree relative.

Q. What is Beightons score?

See Chapter 11, Page 265.

Q. How will you manage the case?

- Patient education and counceling
- Investigations: X-rays of hand
  ECHO to rule out MVP.
- Pharmacology: NSAIDs for pain
- Nonpharmacology:
- PT Exercise: Strengthening exercises
- Modalities: Ice for pain
  Local heat.
- UST: Only if ephiphyseal fusion has occurred
- PO: Shoe modification for pes cavus
- OT: Energy conservation technique
  Joint protection technique.

Q. What are the features of Ehler Danlos?

- Face: Epicanthial fold, flat nasal bridge, prominent ears
- Skin: Hyperextensible, elastic, very thin
  - Poor healing,
  - Cigarette Paper scar
  - Fish mouth wound
  - Purpura
  - Kyphoscoliosis, genu recervatum.

Q. What are its complication?

- Bleeding from gut
- Poor hearing
- Recurrent fall
- Hernia/diverticulum
- Spontaneous pneumonia
- Dissecting aneurysm
- Spontaneous rupture of large arteries
- Mitral valve prolapse
- Recurrent dislocation of patella, thinner hip.

Q. What are the features of pseudoxanthoma elasticum?

- Skin: Loose on neck, axilla, ante cubital fossa, groin
- Yellow pseudoxanthoma plaques
- Plucked chicken appearance
- Occlusive arteriopathy: MI / IHD/PVD
- Blue sclera
- Loose joint
- Hypertention
- Hemorrhage (GI/GU)
- Mitral incompetence
- Hypothyroid
- Inherited deficiency of elastin
- Angiod streaks of retina *(also seen in pagets, Sickle cell anemia, hypophosphatemia)*
- Confirmed by skin biopsy.

Q. What are the clinical features of Marfans syndrome?

- Appearance: Tall, long extremities, arachnodactyly
  pigeon chest, pes excavatum, flat foot,
  genu recurvatum, kyphoscolosis

- Joint: Hypermobility
- Palate: High arched
- Eyes: Iridodenesis, lens dislocation, blue sclera, Retinal detachment
- Lungs: Cystic disease, recurrent pneumonia
- CVS: MVP, coarctation of aorta
- Hernia-Inguinal/Femoral.

Q. Which gene the defect lies?
Fibrillin gene (Chromosome 15 long arm).

Q. Most common cause of death?
Due to cardiovascular causes.

Q. What are the features of Homocyestinuria?
- Marfanoid Features
- Mental retardation
- Osteoporosis
- Recurrent venous thrombosis
- Urine: cyanide nitroprusside test positive.

Q. What are the difference from marfans syndrome?
Lens sublaxation is downward and nasal with presence of mental retardation and recurrent venous thrombosis in homocyestinuria.

Q. What are the features of Osteogenesis imperfect?
- Blue sclera
- Fragile bones
- Deafness from osteosclerosis
- Laxity of legs
- Muscles hypotonia and wasting
- Increased alkaline phosphatase and acid phosphatase
- Urine: Hydroxyl proline
- No specific treatment
- Calcitonin may be tried
- Bone marrow transplant can be done.

BULBAR AND PSEUDOBULBAR PALSY

Q. What are the features of bulbar palsy?
- Tongue flaccid, fasciculation, wasting
- Flaccid dysarthric / indistinctive speech, lacks modulation
- Absent palatal movement
- May be dysphagic with nasal regurgitation.

Q. What are the causes?
- Motor Neuron Disease
- Bulbar syrinx
- GBS
- Poliomyelitis
- Subacute meningitis
- Neurosyphilis.

Q. What is pseudo bulbar palsy?
- Can not protrude tongue, small and spastic
- Donald duck dysarthria—Nasal voice, slurred, high pitch
- Absent palatal movement
- Small tight tongue which cannot be protruded
- Persistant dribbling from mouth
- May be dysphagic with nasal regurgitation
- Increased jaw jerk
- Emotional liability.

Q. What are the causes?
- CVA—Bilateral internal capsule
- Multiple sclerosis
- MND
- Head injury
- High brainstem tumor.

CHARCOT-MARIE-TOOTH DISEASE

Summary

A 35-year-old patient presented with weakness of distal part of both upper and lower limbs for last one year which is gradual in onset slowly progressive in nature. He has pes cavus deformity of bilateral foot with foot drop in bilateral lower limb. His ankle jerk was absent with bilateral flexor planter. His popliteal nerve is thickened without any hypoanesthetic patch in his limbs. This is associated with with sensory loss in distal part of both limbs with wasting of small muscles of the hand. His legs appear like an inverted champagne bottle. He has a high stepping gait. His one brother also suffers from similar type of illness.
P/D: Charcot-Marie-tooth disease.

Q. What is peripheral neuropathy?
Peripheral neuropathy (PN) is damage to or disease affecting nerves, which may impair sensation, movement, gland or organ function, or other aspects of health, depending on the type of nerve affected.

Q. What are the types of HSMN?
- Type I Charcot-Marie-Tooth (CMT) disease
- Type II CMT
- Type III Dejerine–Sottas disease
- Type IV Refsum's disease
- Type V With spastic paraplegia
- Type VI With optic atrophy.

Q. Why is it inverted champagne bottle?
It is due to wasting of the distal musculature of foot and calf muscle hypertrophy.

Q. What is the surprising thing in disability of CMT?
Sometimes degree of disability is slight inspite of severe deformity.

Q. What are the investigations to be done?
- Routine blood
- NCS of all 4 limbs

(Classical clinical feature of peripheral neuropathy with inverted champagne bottle appearance with common peroneal nerve thickening with positive family history clinches the diagnosis of CMT).

Q. How will you manage this case?
- Counseling and patient education
- Pharmacological—Supportive
- Nonpharmacological—Strengthening exercise, maintaining ROM, stretching exercises
- Orthosis AFO (posterior leaf spring).

Other relevant questions on nonpharmacological management is similar to GB syndrome.

COLOSTOMY

Q. What is colostomy?
Colostomy is an artificial outlet for the feces, done either temporarily or permanently by establishing an opening between the skin surface and some portion of colon (large intestine).

Q. What are the types of colostomy?
Based on duration:
a. Temporary:
  1. Done for a period of time to allow a portion of colon to rest or as a first step of a definitive surgery.
  2. Closure can be done after weeks , months ,years.

b. Permanent:
  1. Done as a permanent exit for stool.
  2. Closure never done in future.

Depending on the site of colostomy
1. Ascending colostomy.
2. Transverse colostomy.
3. Descending and sigmoid colostomy.

Other types of colostomy
1. Loop colostomy.
2. Double barrel colostomy.
3. Decompression colostomy.

Q. Write about basic management of colostomy?
- Patient must be well informed about entire procedure and its consequence
- Psychological counseling and support
- Introducing with a person leading a colostomy life
- Appointing a WOC (trained for ostomy management)
- Regular follow-up.

Q. Write salient features of Stoma.
- Stomas are of different shapes and sizes
- Stoma may stick out (a budded stoma) or a flat should be above skin
- Color: Deep red or pink
- Feel: Warm and moist
- Change of shape through-out life with weight gain or loss
- Most noticeable change of shape *6–8 week after surgery*
- Stoma is never painful
- Drop of blood is seen in stoma during washing—it is common
- Stoma has no muscle or sphincter around the stoma so bowel movement cannot be controlled.

Q. What are the types of pouching system?
It is of two types:
- One piece pouches are attached to skin barrier
- Two piece systems are made up of a skin barrier and a pouch that can be taken off and put back on the barrier.

Q. What are the features of a good pouching system?
- Secure, with a good leak proof seal that lasts for up to 3 days
- Odor resistant
- Protective of the skin around stoma
- Nearly invisible under clothing
- Easy to put on and take off.

Q. Write on self image of colostomy patient?
- It may be extremely awkward and depressing for colostomy patient
- Proper counseling pre- and postoperative is best method
- Family support, positive outlook needed
- The situation should be faced courageously and truthfully, this is nothing but consequence of a life saving surgery done for a deadly condition should be properly conveyed to surrounding
- Cleanliness and skillful management will not cause any difficulties to others
- Patient must try to resume previous life at best.

Q. When to change pouching system?

- Some are changed every day, some every 3 days some every week
- If *leakage, itching, burning* occurs any time pouch should be changed
- Over time patients learn when bowel activity remains least which is best time for changing pouch.

Q. How to change pouching system?

- Assembling the supplies—Scissors, measuring guide, wash cloths /wipes, towel, paste.

Preparing wafer or pouch

- Opening is traced on back of wafer and cut out → Snapping the pouch to the wafer and paper backing is removed → Paste is placed on sticky side of wafer around inner edge for minor creases.

Removing the old pouch

- Pouch is gently lifted up on tape while pressing underneath skin.

Cleaning the skin

- Cleaning the skin with wet wash cloth or wipe
- Skin is dabbed dry with soft towel
- Stoma is to be remeasured before applying pouch with a guide
- New sizes are regularly noted *(up to 2 months of surgery stoma size is more frequently noted)*
- Adjust the size as required.

Apply the pouch

- Opening in wafer is centered around the stoma
- Sticky side is applied to skin
- Lower edge is folded up 3 times
- Entire bottom is pinched.

Q. When is medical attention needed?

- Change in color from pink red to purple black
- Excessive continuous bleeding
- Unusual bulging around stoma
- Abdominal pain/cramp lasting for >2–3 hours
- Watery output for >5–6 hours
- Continuous nausea vomiting
- Bad or unusual odor for >1 week
- Blockage/Prolapse/Injury in stoma.

Q. How the pouch is emptied?

- When pouch is 1/2 to 1/3rd filled with stool and air, it is best to empty
- Toilet paper is to be placed to prevent splashing
- Pouch is emptied between legs in sitting position or facing the toilet bowl in standing
- End is cleaned and clip is replaced or Velcro is closed.

Q. What is irrigation of stoma? How is it done?

- *Irrigation is putting water into colon through the stoma to regulate bowel movement*
- It depends on active bowel movement, previous bowel habit, skill of irrigation
- It is done under doctors advice and expert guidance
- The procedure may vary from person to person.

Q. What are the skin protection around stoma?

- Right shape and size of pouch and skin barrier
- Regular change of barrier
- Cleaning the skin with water and pat dry
- Regular shaving (dry) or trimming of hair around stoma
- Testing for sensitivities and allergies of skin barrier, paste by patch testing
- *Do not rub*
- *Do not* rip the pouch or pull the barrier
- *Do not* change pouch more than once daily.

Q. How to manage odor problems?

- Avoid egg, cabbage, broccoli, onions, fish, beans, milk cheese, carbonated drink, alcohol
- Regular eating of small meal in short intervals and no skipping, good chewing
- Odor resistant pouch, secure skin barrier, regular emptying, using deodorant liquid /tablet in pouch and air deodorizer.

Q. How to manage travelling with colostomy?

- Adequate supplies are always kept in cool safe, easy to access place
- Avoid trunk or back window ledge
- Avoid unhealthy food and drink
- While travelling abroad connect with the international association for medical assistance to travelles.

Q. Write on activities of daily living with colostomy?

- Bathing : It will not harm, soap must be cleaned properly
- Eating and digestion: Regular nutritious balanced diet and plenty of water—There is no colostomy diet
- Dressing: Snug undergarments, cotton stretch paint, T-shirt, camisoles gives support, pouch cover absorbs body sweat
- Sports and activities: No restriction for exercise or sports but *contact sports, weight lifting* should be avoided
- Water proof swim suit, secured skin barrier, bike shorts, support costume to be used

- Intimacy and sexuality: No restriction, becomes normal after period of adjustment
- Pregnancy: Colostomy is not a contraindication.

COMPLEX REGIONAL PAIN SYNDROME (CRPS)

Summary

A 65-year-old female presented with gradual onset painful swelling in right wrist and hand for last twenty days, not only that but also there is redness over her hand along with pain in her right shoulder. This episode was preceded by colles fracture which was immobilized in a POP cast for 4 weeks. Her symptoms are not responding with painkillers, antibiotics and a course of paraffin bath.

On examination there is diffuse pain over the wrist and hand with redness, edema and raised temperature. There is allodynia with nail changes. ROM is normal, no sensory deficit, pulse is palpable and no cyanosis.

P/D - CRPS type 1 secondary to Colle's fracture in acute (stage 1) stage in right hand.

Q. What is CRPS?

Disorder characterized by sympathetically-maintained pain and related sensory abnormalities, abnormal blood flow, abnormalities in the motor system, and changes in both superficial and deep structures with trophic changes.

Q. What is the pathogenesis of CRPS?

Abnormal adrenergic sensitivity develops in injured nociceptors, and circulating or locally secreted sympathetic neurotransmitters trigger the painful afferent activity.

- Cutaneous injury activates nociceptor fibers A (central pain-signaling system)
- Central sensitization of pain-signaling system
- Low-threshold mechanoreceptor input develops capacity to evoke pain
- With time, efferent sympathetic fibers develop capacity to activate nociceptor fibers.

Q. What are the types of CRPS?

- CRPS type I = RSD (reflex sympathetic dystrophy)
- CRPS type II = Causalgia—pain limited to a peripheral nerve distribution.

Q. What are the stages of CRPS?

Stage 1 (Acute): burning pain, diffuse edema, severe tenderness, hyperpathia and/or allodynia, increased nail and hair growth, hyperthermia or hypothermia, sweating.

- 3–6 months.

Stage 2 (Dystrophic): Pain becomes more intense and spreads proximally, skin/muscle atrophy, brawny edema, cold insensitivity, nail atrophy, decreased ROM, mottled skin, early atrophy, and osteopenia (late).

- 3–6 months.

Stage 3 (Atrophic): Pain decreases, hand/skin appear pale and cyanotic with a smooth, shiny appearance, feeling cool and dry; bone demineralization progresses with muscular weakness or atrophy, contractures/flexion deformities of shoulder and hand, tapering digits; no vasomotor changes.

Q. What are the precipitating factors?

- Cerebral lesions
- Myocardial infarction
- Infection
- Stroke
- Radiation therapy
- Repetitive motion disorder (e.g., carpal tunnel syndrome)
- Spinal cord disorders
- Surgery
- Trauma (e.g., bone fracture, gunshot and shrapnel wounds).

Q. What is the management?

- Investigation
  - Routine blood (cellulitis)
  - X-ray hand: Shows diffuse blotchy osteoporosis
  - Triple phase bone scan
  - Diagnostic stellate ganglion block
- Pharmacological management
  - Oral steroids: Short course tapering dose
  - Bisphosphonates: Risedronate effective
  - NSAIDS: For pain management
  - Anticonvulsant
  - Calcium supplementation.
- Intervention—Stellate ganglion block: Treatment of choice
- Nonpharmacological
  - PT—ROM exercise
  - Modalities—TENS, paraffin bath (symptomatic).

Q. What is stellate ganglion?

The stellate ganglion is named because of its star-shaped appearance resulting from the union of the inferior cervical ganglion with the first thoracic ganglion. It is located posterior to the junction of the subclavian and vertebral arteries at the C7-T1 level, anterior to the junction point of the C7 vertebral body and its transverse process. The stellate ganglion represents a key relay station for sympathetic nerves from the head and neck as well as from the upper extremity.

Q. How do you block it?

Anterior-to-posterior image guidance is used in placing the tip of a thin, 25-gauge, 3.5 in. spinal needle at the junction of the C7 vertebral body and the proximal transverse process.Confirmation that the needle tip is not in a vascular structure, such as the vertebral artery can be obtained by aspirating and injecting under real-time fluoroscopy 3–4 mL of radiographic contrast (Omnipaque 240 or equivalent). The operator should see local pooling of contrast material, never any vascular runoff.

A slow injection of 5–10 mL of 0.25% bupivacaine is used for temporaryre lief. For permanent neurolysis, 5–10 mL of absolute alcohol is injected slowly under general anesthesia or heavy conscious sedation (3–6% phenol can also be used in similar volumes). Permanent neurolysis should always follow a temporary test with anesthetic.

An effective stellate ganglion blockade will typically produce an ipsilateral Horner's syndrome along with ipsilateral venous engorgement of the ipsilateral upper extremity.

Q. What are the agents used in block?

- 0.2–0.5% bupivacaine (0.5–1%)
- 1–2% lidocaine
- Steroids (optional)
- Phenol (3% phenol in iohexol).

Q. What are the indications of stellate ganglion block?

- Pain from upper face and neck (e.g., herpes zoster, Ménière's disease)
- Pain from upper extremities (e.g., chronic arterial embolic disease, Raynaud's disease, reflex sympathetic dystrophy)
- Hyperhydrosis and post-traumatic shock syndromes of the upper extremity.

Q. What are the contraindications of stellate ganglion block?

- Anticoagulant therapy
- Pneumothorax on contralateral side
- Pneumonectomy on contralateral side
- Recent AMI
- Glaucoma.

Q. What are the complications of Colle's fracture?

- Malunion resulting in dinner fork deformity.
- Median nerve palsy and post-traumatic carpal tunnel syndrome
- Reflex sympathetic dystrophy
- Secondary osteoarthritis, more frequently seen in patients with intra-articular involvement
- Extensor pollicis longus tendon tear.

CONGENITAL TALIPES EQUINO VARUS (CTEV)

Summary

A 5-year-old boy presented with right-sided foot deformity and difficulty to walk since birth. His developmental mile stones are normal without any history of birth asphyxia. His bowel bladder and higher mental function are absolutely normal.

On examination, his right foot is smaller in size with small heel and deep skin crease on back of heel and medial side of sole. There is bony deformity on lateral side of the foot, i.e equino varus deformity. Other neurological examination is essentially normal.

P/D: Congenital talipes equino varus (CTEV)

D/D: Cerebral palsy (CP)

Q. What is hind foot?

Calcaneum and talus forms the hind foot along with subtalar and calcaneocuboid joint.

Q. What is mid foot?

Navicular, cuboid and cuneiform bones form the mid foot along with talonavicular and naviculo cuneiform joint.

Q. What is fore foot?

Metatarsal and phalanges form forefoot along with tarsometatarsal joints and all distal joints.

Q.4 What are the ligaments of ankle?

Primary ligaments of ankle include:

- Medial
  - Deltoid ligament
  - Calcaneonavicular ligament (spring ligament)
- Lateral
  - Syndesmosis
  - Anterior talofibular ligament (ATFL)
  - Posterior talofibular ligament (PTFL)
  - Calcaneal fibular ligament (CFL)
  - Lateral talocalcaneal ligament (LTCL).

Q. Commonest congenital foot deformity?

Congenital talipes equino varus (CTEV).

Q. What are the other congenital foot deformity?

- Talipes calcaneo valgus
- Metatarsus adductus
- Metatarsus varus.

Q. What are the etiology of CTEV?

Multifactorial

- Increases intrauterine pressure - Oligohydramnios, multiple pregnancy
- Ischemia of calf muscles in intrauterine life
- Genetic.

Q. What is primary and secondary club foot?

- Primary is idiopathic from birth.
- Secondary where cause is found and acquired like poliomyelitis, myelodysplasia, Freidreich's ataxia.

Q. How will you manage the case?

Investigation:

- X-ray of foot: AP view (Talo calcaneal angle >35 degree normal decreased in CTEV).
- Management: Manipulation
  Corrective plaster cast preceeding manipulation.

Orthosis: Dennis brown splint (used before child starts walking)
CTEV shoes (Used up to 5 years of age).

Q. Which deformity is corrected first?

(Mneumonic: CAVE)

Cavus followed by **A**dduction and **V**arus then **E**quinus.

Q. What is Dennis Brown splint?

- The brace consists of open toe high-top straight last shoes attached to a bar
- For unilateral cases, the brace is set at 60–70 degrees of external rotation on the clubfoot side and 30–40 degrees of external rotation on the normal side
- In bilateral cases, it is set at 70 degrees of external rotation on each side
- The bar should be of sufficient length so that the heels of the shoes are at shoulder width
- The bar should be bent 5–10 degrees with the convexity away from the child, to hold the feet in dorsiflexion.

Q. What is the protocol for wearing DB splint?

The brace should be worn full time (day and night) for the first 3 months after the last cast is removed then the child should wear the brace for 12 hours at night and 2–4 hours in the middle of the day for a total of 14 to16 hours during each 24-hour period. This protocol continues until the child is 3–4 years of age.

Q. What is the rationale for splinting?

- At the end of casting, the foot is abducted to an exaggerated amount, which should measure 60 to 70 degrees. This degree of foot abduction is required to maintain the abduction of the calcaneus and forefoot and prevent relapse
- The foot will gradually turn back inward, to a point typically of 10 degrees of external rotation
- The medial soft tissues remain stretched out only if the brace is used after the casting
- In the brace, the knees are left free, so the child can kick them "straight" to stretch the gastrosoleus tendon
- The abduction of the feet in the brace, combined with the slight bend (convexity away from the child), causes the feet to dorsiflex. This helps maintain the stretch on the gastrocnemius muscle and Achilles tendon.

Q. What are the surgeries done?

- Soft-tissue release
- Postero medial soft tissue release
- Dwyer's osteotomy
- Evan's operation
- Wedge tarsectomy
- Triple arthrodesis.

Q. How will you manage CTEV generally?

Management of CTEV is discussed in Flowchart 3.1.

CARPAL TUNNEL SYNDROME

Summary

A 45-year-old nondiabetic housewife presented with severe pain and tingling sensation in the palmer aspect of right hand especially aggravating at night and disturbing her sleep. The pain decreased a little bit for a while. She did not have any pain or arthralgia anywhere else. She is a little bit obese but not suffering from any cold intolerance, recent weight gain. She is not using any contraceptive pill.

On examinations, there is paresthesia in medialthree and half fingers with little bit wasting in right thenar muscle. Tinel sign and reverse phallen sign test are positive in right hand. She does not have any joint deformity , large hand or leg. Range of motion of shoulder is full without any pain.

PD: Carpal tunnel syndrome (CTS)

D/D:

- Pronator syndrome
- Diabetic neuropathy
- Cervical radiculopathy.

Flowchart 3.1: CAVE management

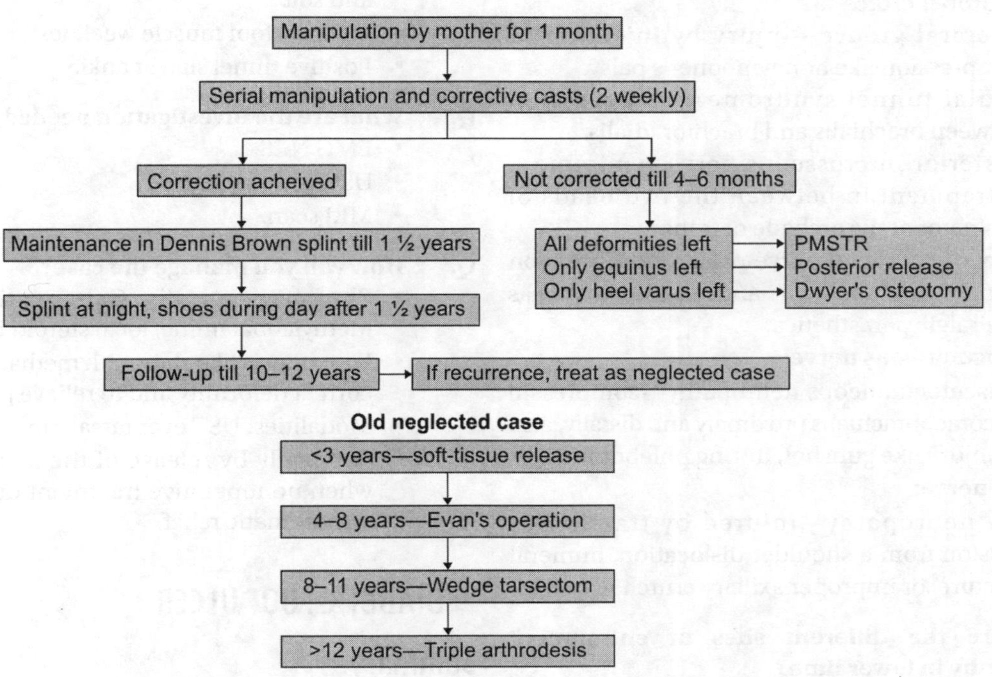

Q. What are the types of nerve injury?

- **Neuropraxia**—Focal conduction block, no axonal damage
- **Axonotmesis**—Axonal damage wth Wallerian degeneration but supporting structure intact
- **Neurotmesis**—Axonal and supporting system damage.

Q. What is entrapment neuropathy?

Entrapment neuropathies refers to isolated peripheral nerve injuries occurring at specific locations where a nerve is mechanically constricted.

Q. What are the normal pressure of carpal tunnel in different position?

- Neutral: 3.48 ± 0.43 mm of Hg
- 90 degree flexion: 9.32 ± 1.06 mm of Hg
- 90 degree extension: 12.68 ± 1.16 mm of Hg

Q. What are the muscle supplied by median nerve after passing through carpal tunnel?

- Lumbricals (1,2)
- Opponens pollicis
- Abductor pollicis brevis
- Flexor pollicis brevis (superficial).

Q. What is cumulative trauma disease?

Cumulative trauma disorders (CTDs) are injuries to the nervous and/or musculoskeletal system caused by repetitive physical tasks, poor posture or biomechanics,vibrations, and/or repetitive forceful exertions.

Q. What are the occupations precipitating CTDs?

- Manual labor
- Office workers
- Typing
- Washing.

Q. What is hand arm vibration syndrome?

Vascular and neuromuscular symptoms caused by high levels of exposure to vibration.

Q. What is ergonomics?

According to the International Ergonomics Association Council of 2000, ergonomics is defined as- "the scientific discipline concerned with the understanding of interactions among humans and other elements of a system, and the profession that applies theory, principles, data and methods to design in order to optimize human well-being and overall system performance.

Q. What are the work modification needed?

- Reduced repetitiveness of tasks
- Limiting use of wrist works.

Q. What are the different sites of entrapment neuropathy in upper limbs?

Radial nerve:

1. Crutch palsy at axilla—Compressed by improper crutch use.
2. At spiral groove—Injury by injection or compression like honeymooner's palsy.
3. Radial tunnel syndrome—Compression between brachialis and brachioradialis.
4. Posterior interosseous nerve syndrome—entrapment in between the two heads of supinator at the archade of frohse.
5. Superficial radial nerve palsy—Compression by tight wristwatch an handcalf, also known as cheiralgia paresthetica.

Musculocutaneous nerve:

1. Musculocutaneous neuropathy—compressin by coracobrachialis proximaly and distally, also by injury like gunshot, during phlebotomy.

Axillary nerve:

Axillary neuropathy—injured by traction or compression from a shoulder dislocation, humeral head fracture, or improper axillary crutch use.

Q. What are the different sites of entrapment neuropathy in lower limb?

- Sciatic neuropathy—Compression by piriformis muscle (piriformis syndrome).
- Lateral femoral cutaneous nerve—Along pelvis Exiting pelvis
- Iliac crest and anterior superior iliac spine
- Peroneal nerve—Fibular neck
- Tibial nerve—Lancinate ligament (tarsal tunnel).

Q. What is tarsal tunnel syndrome?

Entrapment of tibial nerve in tarsal tunnel at ankle.

Q. What are the structures passing through tarsal tunnel ?

- Tibialis posterior
- Flexor digitorum longus
- Tibial artey and vein
- Flexor hallucis longus.

Structures in Carpal tunnel: median nerve and nine flexor tendons:

- Flexor pollicis longus,
- Four flexor digitorum profundus,
- Four flexor digitorum superficialis tendons *the nerve lying superficially and anteroradially in the tunnel.*

Q. What are the precipitating factors of TTS?

- Foot injury
- Pes planus.

Q. What are the clinical signs and symptoms?

- Pain, numbness, tingling sensation in medial heel and sole.
- Intrinsic foot muscle weakness.
- Positive tinnel sign at ankle.

Q. What are the investigation needed?

- EMG NCS
- USG of tarsal tunnel
- MRI scan.

Q. How will you manage the case?

- Pharmacologically: Gabapentin, pregabalin, Methylcobalamine, local steroid infiltration.
- Foot ortosis like shoe with medial arch support to correct deformity and to relieve pain.
- Modalities: UST over tarsal tunnel
- Surgically by release of the laciniate ligament when nonoperative treatment does not provide symptomatic relief.

DIABETIC FOOT ULCER

Summary

A 68-year-old poorly controlled diabetic patient presented with a ulcer in right forefoot for last three months which is not healing with recurrent course of antibiotics and continued dressing of wound. He is on insulin for last two months. Glycemic control became better in last two months.

On examinations there is callous formation over pressure ulcer and the foot is cold with absence of peripheral pulsation. There is 2 × 3 cm ulcer over noted without any sinus formation and discharge under right 1st metatarsal head. There is loss of sensation of light touch, pinprick and vibration stocking distribution.

PD—Diabetic foot ulcer (grade) with peripheral neuropathy with peripheral vascular disease.

Q. What are the common sitess of foot ulcer?

- Forefoot—Diabetic (ball of toes, undersurface of great toe), Hansen's disease
- Midfoot—rare
- Hindfoot—Diabetes, Hansen's disease.

Q. What are the factors responsible for diabetic foot ulcer?

- Altered biomechanics—Due to motor weakness, callous formation
- Sensory neuropathy—Unnoticed injury
- PVD—Decreased perfusion

- Poor glycemic control—Decreased healing ,increased risk of infection
- Maldistribution of pressure—Increased friction
- Illfitting shoes—More chances of injuries
- Smoking.

Q. What are the causes of unhealing ulcer?

Neuropathic ulcers like:

- Hansen's disease
- Tabes dorsalis
- Amyloidosis
- CMT/HSMN.

Q. How can you measure the ulcer?

- Ulcer can be measured using—
- Measuring tape
- Transparent sheet
- Marker pen
- Sterile probe (blunt tip)
- Parameter to be measured—
  - Length
  - Depth
  - Width

Q. How will you assess the ulcer?

For assessment of patient of ulcer -to look for:

- Deformity
- Callous
- Peripheral pulsation for PVD
- Any sensory loss
- Other signs of poor glycemic control.

Q. What are the complications?

- Gangrene
- Wond infection
- Autoamputation.

Q. What investigations you will do?

- Blood—FBS, PPBS, HBA1c, lipidprofile, urea/creatinine, electrolyte
- Wound swab for culture sensitivity
- X-ray—to rule out osteomyelitis
- NCS: For neuropathy
- Doppler ultrasound: To see peripheral arteries
- CT Angio for PVD: If intervention is planned.

Q. How you will you manage the case?

- Good glycemic control with insulin and oral hypoglycemic drugs
- Wound care—regular dressing, local antibiotic
- If wound culture positive—specific antibiotic
- Impaired sensation—Gabapentine, vit B12
- PVD—vasodilator
- Treatment for other complications and comorbidities
- *Total contact casting.*

Q. What are the stages of ulcer?

By Wagner there are 6 stages:

1. Intact skin
2. Superficial ulcer of skin or subcutaneous tissue
3. Ulcers extend into tendon, bone, or capsule
4. Deep ulcer with osteomyelitis, or abscess
5. Gangrene of toes or forefoot
6. Midfoot or hindfoot gangrene

Q. What is TCC?

TCC is a procedure of total casting of foot to augment healing of ulcer by offloading of ulcer area after distribution of weight all over plantar aspect of foot.

Q. How you can do it?

- Proper dressing of wound
- Cast stocking from toes to tibial tuberosity
- Padding of interdigital space and bony prominences
- One layer padding thick by cotton roll
- Offloading of ulcer area by rocker bottom sole
- Casting.

Q. How frequently it should be done?

Weekly to every 3 weeks depending upon ulcer healing status.

Q. What are the Complications of TCC?

- Infection
- Ischemia
- Nail changes like paronychia.

Q. What are the contraindications of TCC?

- Active infection
- Poor foot hygiene
- Ischemia
- Poor compliance
- Refusal of patient.

Q. What are the alternate of TCC?

PTB orthosis.

Q. What are the do's and don't in diabetic ulcer?

Do's:

- Proper foot care
- Always keep the foot dry and free of moisture
- Shake and inspect the shoes before putting in
- Replace or repair the old torn shoes
- Inspect the foot regularly
- Visit doctor if there is callous.

Don'ts:

- Walk in barefoot
- Trying to remove corn/callous by self
- Burn of foot
- Injury to foot.

Q. What are the type of diabetic neuropathy?
- Pure sensory
- Sensory motor
- Diabetic amyotrophy
- Autonomic
- Cranial nerve palsy.

Q. How do you treat diabetic neuropathy?
- Medication—Gabapentin, VIT B_{12}, B_6, analgesic
- Good glycemic control
- Prevention and management of complication
- Sensory reeducation
- Modality like TENS
- Footwear modifications.

Q. What are the other disability in this patient?
Visual impairment.

Q. What are the musculoskeletal problems that may develop?
- Charcot joint
- Autoamputation
- Osteomyelitis
- Muscle weakness,wasting/atrophy.

DUPUYTREN CONTRACTURE

Summary

A 62-year-old diabetic patient presented with gradual onset, slowly progressive tightness of his left palm and slight bending of his left ring finger for last 6 weeks. He is not suffering from any pain anywhere. He did not receive any antitubercular medicines or anti convulsants.

On examinations there is thickening of left palmer fascia with flexion deformity of his left 4th finger. His chest is clear and liver is not palpable. There is no peripheral signs of chronic liver disease.

P/D: A case of dupuytrens contracture in diabetic patient.

Q. What is Dupuytren contracture?
Dupuytren's contracture is a flexion contracture of the hand due to a palmar fibromatosis, in which the fingers bend towards the palm and cannot be fully extended (straightened). It is an inherited proliferative connective tissue disorder that involves the hand's palmar fascia.

Q. What is the pathogenesis of Dupuytren contracture?
Exact pathogenesis is unknown but may be due to repeated trauma or vibration, genetic predisposition and involvement of fibroblast proliferation, and collagen deposition leading to contractures of the palmar fascia.

Q. What is the earliest involvement of Dupuytren contracture?
It first presents as a thickening or nodule in the palm, which initially can be with or without pain. Later in the disease process, there is increasing painless loss of range of motion of the affected fingers. The earliest sign of a contracture is a triangular "puckering" of the skin of the palm as it passes over the flexor tendon just before the flexor crease of the finger, at the MCP joint.
Earliest finger involved is ring finger.

Q. What are the triggering factors in Dupuytren contracture?
Trauma and Vibration.

Q. What are the risk factors of Dupuytren contracture?
- People of Scandinavian or Northern European ancestry
- Men rather than women (men are more likely to develop the condition)
- People over the age of 50
- Smokers
- Thinner people
- Diabetic
- Manual workers
- Liver disease
- Alcoholic
- People with a family history
- People with Ledderhose disease.
- People with epilepsy (possibly due to anti-convulsive medication)
- People with HIV.

Q. How will you manage the case?
- Investigations:
  - CBC, FBS, LFT
  - CXR PA view
  - USG of involved finger.
- Treatment:
  - Counceling
  - Treating the medical cause: Diabetes, Chronic liver disease, Tuberculosis
  - PT: Range of motion exercises
    Stretching exercise (Vigorous stretching should be avoided because it aggrevates the condition)
    Modalities: UST (Effectiveness is debatable as per current evidences)
  - OT: ADL training

- PO: Wrist hand orthosis/Hand orthosis
- Needling
- Radiation therapy
- Collagenase Clostridium histolyticum
- Surgeries.

Q. What is the role of WHO and HO?
Post surgery night time use of extension orthosis.

Q. What are the indications of surgery?
- MCP flexion contracture of 30° or more
- Proximal interphalangeal (PIP) flexion contracture of any degree
- Significant first web space contracture involving the thumb.

Q. Mention the surgeries done in DC?
- Needle fasciotomy
- Open fasciotomy
- Regional fasciectomy
- Segmental fasciectomy
- Dermofasciectomy.

DEEP VEIN THROMBOSIS (DVT)

Summary

A 65-year-old female known patient of quadriparesis due to complete SCI for last two months, presented with sudden-onset painful swelling of her right legs for last three days.

On examination there is tenderness over her right calf muscle, redness, edema of right foot and ankle region. Homans sign is positive. Her respiratory examinations is absolutely normal.

P/D: A case of deep vein thrombosis (DVT) of right leg
D/D: Cellulitis.

Q. What is DVT?
DVT refers to the formation of one or more blood clots (a blood clot is also known as a "thrombus," while multiple clots are called "thrombi") in one of the body's large veins, most commonly in the lower limbs (e.g., lower leg or calf).

Q. What is Virchows triad?
- Endothelial injury
- Abnormal blood flow
- Hypercoagulability

} Clot Formation

Q. How is Homans sign tested?
Pain in the calf with forced dorsiflexion of the foot.

Q. What are the risk factors?
- Age >40 years
- Family history of DVT or PE
- Pelvic fractures or lower extremity fractures
- Immobilization >3 days
- Oral contraceptive pills
- Pregnancy
- Recent surgery.

Q. What is the difference with cellulitis?
In cellulitis:
- Absent Homans sign
- Superficial tenderness only
- Doppler ultrasound negative
- D Dimer negative
- Pyrexia
- Signs of infection present.

Q. What are the complications of DVT?
Pulmonary embolism.

Q. How will you manage the case?
Investigation:
- Routine blood: PT, INR, APTT.
- Doppler ultrasound of both lower limbs venous system.
- D Dimer (as screening).
- CXR (to rule out PE).

Management:
- Prophylaxis: DVT Stockings.
- Low molecular weight heparin.
- Active foot and ankle exercise

Therapeutic:
- LMWH followed by Warfarin: Target INR: 2.5–3.

Q. What is the dose of LMWH?
- Preventive: 40 mg S/C once daily.
- Therapeutic: 1 mg/kg/bw Stop when INR >2.5.
- Reduced dose in renal and hepatic dysfunction.

Q. What is dose of warfarin?
Bolus dose followed by maintainance dose
(Normally 10 mg on day 1, 10 mg on day 2 and 5 mg on day 3 repeat INR)
(Elderly: 5 mg ---- 5 mg---- check INR).

Q. How many days should anticoagulation be continued?
- Distal DVT: 3 months
- Proxymal: 6 months
- Recurrent DVT: 6 months
- PE: 6 months.

Q. What are the drugs that interact with warfarin?
Drugs that potentiate warfarin (O DEVICES) acts on *CYP2C9:*

- Omeprazole
- Disulfiram
- Erythromycin
- Valproate
- Isoniazid
- Ciprofloxacin and cimetidine
- Ethanol (acutely)
- Sulphonamides.

Drugs that decrease the effectiveness of warfarin (PC BRAS):
- Phenytoin
- Carbamazepine
- Barbiturates
- Rifampicin
- Alcohol (chronic use)
- Sulphonylureas.

Q. What is the antagonist of warfarin?
Vitamin K.

Q. If patient continues to bleed?
Infuse FFP.

Q. What are the signs and symptoms of PE?
Symptoms:
1. Dyspnea (most common).
2. Pleuritic chest pain.
3. Hemoptysis.
4. Cough.
5. Diaphoresis,.
6. Shock.
7. Loss of conciousness.

Signs:
1. Tachypnea, RR >20/min (MC).
2. Tachycardia HR >100/min.
3. Hypotension.
4. Low-grade fever.
5. Engorged neck veins.
6. Accentuated p2.
7. Sometimes paradoxical bradycardia.
8. Pleural rub.
9. Inspiratory crackles.
10. Cyanosis.
11. 4th heart sound.
12. Signs of RHF.

Q. What investigations will you suggest for PE?
- Chest X-ray for Westermark's sign
  - Hampton's hump
  - Palla's sign
  - ABG: Type I respiratory failure
  - Investigation of choice: CECT scan of chest.

Q. What is the treatment of choice for recurrent PE in DVT patient who are not fit for warfarin?
IVC filter.

Q. Salient features of DVT stocking?
- Types:
  - Elastic stocking
  - Pneumatic compression stocking.
  - Sequential compression.
- Pressure
  - Maximum at ankle and minimum at thighs.
  - Role in prevention.
  - No role as therapeutic measure.

DYSPHASIA

Summary 1

A 65-year-old hypertensive right-handed male presented with nonfluent telegraphic speech after stroke. Sometimes he is facing difficulty to find words but his comprehension is intact and higher function is also quite normal. His ability to repeat word is also impaired.

Summary 2

A 70-year-old diabetic right-handed female patient presented with fluent unintelligible speech after an episode of stroke. She is using words in wrong order and sometimes is mixing nonexistent words or phrases. While she attempts repetition it results in paraplegic distortion and irrelevant insertion. On evaluation comprehension is severely affected.

P/D: Case 1: Broca's dysphasia
Case 2: Wernicks dysphasia.

Q. What is aphasia and dysphasia?
Aphasia is an acquired communication disorder caused by brain damage, characterized by an impairment of language modalities: Speaking, listening, reading and writing. It is not the result of a sensory deficit, a general intellectual deficit or a psychiatric disorder.

Q. What is aphonia?
Aphonia is the inability to produce voice.

Q. What is anomic aphasia?
Anomic aphasia (also known as dysnomia, nominal aphasia, and amnesic aphasia) is a type of aphasia where an individual has consistent inability to produce words for things that they want to talk about (particularly nouns and verbs).

Q. What are the different types of dysphasia?

Fluent	*Nonfluent*
Wernicke's	Broca's
Transcortical sensory	Mixed transcortical
Conduction	Global
Anomia	Transcortical motor.

Q. What is neologism?

A newly coined word or expression.

Q. What is paraphasia?

A type of language output error commonly associated with aphasia, and characterized by the production of unintended syllables, words, or phrases during the effort to speak.

Q. What is echolalia?

It is defined as the unsolicited repetition of vocalizations made by another person (by the same person is called palilalia).

Q. Which part of brain is affected in different types of dysphasia?

- Wernicks: Posterior part of superior temporal gyrus
- Broca's: Posteroinferior frontal lobe
- Global: Entire perisylvian region (MCA territory)
- Anomic: Angular gyrus region
- Conduction: Archuate fasciculus or insula
- Transcortical motor: Frontal lobe, anterior superior to brocas area or subcortical region deep to brocas
- Transcortical sensory: Posterior inferior temporal lobe.

Q. What is dysarthria?

Dysarthria is speech disorder resulting from disturbances in muscular control over the speech mechanism due to damage of central or peripheral nervous system.

Q. Which part is affected?

7th and/or 12th cranial nerve involvement in hemiplegic patients.

Q. What are the types of dysarthria?

- Flaccid dysarthria
- Spastic dysarthria
- Ataxic dysarthria
- Hypokinetic dysarthria
- Hyperkinetic dysarthria
- UMN dysarthria
- Mixed dysarthria.

Q. What are the standard questions to ask for assessment?

1. Ask patient's name: No voice: Aphonia
   Global aphasia.
2. Ask patient his address: Relevant answers: Normal
   Non relevant: Paraphasia + neologism ..→ Wernicks dysphasia.
3. Ask patient to repeat any word: Absent in Brocas, Wernicks, global and conduction.
4. Ask patient to name a pain or tie?: Not able to name but can repeat words like constitution is: ANOMIC.
5. Ask patient to say British constitution: Can't say: DYSARTHRIA.
6. Give a small command writing in paper : Can understand plus fluent speech: Wernick/ Transcortical sensory.
7. Not answer words but can write: Global.
8. Give a verbal command: Can answer on paper: APHONIA.

Q. How will you treat dysphasia?

- Speech therapy
- Melody intonation technique

Q. How will you approach a case of dysphasia?

Approach for case of dysphasia is given in Flowchart 3.2.

ERB'S PALSY

Summary

A one-year-term baby presented with weakness and lack of movement of her right arm after birth. Her hand is hanging in medially rotated position with pronated arm and wrist in extension giving the appearance of "waiters tip" posture. She has lower motor neuron type of weakness in shoulder muscle and biceps. There is a gross sensory changes in her proximal part of right upper limb. Her developmental milestones are otherwise normal. She sometimes suffers from muscle cramps of right upper limb. Her mother noted a bit of improvement in right arm in last few months.

P/D: A case of Erb's palsy.

Q. What is Erb's palsy?

Erb's Palsy is a common birth injury resulting due to paralysis to the upper brachial plexus involving C5–C6 +/- C7 roots.

Q. What are the common clinical features ?

- Weakness in one arm
- Arm is bent at elbow and held against body
- Decreased grip strength in hand of the affected side

Flowchart 3.2: Approach in a case of dysphasia

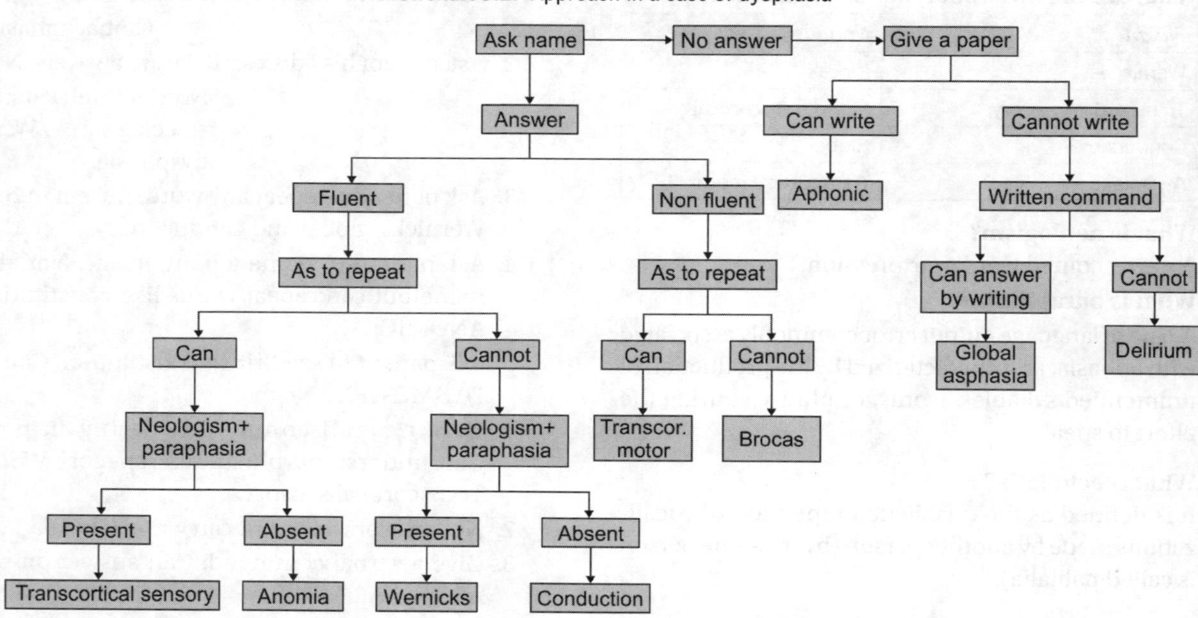

- Numbness in arm
- Impaired circulatory, muscular and nervous development
- Partial or total paralysis of the arm.

Q. What type of injury?

LMN type of injury.

Q. What is Erb's point?

It's the junction of C5 C6 root, anterior and posterior division of superior trunk and two nerves, nerve to subclavius and suprascapular nerve.

Q. What are risk factors for Erb's palsy?

- Excessive pulling on the shoulders during a head first delivery pressure on the infant's raised arms during a feet first delivery.
- Using extraction tools like forceps during delivery.
- Second stage of labor lasting over an hour.
- Large infant size.
- Excessive maternal weight gain.

Q. How will you manage the case?

- Education and councelling of parents.
- Pharmacological: Vit B_{12}
- Nonpharmacological: Exercise: AROM exercises, strenghthening exercises.
- Modalities: Electrical stimulations to the muscle supplied.
- Orthosis: Balanced forearm orthosis.

Q. What are the prognostic factors?

- Early diagnosis
- Neuropraxic injury.

Q. What are the surgical procedures that can be done?

- Surgery may help children who do not recover by the age of 5 months.
- Nerve surgery is most effective when it is done between the ages of 5 and 12 months and becomes less effective after 1 year.
- Nevertheless, surgical correction for permanent disability or deformity can be performed in the school-aged child where necessary.

Q. What is Klumkes paralysis?

This injury involves the C8–T1 nerve roots or lower trunk.

Q. What are the clinical features?

The patient may have wasting of the small hand muscles and a claw-hand deformity (lumbrical weakness). The shoulder girdle muscle function is preserved.

Q. How will you differentiate between the two?

Differentiate between Erb's palsy and Klumke's paralysis have been given in Table 3.5.

Table 3.5: Differentiate between Erb's palsy and Klumke's paralysis

Features	*Erb's Palsy*	*Klumke's paralysis*
Level	C5-C6 nerve roots	C8–T1 nerve roots
Shoulder	At side of body	Normal
Arm	At side of body	Normal
Forearm	At side of body	Normal
Hand	Normal	Claw hand

ERYTHEMA NODOSUM

Summary

A 20-year-old young female patient presented with diffuse, red, raised lesion 2–6 cm in diameter over both legs for last five days. She also complained of recurrent polyarthralgia on NSAIDs and under clinical evaluation. She has recent episode of coughs and fever for last few months.

PD: A Case of erythema nodosum probably due to sarcoidosis.

Q. What is erythema nodosum?

It is a reacting pattern of various disease, infection or drugs presenting as painful, erythematous, nonulcerative lesion mainly appearing over shin.

Q. What are the etiologies?

- Sarcoidosis
- Streptococcus infection
- Tuberculosis
- Rheumatoid arthritis
- Drugs—sulfonylureas penicillin, OCP, salicylates, barbiturates
- Others—Ulcerative colitis, chrons disease, Hansen's disease, idiopathic.

Q. What are the history supporting panniculitis?

- Weight loss
- Fatigue
- Erythematous or pigmented tender firm nodule.

Q. How you treat the patient of EN?

- Stop culprit drugs
- Skin care and tropical steroid
- Treatment of underlying cause.

Q. What is sarcoidosis?

Sarcoidosis is a multisystem inflammatory disease of unknown etiology that mainly affects the lungs and intrathoracic lymph nodes characterized by noncaseating granulomas of affected organ.

Q. What are the clinical features of sarcoidosis?

- Around 5% cases are asymptomatic.
- Systemic features—Fever, weight loss, anorexia, fatigue, weight loss

Acute Sarcoidosis:

Lofgren's syndrome, an acute presentation consisting of:

- Fever
- Arthralgia
- Erythema nodosum
- Bilateral hilar adenopathy.

Heerford's syndrome :

- Anterior uveitis
- Fever
- Parotid enlargement
- Facial palsy

CHRONIC SARCOIDOSIS

Lung—Dyspnea, cough, chest discomfort, wheezing, bilateral hilar lymphadenopathy, interstitial lung disease, pleural effusion.

Skin—

- Erythema nodosum
- Lupus pernio
- Violaceous rash over the cheeks or nose
- Osseous involvement may be present
- Maculopapular plaques.

Eye—

- Anterior or posterior granulomatous uveitis
- Conjunctival lesions and scleral plaques
- Ocular involvement may lead to blindness if untreated.

CVS—

- Heart failure from cardiomyopathy
- Heart block and sudden death

Musculo skeletal—

- Myalgia.
- Muscle weakness.

CNS—

- Headache
- Cranial-nerve palsies: 7th cranial nerve
- Ataxia
- Weakness of muscle
- Seizures
- Cognitive dysfunction

Gastrointestinal—

- Spleenomegaly
- Cholestatic syndrome
- Portal hypertension with variceal bleeding
- Hepatopulmonary syndrome with refractory hypoxemia
- Cirrhosis leading to liver failure occur in 1% of patient.

Q. What are the investigations needed?

- **Blood**—Serum ACE, calcium, ALP
- **Kveim test**
- **Chest X-ray:** For hilar lymphadenopathy.
- **CECT** of thorax, if needed

- **Biopsy of lymph node:** Histopathology: Noncaseating granulomatosis.

Q. How will you treat the case?
- NSAIDs
- Steroids—Prednisone
- Nonsteroid drugs—
  - Chloroquine and hydroxychloroquine
  - Cyclophosphamide
  - Azathrioprine
  - Chlorambucil
  - Cyclosporine
  - Infliximab
  - Tetracycline
  - Thalidomide.
- Other symptomatic treatment of organ involvement
- Prognosis good in pregnancy.

FOOT DROP

Summary

A 35-year-old farmer presented with right-sided gradual onset foot drop with hypoanesthetic patches over lateral half of right leg and lateral aspect of foot. He was treated with combined daily medication and once a month medication for few months. But he is still struggling to do his regular work and walks with high steppage gait. His power of tibialis anterior and extensor hallucis longus is 0/5.

P/D: A case of right-sided foot drop secondary to Hansen's disease.

D/D: Common peroneal nerve palsy of other etiology.

Q. What are the causes of foot drop?
- Tourniquet palsy
- Peripheral neuropathy like diabetes
- Trauma to common peroneal nerve
- Hansen's disease
- Lumbosacral plexopathy
- L5 S1 radiculopathy.

Q. Why do you say this as Hansen's disease?
- Hypoanesthetic patch
- Nerve thickening.

Q. How do you classify Hansen's disease?

According to WHO, it can be classified as:
- Paucibacillary
- Multibacillary.

According to Ridley–Jopling, it can be classified as:
- Tuberculoid leprosy (TT)
- Borderline tuberculoid leprosy (BT)
- Borderline leprosy (BB)
- Borderline lepromatous leprosy (BL)
- Lepromatous leprosy (LL).

Q. What investigations will you do?
- NCS
- Nerve and skin biopsy
- Routine blood.

Q. What is the management?
- Counseling
- Pharmacological—Dapsone, rifampicin
- Nonpharmacological
  - Physical therapy:
    - Maintaining ROM
    - Strengthening exercise
    - Modalities—E/S to ankle dorsiflexors
  - Orthosis—AFO (PLS)
  - Occupational therapy—Gait training, sensory reeducation, foot care.
- Surgery
  - Tendon transfer from Tibialis posterior to tibialis anterior.

Q. Write about multi-drug therapy regimen in leprosy.

MB (Multi Bacillary) leprosy:
- Rifampicin: 600 mg once a month
- Clofazimine: 300 mg once a month, and 50 mg daily
- Dapsone: 100 mg daily
- Duration: 12 months (12 blister packs)

PB (Pauci Bacillary) leprosy:
- Rifampicin: 600 mg once a month
- Dapsone: 100 mg daily
- Duration: Six months (six blister packs).

Q. What is the management option for flail ankle?

Ankle arthrodesis.

Q. What are the advantages and disadvantages of Arthrodesis?

Disadvantage
- No movement possible
- Abnormal gait pattern.

Advantage
- Done where replacement failed
- Can be done in neuropathic joint.

Q. What are the pathological changes in Hansen's disease?

Macrophages and Schwann cells filled with organisms and debris (foamy cells) appear in the epineurium, endoneurium, and perineurium. In the perineurium, foamy macrophages infiltrate and separate individual layers, fibroblasts and perineurial cells proliferate, and collagen is deposited. This produces onion-skinning of the nerve fascicles. Proliferation of connective tissue (peri- and endoneurial fibrosis) is not as prominent as in tuberculoid (TT) disease.

Q. What are sites of trophic ulcer in Hansen's disease?
- Base of 5th metatarsal head
- Heel.

Q. What are the measurement criteria for ulcer?
- Length
- Breadth
- Depth.

Q. What is the management of ulcer?
- Wound care
- Sensory reeducation
- Foot care
- Shoe modification (MCR)
- Total contact casting (TCC).

FRIEDREICH ATAXIA

Summary

A 14-year-old boy presented with pes cavus high-arched palate, intention tremor and head shakes. He had few episodes of fall due to ataxia. On examination there is dysarthria, nystagmus though slow and course. There is bilateral dysdiadokinesia and heel shin test positive with persistently diminished vibratory sense up to the knee. His knee and ankle jerk is absent with extensor planter bilaterally. So I think he is suffering from Friedreich ataxia.

Q. What are the D/Ds of absent ankle jerk and bilateral extensor planter?
- Friedreich ataxia
- MND
- Demyelinating disease
- Sub acute degeneration of cord (SACD)
- Neurosyphilis
- Mixed lesion (compressive myelopathy with L5,S1 LMN palsy).

Q. What are the other clinical features of Friedreich ataxia?
- Cardiomyopathy
- Early osteoarthritis
- Higher function—Dementia
- Diabetes mellitus.

Q. What is the inheritance pattern of Friedreich ataxia?
- Autosomal recessive
- Mutation in chromosome 9
- The particular genetic mutation (expansion of an intronic GAA triplet repeat in the FXN gene)
- Reduced expression of the mitochondrial protein frataxin.

Q. What are the close differentials?
- Bassen—Kornweigs syndrome (Abetalipoproteinemia)
- Refsum's disease (accumulation of phytanic acid due to deficiency of lipid alpha oxidase)
- Roussy levy syndrome (a variety of HSMN).

Q. What is the progression of the disease?
Usaually slowly progressive.

Q. What is the management?
- Investigation:
  - Blood—FBS, PPBS
  - Eye examination
  - ECHO
  - Vit B_{12} level—for SACD
  - VDRL
  - MRI Brain.
- Counseling
- Pharmacological: Not effective
- Physical therapy:
  - Maintaining ROM
  - Frenkel exercise.
- Occupational therapy:
  - Gait training.
- Orthosis:
  - Shoe modification for pes cavus.

KLIPPEL-FEIL SYNDROME

Summary

A 16-year-old female presented with limited range of motion of neck due to short and webbed neck. She has a low hair line. There is no definite tenderness on cervical spine or radiculopathy on neurological examination.
P/D: Klippelfeil syndrome.

Q. What are the other associations of Klippelfeil syndrome?
- Cervical vertebrae fusion
- Hearing problem
- Scoliosis
- Spina bifida
- Anomalies of the kidneys and the ribs

- Cleft palate
- Dental problems
- Respiratory problems
- Heart malformations
- Short stature
- Duane syndrome
- Sprengel's deformity.

Q. What are the other causes of webbed neck?
- Turner syndrome
- Noonan syndrome
- Pseudoxanthoma elasticum
- Multiple pterygium syndrome.

Q. Why is she not suffering from Turner syndrome?
Since there is absence of features like:
- Short stature
- Short metacarpal
- Coarctation of aorta
- Shield chest
- Increased carrying angle.

Q. Which is the key point of diagnosis?
Limited ROM of cervical spine is very specific.

Q. How will you manage the case?
- Pharma: Nil
- Nonpharma: Councelling and patient education
  - Exercise: Range of motion of neck
  - Modalities: If any pain heat therapy can be given
  - Orthosis: Generally not indicated.

LATERAL EPICONDYLITIS

Summary

A 40-year-old nondiabetic, euthyroid housewife is suffering from subacute pain over her right elbow for last 2 months which was not responded with analgesics and rest. She is not suffering from any other joint pain or swelling.

On examination there is tenderness over her right lateral epicondyle without any synovitis, effusion or bony deformity of elbow. Cozens sign is positive.

P/D: A case of right-sided lateral epicondilytis.

Q. What is the other name of lateral epicondilytis?
Tennis elbow.

Q. Why is it named so?
Because it is commonly seen in tennis players, but may be seen in any other sports involving racquet or even in individuals who use their forearm vigorously.

Q. Mention the tendons that originates from lateral epicondyle?
Common extensor tendon which serves as the upper attachment (in part) for the superficial muscles that are located on the posterior aspect of the forearm:
- Extensor carpi radialis brevis
- Extensor digitorum
- Extensor digitiminimi
- Extensor carpi ulnaris.

Q. How will you perform Cozens test?
Stabilize the patient's elbow in 90 degrees of flexion with one hand while palpating over the lateral epicondyle. The other hand positions the patient's hand into radial deviation and forearm pronation while the patient is asked to resisted wrist extension in this position against manual resistance. The test is considered positive if it produces pain or reproduction of other symptoms in the area of the lateral epicondyle.

Q. What are the risk factors of TE?
Activities that involve repeated movements of the forearm, wrist, and fingers. This includes grasping and twisting arm movements, such as carpentry, plumbing, lifting objects or gardening and sports (such as racquet sports, throwing sports, or swimming).
- Improper techniques while doing movements, such as gripping a handle or twisting an object
- Improper equipment for work, daily activities, and sports, such as using a hammer or a tennis racquet with a grip that is the wrong size for your hand
- Age tennis elbow is most common in people who are in their 40s
- History of tendon injuries.

Q. What will you suspect if bilateral or recurrent TE?
- Diabetis mellitus
- Hypothyroidism
- Crystal disease
- Collagen vascular disease
- Enthesopathy.

Q. What are the differential diagnosis?
- Cervical radiculopathy
- Elbow and forearm overuse injuries
- Little league elbow syndrome
- Plica syndrome
- Radial nerve entrapment.

Q. How will you manage this case?
- Counceling and patient education
- Investigations: Blood, CBC, FBS, TFT, ESR, CRP
- RF, Anti CCP, HLAB27, ANF : If any other joint pain
- X-ray of elbow

- USG of elbow to rule out tear or injury of extensor group of muscles.

Pharmacological: NSAIDS—Topical and oral
Intervention: Steroid along with lignocaine
Platelet-rich plasma
Hyaluronic acid.
Nonpharmacological: Orthosis: Tennis elbow band.
Exercise: Eccentric strengthening of wrist extensors.
Modalities: Ice compression
UST over lateral epicondyle
LASER on lateral epicondyl
OT Work station modification.

Q. What is resistant TE?
It is radial tunnel syndrome which mimics tennis elbow.

Q. Where should TE band be placed?
Upper border of band two inch below lateral epicondyle.

Q. What is golfer's elbow?
It is medial epicondylitis.

Q. Why is it called so?
Since it is seen in golfers who mainly use their wrist flexors, hence more chance of cumulative trauma to origin of flexor muscles on medial epicodyle.

Q. What are the clinical features of Olecranon bursistis?
- Pain
- Swelling
- Restricted ROM
- If infected there is redness and tender, fever, discharge.

Q. What are the investigations to be done?
- Routine blood
- Uric acid
- Fluid analysis
- USG
- X-ray of elbow joint.

Q. How will you manage the case?
- Ice compression
- NSAIDs
- Avoidance of exaggerating factors
- Aspiration and steroid injection (if there is no improvement)
- Treat systemic disease.

MOTOR NEURON DISEASE (MND)

Summary

A 60-year-old male presented with right upper limb wasting and weakness with diminished jerks. He is also complaining of thinning and decreased grip of his hand for last six months. On examination, he has fasciculation in right hypothenar and deltoid muscles. His right lower limb gross motor power is 4/5 with spascity and increased jerks with extensor planter.
So, I think this is a case of MND.

Q. What are the differentials ?
- Cervical myelopathy
- Syringomyelia
- Spinal muscular atrophy (SMA).

Q. What is MND?
This is a disease of unknown etiology which leads to degeneration of anterior horn cells of the spinal cord, motor nuclei of cranial nerves, and the corticospinal and corticobulbar pathways. The disease is characterized by insidious onset with a steady progressive course.

Q. What are the types of MND?
- Amyotrophic Lateral Sclerosis (ALS)
- Primary lateral sclerosis (PLS)
- Progressive muscular atrophy (PMA)
- Progressive bulbar palsy (PBP)
- Adult-onset, progressive spinal muscular atrophy (SMA)
- X-linked, recessive spinobulbar muscular atrophy (SBMA).

Q. How will you diagnose MND?
Diagnosis of MND have been discussed in Flowchart 3.3.

Q. What is the age of onset of ALS?
40–60 years.

Q. How will you manage this patient?
- Counselling
- Nutrition
- Investigation:
  - NCS
  - MRI of spine (to rule out syrinx, demyelination)
  - CSF study
- Pharmacological:
  - Riluzole

Flowchart 3.3: Diagnosis of MND

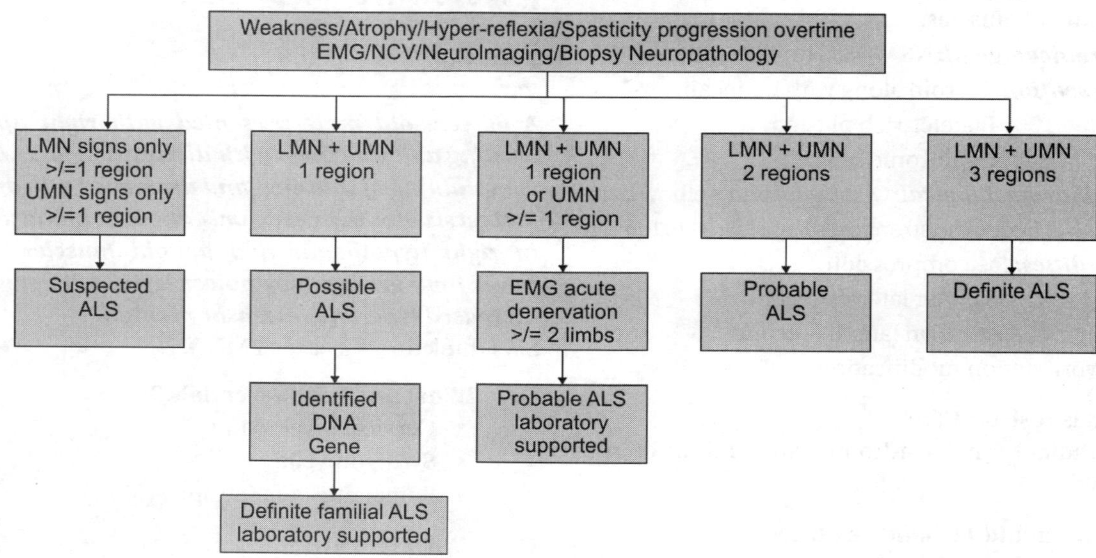

- Nonpharmacological:
  PT
  - ROM exercise
  - Strengthening exercise
  - Breathing exercise

  Occupational therapy—Gait training
  Home modification
  Assistive and adaptive device
  - Wheelchair.

Q. What are the causes of bilateral small muscle wasting of hand?

- Anterior horn cell disease involving C8 and T1
- MND
- Post polio residual paralysis (PPRP)
- Syringomyelia
- Hereditary sensory motor neuropathy (HSMN)
- C8/T1 root lesion
- Brachial plexus causes:
  - Cervical rib
  - Pancoast tumor
  - Trunk injury
- Disuse atrophy due to arthritis.

MULTIPLE SCLEROSIS

Summary

A 26-year-old female patient presented with sudden-onset quadriplegia with gross motor power of 2/3 in both upper limbs and 3/5 in both lower limbs. She was also suffering from little bit of incontinence of bladder. There is no loss of sensory changes noted. She had history of right-sided nystagmus, irritability and fall to her right side while going upstairs that episode recovered completely. She also had previous episode of left-sided 7th cranial nerve palsy which was also resolved.

On examination, she is suffering from spastic quadriparesis with temporal pallor on fundoscopic examination.

P/D: Demylenating disease probably multiple sclerosis

D/D: Devics disease
Vasculitis.

Q. What is multiple sclerosis?

An chronic inflammatory disease in which the fatty myelin sheath around the axons of the brain & spinal cord (CNS) are damaged, leading to demyelination & scarring (gliosis) as well as a broad spectrum of signs and symptoms.

Q. What are the types of Multiple sclerosis?

- Relapsing remitting (RRMS)
- Secondary progressive (SPMS)
- Primary progressive (PPMS)
- Progressive relapsing (PRMS).

Q. Differentiate between multiple sclerosis and Devics disease?

Presence of optic neuritis and transverse myelitis favors Devics disease.

Q. What are the signs of multiple sclerosis?

Any combination of neurological signs and symptoms can occur in multiple sclerosis.

Q. What is the clinical feature of multiple sclerosis?

- Cranial nerves: 5th, 7th
- Eye: Diplopia on lateral gaze

- Pyramidal features: Muscle cramping secondary to spasticity
- Extrapyramidal features: Charcot triad of dysarthria, ataxia, and tremor
- Others :
  - Sensory loss (i.e., paresthesias)—Usually an early complaint
  - Cerebellar symptoms
  - Optic neuritis
  - Trigeminal neuralgia—Bilateral facial weakness or trigeminal neuralgia
  - Facial myokymia (irregular twitching of the facial muscles)—May also be a presenting symptom
  - Heat intolerance
  - Pain
  - Subjective cognitive difficulties
  - Depression.

Q. What is Lhermitte's phenomenon?

Lhermitte's phenomenon is an electrical sensation that runs down the back and into the limbs. The sensation can feel like it goes up or down the spine. In many patients, it's elicited by bending the head forward.

Q. What is Uhthoff's phenomenon?

It is the worsening of neurologic symptoms in multiple sclerosis (MS) when the body gets overheated from hot weather, exercise, fever, and water. It is possibly due to the effect of increased temperature on nerve conduction. With an increased body temperature, nerve impulses are either blocked or slowed down in a damaged nerve but once the body temperature is normalized, signs and symptoms may disappear or improve.

Q. When benign course are likely ?

- Pure sensory
- Infrequent after hypnosis
- Optic neuritis
- Benign clinical symptoms at onsey.

Q. What are the causes of compressive myelopathy?

See chapter with SCI.

Q. How will you manage this case?

Investigations:

- MRI: Multiple bilateral lesion
- CSF: Oligoclonal band

Symptomatic treatment:

- Baclofen—spasticity
- Amitryptiline
- Muscle relaxants
- Oxybutinine, CIC—Bladder.

Specific treatment

- Interferon beta
- Copaxone
- Plasmapheresis.

Nonpharmacological

- See SCI.

Q. What is the prognosis?

- Most patients ultimately experience progressive neurologic disability
- Median time until a cane—20 years from the time of symptom onset and 30 yrs until wheelchair use
- The median survival time from onset is approx 10 yrs shorter than age-matched control
- Many patients might remain stable, progress only minimally in over a decade of living with the disease.

Q. What are the effects of plasmapharesis?

- Short-term effect
- Works best in men and if started within 20 days of onset of symptoms

Q. What is the role of exercise?

- Exercise has a beneficial effect on MS disability and quality of life
- Aerobic training improves maximum exercise capacity for ambulatory MS individuals, while inactivity makes it worse
- Every exercise prescription should be tailored to meet individual circumstances
- 3 sets of 10 repetitions, 2 muscles/limb, 2 limbs/ session
- Specific muscle training is recommended for improving focal weakness
- To improve gait, exercise must include standing and walking.

MUSCULAR DYSTROPHY

Summary

A 13-year-boy presented with gradual-onset progressive weakness of his both upper limbs and lower limbs. In early childhood he had several episodes of fall. His elder brother is already dependent on mobility due to similar types of weakness. He is also facing difficulty to climb stairs now-a-days.

On examination his proximal muscle power is 3/5 in upper limb and 2/5 in both lower limbs with wasting of

quadriceps. He has pseudohypertrophy of calf muscles and buttocks and has waddling gait. Gower sign is positive

P/D: Beckers muscular dystrophy

D/D: Duchenne muscular dystrophy

Q. What is muscular dystrophy?

Muscular dystrophy (MD) is a group of muscle diseases that weaken the musculoskeletal system and hamper locomotion and characterized by progressive skeletal muscle weakness, defects in muscle proteins, and the death of muscle cells and tissue.

Q. What is pseudohypertrophy?

The condition in which fat and fibrous tissue infiltrate muscle tissue, causing eventual weakening of the respiratory muscles and the myocardium.

Q. What are the common sites of pseudo hypertrophy?

- Gastrocnemius soleus
- Glutei
- Brachioradialis
- Deltoid.

Q. What are the chances of inheritance?

- If mother carrier and father normal—25%
- If father suffering and mother normal—nil (but all girls carrier).

Q. What are the chances of mental retardation in muscular dystrophy?

1/3rd in BMD and DMD.

Q. What is Gower's sign?

Difficulty in rising from floor due to hip and knee extensor weakness.

Q. Why there is waddling gait?

See gait.

Q. What are the difference between BMD and DMD?

Difference between BMD and DMD have been disscussed in Table 3.7.

Table 3.7: Difference between BMD and DMD

	DMD	*BMD*
Age of onset	<5 years	Early adolescence
Scoliosis	Severe and progressive	Usually mild
Wheelchair bound	Early adolescence	Late adolescence
Pulmonary dysfunction	Severe	Mild
Cognitive involvement	Frequent	Unusual
Life expectancy	27 years (approximate)	60 years (approximate)
Dystrophin	Completely absent	Faulty/Segmental

Q. What are the clinical features of FSMD?

- Early adulthood onset
- Facial weakness
- Difficult eye closure
- Expressionless face
- Scapular stabilizer weakness.

Q. How will you manage the case?

Investigation:

Blood: CPK and aldolase

NCS and EMG (to see myopathic changes)

Q. What are the types of muscular dystrophy?

Types of muscular dystrophy have been discussed in Table 3.6.

Table 3.6: Types of muscular dystrophy

Type	*Inheritance*	*Gene*	*Age of onset*	*Clinical feature*
Duchenne Muscular Dystrophy	X linked	Dystrophin	<5 years	Proximal weakness, Gower's sign, Pseudohypertrophy
Becker Muscular Dystrophy	X linked	Dystrophin	Early adolescent	Same
Limb Girdle Muscular Dystrophy	AD/AR	Myotilin, laminin A/C, caveolin-3	Variable	Slowly progressive, proximal weakness greater than distal
Facioscapulohumeral Muscular Dystrophy	AD	DUX4 (deletions of D4Z4 repeats)	Early adulthood	Shoulder girdle weakness Facial weakness Difficult eye closure but no ptosis Expressionless facies
Emery-dreifuss Muscular Dystrophy	X linked	Emerin, Lamenin	Variable	Elbow contracture, rigid equinus, neck contracture. Scapular and peroneal involvement
Congenital Muscular Dystrophy	AR	Merosin	Infants	Severe contractures

Muscle biopsy (to see dystrophin protein)
Genetic study.

Management: Councelling and patient education
Goal setting
Steroids (low dose).

Nonpharmacological:

PT: Submaximal strengthening, preventing contracture, maintaining ROM

OT: Gait training.

Electrical Stimulation: To affected muscles.

Q. What is role of steroid?
It is a double-edge sword. In low doses it delays wheelchair dependency by 2 years. In high and prolonged doses it itself causes myopathy.

Q. Why is submaximal exercise recommended?
To prevent fatigue and prevent structural disintegration of muscle fibers.

Q. What type of muscle fibre is affected in DMD?
Fast muscle fibres are preferentially affected.

Q. EMG detects which muscle fibers?
Type 1a.

Q. What is the prognosis and life expectancy in BMD and DMD?
- Prognosis is very poor in DMD, wheelchair bound by 12 years.
- DMD—Late teens
- BMD—4th–5th decade.

Q. What is the commonest cause of death?
Pulmonary infection.

MYASTHENIA GRAVIS

Summary

A middle-aged female patient presented with bilateral ptosis accentuated by upward gaze along with diplopia, lack of facial expression and generalized facial weakness seen mainly at the end of the day.

His voice is becoming shallow with nasal intonation in the afternoon. Not only that but also she has proximal muscle weakness which is worsening after repeated activities.

P/D: A case of myasthenia gravis

Q. How do you confirm your diagnosis?
By Edrophonium test.

Q. What are the clinical features of myasthenia gravis?
- Diurnal variation of weakness
- Decreased swallow and chewing
- Nasal speech
- Normal reflexes and sensory findings
- Jaw supporting sign—Supports weak jaw especially after prolonged talking.

Q. What are the associated immune disorders?
- Thyrotoxicosis
- Hypothyroid
- Rheumatoid arthritis
- Systemic lupus erythematosis
- Diabetis mellitus
- Sjogren
- Sarcoid.

Q. How will you manage this case?
- Investigations: Edrophonium test
  Lung function test—
  Vital capacity (PFT)
- Chest X-ray: To see mediastinal mass
- CT scan: To see for thymoma
  Thyroxine level
  ANA, RF
- NCS: Repeated nerve stimulation (see electrodiagnostics)
- Treatment:
- Pharmacological → If symptomatic: Anticholinergic
  Pyridogostigmin
- Definite management:
  - Immunosuppressant
  - Steroid
  - AZT (azathioprine)
  - Cyclosporin
  - Plasmapheresis.
- Nonpharmacological: Deep breathing exercise
  Maintaining ROM.

Q. What are the diseases which have diurnal variation?
- Botulism
- Lambert Eaton syndrome.

Q. What are the drugs causing MG?
- D Penicillamine
- Aminoglycosides.

Q. What is the difference between cholinergic crisis and myasthenia crisis?

- A small amount of tensilon is infused through the IV line, and the dose is gradually increased while the examiner observes for signs of improved muscle strength (indicating a myasthenic crisis) or worsening muscle weakness (suggesting a cholinergic crisis)
- If the test confirms a myasthenic crisis, the drug neostigmine is given immediately. If having a cholinergic crisis, the drug atropine is administered.

Q. What is the role of thymectomy?

- Beneficial in 85% cases
- 35% drug free remission

Q. What is the grading system of Severity of MG?

Ossermans grade..............see scale.

OSTEOARTHRITIS

Summary

A 65-year-old diabetic lady from middle economic class presented with painful swelling of both knee for last 2 years which was gradual in onset and slowly progressive. She is facing difficulty to perform her normal daily activities. She stays in 1st floor of her apartment. She also was complaining of mild pain in her DIP joints bilaterally.

On examination she has symmetrical hand deformity with sublacation of both 1st CMC Joint. Heberdan nodule was noted on her DIP joints. Her knee joint is tender with mediolateral instability and has genu varus deformity of her knee on standing.

P/D: Generalized OA.

Q. What type of disease is OA?

It falls under degenerative disease and defined as a chronic degenerative disorder of multifactorial etiology characterized by loss of articular cartilage, hypertrophy of bone at the margins, subchondral sclerosis and range of biochemical and morphological alterations of the synovial membrane and joint capsule.

Q. What are the types of OA?

It can be classified into:

a. Generalized

b. Local : Most common joint involvement in Indian population: Knee

Most common involvement in western population: Hip

A. Primary

B. Secondary

(i) Congenital and developmental disorders, bone dysplasias.

(ii) Post-surgery/injury—meniscectomy.

(iii) Endocrine—Diabetes mellitus, acromegaly, hypothyroidism, hyperthyroidism, hyperparathyroidism, Cushing syndrome.

(iv) Metabolic—Hemachromatosis, ochronosis, Marfan syndrome, Ehler-Danlos syndrome, Paget disease, gout, pseudogout, Wilson's disease, Hurler disease, Gaucher disease.

(v) Rheumatologic—Rheumatoid arthritis.

(vi) Neurological—Charcot joints.

(vii) Hematological—Hemoglobinopathies.

(viii) Iatrogenic—Intra-articular steroids.

Q. How will you manage the case?

- Lifestyle modification: Decrease weight, avoid squatting climbing stairs
- Investigations: Routine blood: CBC, ESR, CRP, LFT, creatinine.
- X-ray: Bilateral knee standing AP and lateral 30 degree flexion.
- Synovial fluid analysis : if swelling

Nonpharmacological: PO: Brace (flexible hinged knee orthosis)

Medications: Intra-articular injection

Disease modifiers: Diacerin
Glucosamine
S adenosine methionine

Intra-articular hyaluronic acid (IA HA)

Intra-articular platelet rich plasma (IA PRP)

Nonpharmacological:

Exercise: Isometric quadriceps and hamstring strengthening
Isometric vastus medialisobiquus strengthening
Patellar mobilization exercise
Gravity eliminating knee range of motion
Multi angle quadriceps strengthening
Active ankle foot exercise

Modalities: Ice compression
UST
TENS
Faradic stimulations

OT: Joint protection technique.

PO: Shoe modification.
Hinged-knee orthosis.

Surgery: Total knee replacement (TKR).

Q. Describe the DMOAD?

Various DMOAD have been discussed in Table 3.8.

Table 3.8: Various DMOAD

	Mechanism of action	*Dose*	*Side effects*	*Contraindication*
Diacerin	Act via inhibition of interleukin-1β	50 mg bid	Diarrhea, yellow coloring of urine, nausea	Pregnancy, lactation. Hypersensitivity to anthraquinone derivatives
Glucosamine	Act as a substrate of collagen, stimulating cartilage synthesis	900–1500 OD (max 2000 per day)	Nausea, diarrhea, constipation; stomach pain, gas, bloating; hair loss; or puffy eyelids	
Calcitonin	Its inhibition of subchondral bone turnover may be chondroprotective and, therefore, it may inhibit the structural disease progression of OA	Intra-nasally 2 puff every day, alternate nostrils at alternate day	Runny nose, nose bleeds, nasal irritation, dry nose with crusting, headache, dizziness, nausea, vomiting, loss of appetite, stomach pain, flushing of the face, skin rash or itching	Allergy
Doxycycline	Inhibition of type XI cartilage degradation, inhibition of collagenase activity Metalloproteinase inhibitor	100 mg BD	Stomach upset, diarrhea, nausea, or vomiting, photosensitivity, increased ICP, bone marrow suppression, blindness	Children, pregnancy, lactating mother

Q. What is radiological grading of OA knee?

See Chapter 11.

Q. What is PRP?

PRP is a fraction of whole blood containing concentrated growth factors and proteins and generally has a higher concentration of platelets compared with baseline blood.

Q. How is it prepared?

Step 1. 27 mL of venous blood sample is drawn into three 10-mL vacutainer tubes containing 1 mL of 0.106 M sodium citrate.

Step 2. The samples are thoroughly mixed with anticoagulant with the blood. An aliquot is removed to determine the initial platelet count.

Step 3. The sample is then centrifuged for 15 mins at 3200 rpm at resulting in three layers:
The inferior layer (erythrocytes)
The intermediate layer (leukocytes)
The superior layer (plasma).

Step 4. The buffy coat layer together with the plasma layer is collected and centrifuged for another 10 mins at 1500 rpm to separate the leukocytes.

Step 5. The plasma layer is collected, and the third centrifugation step at 3200 rpm for 10 mins is performed to obtain a two-part plasma: The upper part consisting of platelet-poor plasma and the lower part consisting of PRP.

Step 6. The platelet-poor plasma is first discarded to avoid its mixing up with the PRP. The tubes are shaken vigorously for 30 secs to suspend platelets.

Q. What is its efficacy?

Various studies point efficacy of it is at par with high molecular weight hyaluronic acid.

Q. What is the indication of TKR?

- Severe arthritis with or without significant deformity
- Osteonecrosis with subchondral collapse of a femoral condyle
- Severe pain from OA occurring in chondrocalcinosis and pseudogout
- Severe patellofemoral arthritis in an elderly patient
- Deformity with moderate arthritis
- Marked deformity of the knee, such as genu varum or valgum
- Gross instability or limitation of motion and functional abilities
- Failure of nonoperative management or a previous surgical procedure.

Q. What are the contraindications of TKR?

Absolute:

- Recent or current knee sepsis
- Remote source of ongoing infection
- Extensor mechanism discontinuity or severe dysfunction
- Recurvatum deformity secondary to muscular weakness
- Presence of a painless, well-functioning knee arthrodesis.

Relative:

- Unfit for surgery
- Significant PVD
- Psoriasis within the operative field
- Neuropathic arthropathy
- Morbid obesity
- Sepsis or systemic infection
- Painful solid knee fusion
- Severe osteoporosis
- Debilitated poor health.

Q. How will you rehabilitate the patient after TKR?

Immediate postoperative period:

- Two-handed assistive device (walker or axillary crutches)—for gait
- Adaptive equipment for bathing dressing
- Exercise—
  - Ankle pumps.

First Stage: 1st week (Table 3.9)

Second Stage (1–4 weeks)

- Low resistance dynamic exercise
- Aquatic-based exercise
- Ambulation—with a two-handed or single-handed device if they are fully weight bearing
- Should be independent in all basic ADL
- Electrical stimulation to quadriceps and Hamstrings
- Soft-tissue mobilization.

Third Stage (4–8 weeks)

- Available ROM should be 0°–115°
- Dynamic resistance exercise
- OKC and CKC and dynamic balance exercise
- Advance to a single-handed device or no device for ambulation and at different speeds and on different terrain
- Independent in negotiating stairs.

Final Stage (8–12 weeks)

- Return to preoperative exercise regimen
- Recreation activities
- Kneeling.

Table 3.9: Postoperative rehabilitation

Postoperative day	*Exercise*	*Mobility*	*Ambulatory*
0	Deep breathing exercise Incentive spirometer Quadriceps and gluteal sets Straight leg raise Hip abduction Ankle pump Education on continuous passive motion machine		
1	Lower extremity static resistance exercise Continuous passive motion	Bed mobility Bed to chair transfer with knee immobilizer	
2	Continue previously described exercise Straight leg raise with knee immobilizer Upper extremity strengthening	Continue bed mobility and transfer Begin toilet transfer	Assisted ambulation in room, partial weight bearing or weight bearing as tolerated
3	Sitting full arc motion flexion and extension in conjunction with supine passive flexion and extension	Decreased assistance in basic transfer	Independent ambulation with walker or crutches in room, partial weight bearing as tolerated with knee immobilizer. Trial of ambulation in corridor, possibly practice negotiating 2–4 stairs. Education on joint protection and energy conservation techniques. Independent toileting and grooming
4	Continue previously described exercise with increased intensity Active assistive ROM exercise and quadriceps Hamstrings self stretch	Independent in basic transfers	Gait training to improve pattern and endurance. Discontinue knee immobilizer (if quadriceps strength is greater than 3/5)
5–6	Continue previously described exercise transition from passive to active assistive range of motion exercise		Independent ambulation with assistive device Begin stairs with railing, cane as needed

Q. What is PFJPS?

Patellofemoral joint pain syndrome (PFJPS) is the non inflammatory anterior knee pain due to increased patella femoral joint reaction stress.

Q. What is PFJRF?

It is the resultant force generated within the patella femoral compartment due to vector force laterally by VMO, MCL, medially by LCL and posteriorly by patella.

Q. What is PFJRS?

It is PFJRF/ contact area between patella and femur. Maximum in full flexion (contact area is minimum). Minimum in full extension (contact area is maximum).

Q. Which radiological parameter correlate with PFJRS?

Q angle.

Q. What is Q angle?

Q angle is the angle formed by a line drawn from the anterior superior iliac spine to mid point of patella and a second line drawn from mid point of patella to tibial tubercle:

- 3.5 ± 4.5° is considered as normal Q angle for healthy subjects between the ages of 18 and 35 years
- The Q angle for women is 4.6° greater than that for men due to the presence of a wider pelvis, increased femoral anteversion, and a relative knee valgus angle.

Q angle is increased in:

- Genu valgum
- Increased femoral anteversion
- External tibial torsion
- Laterally positioned tibial tuberosity
- Tight lateral retinaculum.

Q. What is the main management of PFJPS due to increased Q angle?

Patellar taping.

Q. How is taping done?

Originally introduced in 1984 by Jenny McConnell.

Primary goal—To pull the patella away from the painful area thus normalizing Q angle to reduce pain

Mode of application:

- *Clean the area with an alcohol swab*
- *Palpate the patella*
- *Apply white cover strip*
- *Apply McConnell tape (also known as leukotape)*
- *Corrects mal-alignment of the patella.*

Q. What are the clinical features of PFJPS?

- Anterior knee pain—most common
  - The pain most often manifests during activities that require knee flexion and forceful contraction of the quadriceps (eg, during squats, ascending/descending stairs)
  - Pain may be exacerbated by sitting with the knee flexed for a protracted period of time, such as while watching a movie, hence leading to the terms "theater sign" and "movie-goer's knee".

Main precipitating factor: OVER USE AND OVER LOADING.

Q. What is varus correcting orthosis?

See orthosis.

Q. What are the shoe modifications done in varus and valgus deformity?

- Lateral wedge raise: For varus
- Medial wedge raise: For valgus.

PAGETS DISEASE

Summary

A 75-year-old male patient presented with difficulty to walk due to bowed tibia for last ten years. He is also suffering from hearing loss for last one year and thats why using hearing aids.

On examinations he has enlarged skull with warm legs without joint tenderness or synovitis. He is also having kyphosis due to loss of height.

P/D: Bowed tibia due to Pagets disease.

Q. What are causes of bowed tibia?

True bowing:

- Pagets (normally unilateral)
- Rickets (bilaterally symmetrical).

Apparent bowing:

- Secondaryt periosteitis
- Congenital syphilis (anterior bowing).

Q. What are the salient features of Pagets?

- 3% individuals on 40 years age, 10% on 70 years age
- Often asymptomatic
- Bone pain, headache, tinnitus
- May represent like slow virus infection, e.g. paramyxovirus.

Q. What are the complications of Pagets?

- Deafness (secondary to ossicles involvement)
- Optic atrophy

- High-output cardiac failure
- Pathological fracture
- Urolithiasis
- Sarcoma <1%

Q. What are the biochemical changes seen in Pagets?
- Highly raised alkaline phosphatase
- Normal calcium and phosphate
- Raised uric acid
- Raised ESR.

Q. What is the X-ray finding in Pagets?
- Transverse lucent areas
- Osteoporosis circumscripta
- Enlargement of the bones
- Expanding lytic changes, the "blade-of-grass" lesion
- Thickened cortices
- A coarse trabecular pattern
- Sclerotic changes.

Q. What are the treatments available for pagets?

Pharmacological:

1. Bisphosphonates:
   - Etidronate—orally administered at a dose of 5 mg/kg/day for 6 months and may bereinstituted after 6 months.
   - Pamidronate—parenteral therapy at 30 mg/day as a 4-hour infusion on 3 sequential days.
   - Alendronate for 6 months.
   - Risedronate—Orally administered for 3 months. Patients who have become resistant to etidronate appear to respond to risedronate.
2. Calcitonin: Usually initial 6 months course.

Nonpharmacological:
- Patient education and councelling
- Range of motion exercises
- Strengthening exercises

OT: Joint protection technique
Energy conservation technique.

PARKINSONISM

Summary

A 75-year-old gentleman presented with expressionless facies along with monotonous speech and slowness in movement in his right half of body which has gradually and slowly progressed in last one year. He has difficulties to initiate to walk along with festinating gait and sluggish movement with continuous involuntary rolling movement of his thumb. He is unable to stop quickly when asked to do and he has a history of few falls recently.

So this is a case of Parkinson's disease.

Q. What is the difference between Rigidity and Spasticity?

Difference between rigidity and spasticity have been discussed in Table 3.10.

Table 3.10: Difference between rigidity and spasticity

Spasticity	*Rigidity*
Velocity-dependent increase in tone	Velocity-independent increase in tone
Always in UMN lesion	In extrapyramidal lesion
Usually clasp-knife in nature	Usually is lead pipe or cog wheel type
Jerks are brisk	Jerks are normal
Plantar extensor	Plantar flexor
No tremors	Associated with tremors
E.g. CVA, SCI	E.g. Parkinsonism

Q. What is the classical triad of PD?
- Static tremor—4–6 Hz
- Rigidity
- Bradykinesia.

Q. Classify rigidity?
- **Lead pipe:** Uniform resistance present throughout the entire range of passive movement and is mostly seen in legs and trunk
- **Cogwheel:** Fluctuant resistance to passive movement due to presence of static tremor and is best seen in wrist joint.

Q. Classify tremor?

According to posture:
- Static tremor—At rest, eg parkinsons disease
- Kinetic (action) tremor—Appears in precise movements and disappears at rest, eg anxiety, thyrotoxicosis, salbutamol, chronic alcoholism
- Intention tremor—Appears at goal point of activity, absent at rest and beginning, e.g. cerebellar disease
- Flapping tremor—In encephalopathies.

According to amplitude:
- Fine tremor
- Coarse tremor.

Q. Difference between bradykinesia and hypokinesia?
- Hypokinesia is poverty of movement.
- Bradykinesia is slowness of movement.

Q. Difference between Parkinsonism and Parkinson's disease?

Parkinsonism is the syndrome complex which can be due to any insult to the basal ganglia region. Parkinsons disease is idiopathic variety of Parkinsonism.

Q. What are the other causes of Parkinsonism?

- Atherosclerotic
- Vasculitis
- Postencephalitic
- Traumatic
- Drug induced
- Toxic
- Anoxic
- Neurosyphilis
- SOL.

Q. What are the other features of Parkinsonism?

- Seborrhic dermatitis
- Motor
  - Gait
  - Movement initiation and execution
  - Bradykinesia, tremor, rigidity
- Sensory/pain
- Autonomic dysfunction
  - Orthostatic hypotension
  - Constipation
- Cognitive
  - Difficulty in switching from one task to another
- Behavioral and affective
  - Depression, anxiety
  - Psychotic features, such as hallucination
- Gastrointestinal
  - Dysphagia
  - Constipation
- Bladder dysfunction
- Sexual dysfunction.

Q. What is the management of Parkinsonism?

- Investigation—Routine blood, CT scan brain, MRI (vasculitis, SOL), PET scan if needed
- Pharmacological
  - A. Drugs affecting brain dopaminergic system
    - (a) Dopamine precursor : Levodopa (l-dopa)
    - (b) Peripheral decarboxylase inhibitors: Carbidopa, benserazide.
    - (c) Dopaminergic agonists: Bromocriptine, ropinirole, pramipexole
    - (d) MAO-B inhibitor: Selegiline
    - (e) COMT inhibitors: Entacapone, tolcapone
    - (f) Dopamine facilitator: Amantadine.
  - B. Drugs affecting brain cholinergic system
    - (a) Central anticholinergics: Trihexyphenidyl, procyclidine, benztropine
    - (b) Antihistaminics: Orphenadrine, promethazine
  - C. Supportive drugs for constipation, etc
- Nonpharmacological:
  - A. Physiotherapy—
    - Maintaining ROM
    - Stretching exercise
    - Relaxation exercise
    - Strengthening exercise
  - B. Occupational therapy—
    - Arm and hand therapy
    - Handwriting aids
    - Home modification information
    - Driver evaluation and vehicle modification information
    - Cooking and homemaking adaptations
    - Eating and dinnerware adaptations
    - Ways to make the most of your energy
    - Computer modifications
    - Workplace or work equipment modifications
    - Leisure skill development
    - Manual or electric wheelchair use
    - Bathtub and toilet equipment use
    - Dressing and grooming aid.
  - C. Psycological counselling for depression, etc.
  - D. Home modification.
  - E. Resettlement in home with appropriate assessment of caregiver specially in advances PD patients.

Q. What is parkinsonism plus syndrome?

The Parkinson's plus syndromes include multiple system atrophy (MSA), progressive supranuclear palsy (PSP), and diffuse Lewy Body disease (DLBD). **MSA** is characterized by urinary incontinence, reduced sweating, and orthostatic hypotension. **PSP (Steel Richardson Syndrome)** is characterized by no voluntary movement of the eyes, a marked change in personality, marked gait difficulty and those affected tend to have frequent falls specially while walking downstairs due to supranuclear palsy. **DLBD** is characterized by a marked decline in intellectual function, visual hallucinations, and signs of bradykinesia, rigidity, and possibly rest tremor.

PERIPHERAL NERVE INJURY

Summary

This 30-year-old male industry worker presented with weakness and inability to grasp objects for last two months after a glass cut injury proximal to the wrist of right hand. Initially an operation was done to connect

his nerve endings followed by wound care management. Now his wound is healed, a bit of scar hypertrophy is seen. There is weakness of his right thenar muscles, first and second lumbricals. ROM of the wrist and fingers are slightly restricted. The power and pincer grip is quite weak but lateral grip is relatively normal. He received a letter recently from his company to explain his long leave from job, that is why he is quite worried at this moment.

P/D: A case of right-sided median nerve injury at forearm.

Q. Classify the different types of nerve injury?
See scales.

Q. What are the types of nerve repair available?
- Nerve repair
- Nerve graft
- Nerve transfer.

Q. How will you differentiate a nerve injury from a tendon injury?
- In tendon injury - No sensory loss
- No changes in NCS.

Q. What is Wallerian degeneration?
Wallerian degeneration is a process that results when a nerve fiber is cut or crushed, in which the part of the axon separated from the neuron's cell body degenerates distal to the injury. This is also known as anterograde or orthograde degeneration.

Q. How is the nerve regeneration pattern?
Following nerve injury, the nerve will try to repair itself by sprouting regenerating nerve units. These regenerating units will then try to grow down the nerve to reinnervate muscle or skin. If they make a correct connection, motor nerve to muscle or sensory nerve to skin, then recovery of muscle function and skin sensation will occur. If however, the regenerating nerve fibers do not make a correct connection then no recovery will occur.

Q. What is the impact of median nerve injury at forearm?
Weakness of all median nerve innervated muscles except pronator teres.

Q. How can you assess level of injury clinically?
By assessing the power of supplied muscles. Muscles proximal to the level of injury should be spared like Pronator teres spared in forearm injury.

Q. What is total claw?
Caused by combined median and ulnar nerve injury.

Q. What is intrinsic plus and minus hand?
Intrinsic plus hand: Flexion of MCP joints with IP joint extension and thumb adduction.

Intrinsic minus hand: Hyperextension of MCP joints with IP joint flexion.

Q. How electrophysiological assessment helps in management of peripheral nerve injury?
See chapter on electrodiagnostics.

Q. How will you manage this patient?
- Pharmacological—SSRI (for depression), vitamin B_{12}
- Nonpharmacological
  - Orthosis—Opponens splint
  - Modality—Electric Stimulations to thenar muscles
  - Exercise therapy—Maintaining ROM, Scar tissue mobilization
  - Occupational therapy—ADL training, Vocational therapy, Retraining.

Q. What is the maximum time duration of improvement?
2 years.

Q. What will you do if deficit persists beyond 2 years?
- Nerve transplant
- Tendon transfer.

Q. What is tenodesis effect of wrist?
Moving the wrist in extension or flexion will allow the ability of the fingers to curl or grip. It is easier to straighten or release when the wrist is flexed.

Wrist extension tenodesis effect: Stronger grip while wrist in extension.

Q. What are the basic principles of tendon surgery?
1. All joints on which the transfer is to work should have full passive range of motion.
2. Transfer should not cause loss of an essential muscle function.
3. Any muscle looses at least 1 grade of strength with transfer.
4. Muscle excursion should be matched, taking into account 2–3 cm tenodesis action with wrist motion—usually contraindicates wrist fusion for paraplegics.
5. Take into account the effect of remaining joint motion on the force generated by the transfer.
6. Avoid acute angulation of the transferred tendon.
7. Usually attach transferred muscle to the tendon of the motor end to end if no native recovery anticipated; end to side if recovery anticipated.

Q. What is the sequence in repair?
Artery → nerve → tendon.

PERIPHERAL VASCULAR DISEASE

Summary

A 55-year-old diabetic hypertensive patient presented with gradual onset progressive both leg pain for last six months associated with nocturnal calf pain. His walking distance is diminishing day-by-day. He had previous episodes of angina four months back.

On examinations both legs are cold and skin is atrophic, shiny and hairless. There is no palpable pulse below femoral artery. Capillary feeling time of nail bed is also increased. There is no gangrene or ulcer in hand or feet.

P/D: Peripheral vascular disease in diabetic and hypertensive patient.

Q. What is peripheral vascular disease?

Peripheral vascular disease (PVD) refers to diseases of blood vessels outside the heart and brain. It's often a narrowing of vessels that carry blood to the legs, arms, stomach or kidneys.

There are two types of PVD:

- Functional PVDs don't involve defects in blood vessels' structure (The blood vessels aren't physically damaged) These diseases often have symptoms related to "spasm" that may come and go
- Organic PVDs are caused by structural changes in the blood vessels. Examples could include inflammation and tissue damage.

Q. What are the clinical features?

- Intermittent Claudication
- Calf pain
- Venous ulceration
- Gangrene.

Q. What is Burger's test?

Buerger's test is used in an assessment of arterial sufficiency. The vascular angle, which is also called Buerger's angle, is the angle to which the leg has to be raised before it becomes pale, whilst in supine decubitus. In a limb with a normal circulation the toes and sole of the foot stay pink even when the limb is raised by 90 degrees. But in an ischemic leg, elevation to 15 degrees or 30 degrees for 30–60 seconds may cause pallor. A vascular angle of less than 20 degrees indicates severe ischemia.

Q. What is ABPI?

The ankle-brachial pressure index (ABPI) or ankle-brachial index (ABI) is the ratio of the blood pressure at the ankle to the blood pressure in the upper arm (brachium). Compared to the arm, lower blood pressure in the leg is an indication of blocked arteries due to peripheral artery disease (PAD). The ABPI is calculated by dividing the systolic blood pressure at the ankle by the systolic blood pressure in the arm (Table 3.11).

Table 3.11: ABPI value and their interpretation

ABPI value	*Interpretation*
Above 1.2	Abnormal Vessel hardening from PVD
1.0–1.2	Normal range
0.90–0.99	Acceptable
0.80–0.89	Some arterial disease
0.50–0.79	Moderate arterial disease
Under 0.50	Severe arterial disease

Q. What is normal capillary filling time?

Less than 2 secs.

Q. How will you manage this case?

Patient education and counselling

Lifestyle modification—Smoking cessation

Investigation:

- Blood—FBS, lipid profile, TSH, urea, creatinine, HbA1C
- Doppler USG of both lower limbs
- ECG
- ECHO
- Angiography if needed.

Pharmacological:

- Aspirin
- Vasodilator: Ca channel blocker
- PG infusion
- Angioplasty.

Nonpharmacological:

- Buerger's exercise
- ROM exercises.

Q. What is Burger's exercise regimen?

Specific exercises intended to improve circulation to the feet and legs. The lower extremities are elevated to a 45–90 degree angle and supported in this position until the skin blanches (appears dead white).

The feet and legs are then lowered below the level of the rest of the body until redness appears (care should be taken that there is no pressure against the back of the knees).

Finally, the legs are placed flat on the bed for a few minutes. The length of time for each position varies with the patient's tolerance and the speed with which color change occurs.

Usually, the exercises are prescribed so that the legs are elevated for 2–3 minutes, down 5–10 minutes, and then flat on the bed for 10 minutes.

Q. What are the complications of peripheral vascular disease?
- Ulcer
- Gangrene
- Auto amputation.

Q. What is the other name of Burger's disease?
Thromboangiitis obliterans (TAO).

Q. What are the salient points?
- Nonatherosclerotic segmental vasculitis that affects small and medium-sized arteries and veins of the extremities
- 20–40 years male
- Strongly associated with tobacco exposure.
- Moderate to heavy smoker
- Autoimmunity triggered by smoking
- Raynauds phenomenon
- Migratory thrombophlebitis
- Treatment: Stop smoking, Burgers exercise, others same.

Q. What is Leriche's syndrome?
- Weak or abnormal femoral pulse
- Asymmetrical
- Bruit over lower abdomen and femur
- Claudication of buttock, thigh and calf
- Atrophy of limbs and buttocks
- Impotency.

D/D: Sciatica/ radicular pain.

POST BURN CONTRACTURE

Summary

A 35-year-old female patient presented with limited range of motion and pruritus over her right upper limb and chest after a burn injury. Fifteen day back she had an accidental burn injury while working in her kitchen. There after she had been treated in burn care unit with dressing and fluid management. Now the wound is almost healed with limited range of motion of right shoulder and elbow. She is severely depressed at this moment.

P/D: Post burn contracture.

Q. What is burn?
Burn is an injury to skin or flesh, deeper tissues due to heat, electricity, chemical, friction or radiation.

Q. What are the types of Burn?
Depending on:
- *Depth*: First degree, second degree, third degree
- *Cause*: Thermal, chemical, electrical, radiation, non-accidental, cement burn
- *Severity*: Mild, moderate, severe.

Q. What are the causes of burn?
See above.

Q. Classify burn according to severity?
See above.

Q. What is the rule of 9 in burn?
Body is divided into eleven 9% areas :
- Head and neck
- Anterior chest
- Abdomen
- Upper back
- Lower back
- Right arm
- Left arm
- Right leg anterior part
- Right leg posterior part
- Left leg anterior part
- Left leg posterior part.

11 parts × 9 = 99% **Rest 1% = Genitals**

Q. What is palm method?
The area of the patients hand is taken as 5%.

Q. How will you manage this patient?
- Councelling
- Goal setting
- Investigations:
  - Blood: Electrolytes
  - X-ray: Shoulder
  - Lung function test.
- Medical management:

Wound dressing:
1. Biological dressing—autograft (STSG/FTSG), homografts, xenografts.
2. Synthetic dressing
3. Cultured epithelial autocytes (CEA)
   - Anti depressant
   - Analgesics
   - PPI for gastric ulcer (curling ulcer)
   - Calcium and vit D3 supplementation
     - Nonpharmacological.

A. Positioning (Table 3.12)

Table 3.12: Positioning in burn patents

Region	Preferred position	Positioning devices
Neck	Slight extension	Neck collar Splint that conforms to the neck No pillows under the head
Axilla	Horizontal adduction, 15 degrees Abduction, 80 degrees	Airplane splint Wedge to positioning to abduction If rest of upper extremity involved Can support upper extremities: Bedside table Side boards/bedside extensions
Elbow	Extension 5 degrees	Elbow extension splint
Forearm	Supination	
Wrist	Neutral or slight extension	Wrist cock-up splint Part of resting hand splint
Hand	Wrist: Slight extension MCP: 70–80 degrees flexion IP joints: Full extension Abducted from palm Thumb opposition	Resting hand splint Soft web spacers Intrinsic plus hand splint C bar for thumb
Chest and trunk	Neutral with level hips	Figure of eight device to reduce protraction
Hip	Neutral extension Abduction 20 degrees	Wide soft straps to avoid frog leg position especially in children
Knee	Extension	Knee extension splint, immobilizer
Ankle	90 degrees That is neutral Dorsiflexion, plantar flexion Inversion/Eversion	Posterior shell with ankle in neutral
Foot	Neutral forefoot Supination/Pronation; toes extended	

B. Edema control:
- Upper extremity and hand suspended above patient's head in acute stage
- Resting hand splint with inclusion of wrist
- Compression gloves
- Active range of motion exercise.

C. Physiotherapy:

Exercise therapy:
- Breathing exercises
- Trunk mobilization
- Passive - active assisted - active full ROM
- Active exercise in lower limbs
- Gentle ROM on 3rd–5th day after grafting
- Early active antigravity exercise
- ROM to all body parts up to one joint proximal and one joint distal to grafting
- Gentle passive stretching and active ROM—2–3 times/day
- Daily slow and sustained stretching
- Strengthening exercises
- Aerobic exercise—cycling or rowing ergometry, treadmill walking, stair climbing
- Endurance and co-ordination training
- Facial exercise programme

Modalities: Electrical stimulation:

UST: Scar mobilization
Increase range of motion
Decrease hypertrophy
Paraffin bath
Continuous passive motion (CPM)

Hydrotherapy: For hydrolysis of adherent scar tissue

D. Occupational therapy: ADL training
IDL training.

E. PO: Splint: See prosthesis section (Hyperabduction splint for upper limbs).

Q. What is pre-hospital care of burn management ?

Pre-hospital care or on-site management" implies the management at the site of the trauma and constitutes the major part of the first aid. It begins at the scene of the accident and concludes when specialized/institutional medical care is obtained.

- Stop the burning process
- Patient removed from source
- Rescuer's safety
- Primary assessment of airway, breathing and circulation
- Remove metallic accessories
- Early cooling by direct water with caution for hypothermia
- In case of chemical burn, clothes removed, skin brushed, irrigation with water
- In electrical burn, current source is cut off, use of nonconductor to separate the source
- Elevation
- Oxygen
- Initiation of fluid resuscitation.

Q. What are the criterias to transfer to burn center?

- 2nd degree burns >10% TBSA
- 3rd degree burns

- Burn involving face, hands, feet, genitalia, perineum, major joints
- Chemical burns
- Electrical burns including lightning injuries
- Any burn with concomitant trauma
- Inhalation injury
- Patients with preexisting medical disorders
- Hospitals without qualified personnel or equipment
- Patient needing extensive reconstruction.

Q. What are the factors for acute management?
- Depth
- Extent (TBSA)
- Location
- Age
- Preexisting illness
- Inhalation injury
- Associated trauma.

Q. How much fluid should be infused?
As per the guidelines (Table 3.13).

Table 3.13: Fluid infused in burn

	Amount	*Time duration*	*Type of fluid*
Clincinnati Shriners Burns Hospital	4 mL × kg × % TBSA burn + 1500 cc × m^2 BSA	1st 8 hours 2nd 8 hours	Lactated Ringer's + 50 mg $NaHCO_3$ Lactated Ringer's
		3rd 8 hours	Lactated Ringer's + 12.5 g albumin
Galveston Shriners Burns Hospital	5000 mL/m^2 BSA burn + 2000 mL/m^2 BSA		Ringer's lactate + 12.5 g albumin

Q. Which fluid is to be used?
- <40% TBSA and patients with no pulmonary injury can be resuscitated with isotonic crystalloid fluid
- Burns of >40% TBSA and with pulmonary injury, hypertonic saline in the first 8 hours post burn, then Ringer's lactate in the following hours
- In pediatric and elderly, a lower hypertonic concentration—180 mEq/L helps avoiding complications.

Q. What is Evans formula?
The Evans formula was the first burn resuscitation formula based on body surface area damage and body weight, described in 1952. It was the standard burn care formula for years. Evans formula: normal saline at 1 mL/kg/% TBSA burn "colloid at 1 mL/kg/% TBSA burn. For second 24 hours, give half of the first 24-hour requirements " D5W (dextrose 5% in water) 2000 mL.

Q. What are the things to monitor?
- Intake/output/balance
- Electrolytes: Na, K
- Renal and hepatic parameters.

Q. Dressing of wound?
- Should be started after the initial phase of resuscitation
- Burn wound should be handled with powder free gloves
- Initial treatment involves cleansing of wound
- After wound cleansing dressing with topical agent should be done
- Full-thickness and deep dermal burns need antibacterial dressings to delay colonisation prior to surgery
- Superficial burns will heal and need simple dressings
- An optimal healing environment can make a difference to outcome in borderline depth burns.

Q. What is the current formula for nutritional supplement?
- Curreri formula age: 16–59 years: (25)W + (40) TBSA
  Age 60+ years: (20)W + (65) TBSA
- Sutherland formula Children: 60 kcal/kg + 35 kcal/% x TBSA
  Adults: 20 kcal/kg + 70 kcal/% x TBSA
- Protein needs—Greatest nitrogen losses between days 5 and 10
  20% of kilocalories should be provided by proteins
- Davies formula children: 3 g/kg + 1 g% x TBSA
  Adults: 1 g/kg + 3 g% x TBSA.

Energy requirement and component of total parenteral nutrition—
- 1800kcal+ 20% for a 60 kg wt person
- 75% carbohydrate (70D) + 25% fat (10–20%)
- 2/kg protein (10–15%)
- Electrolyte + trace elements
- 20mL/h
- Increase every 4–6 hr up to 120mL/h
- Monitor—glucose, BUN, electrolyte, creatinine, LFT.

Q. How to control infection in burn patient?
- Burn patients are immunocompromised
- That's why susceptible to infection
- Sterile precautions must be rigorous
- Swabs should be taken regularly
- A rise in white blood cell count, thrombocytosis and increased catabolism are warnings of infection
- Prophylactic antibiotics are not indicated in the early post-burn period.

Q. What are the other complications?

- Orthopedics:
  Contracture
  Delayed bone growth
  - Vit D
  - Bisphosphonate.

  Heterotopic ossification
  - 5 weeks to 3 months after injury
  - Elbow most common
  - NSAIDs
  - Oral bisphophonate
  - Post op radiation.

  Kyphoscoliosis
- Dermatologic
  Pruritis
  - Topical moisterizer
  - Oral and topical antihistamines and prudoxin, a TCA
  - Topical anesthetic.

  Hypertrophic scar
  - Silicone gel
  - Intralesional steroid injection with triamcinolone
  - Excision and steroid injection
- Catabolic state
  - High carbohydrate, high-protein diet
  - Recombinant human growth hormone
  - Low-dose insulin infusion
  - Synthetic testosterone analog (oxandrolone)
  - B-blockade.
- Psychosocial issue
  - Post-traumatic stress, depression, anxiety, sleep disorders.

Q. What is the role of splinting?

- Facilitating proper positioning
- Preventing joint contractures
- Protecting skin grafts or fragile wounds
- Assisting desired motion
- In the post acute period to prevent contractures until the tissue length is stabilized, after surgical release of a contracture.

Q. What are the different types of splint in burn?

See above.

Q. What is the role of serial POP casting?

- Long duration of stretch with minimal force
- Protection of exposed tendons
- Mechanical forces to remodel scar
- Cost-effective
- Treatment useful in children and noncompliant patients
- Treatment option when an open wound is present.

Q. What are the surgeries done in burn?

- Z-plasty
- Skin graft
- Local skin flaps
- Local muscle flaps
- Fasciocutaneous flaps
- Free flaps
- Cross limb flaps.

Axillary contracture

- Five flap releases—tight bands formed near unburned skin.
- Local flaps—if anterior or posterior axillary fold contractures are present.
- Fasciocutaneous flap procedures—contractures that are broader and involve the entire axilla.

Q. What are the issues in pediatric burn?

- Unable to co operate
- Not understand long term goal
- Lack of hand dexterity
- Bandage removal and dislodging common
- Difficulty in positioning, splinting and fitting of compression garments
- Exercise:
  - Nesting blocks to enhance hand function
  - Wheelbarrow walking or crab walking
  - Bicycling, soccer ball kicking
  - Hand-held computer games
  - Theraband and therapy putty.
- Small children—static splint or serial casting
- At 3 or 4- adjustable three point splints
  - Dynamic ankle splints
- Hand of infant—splinted flat with wrist in extension, fingers extended and abducted and thumb in extension and abducted radially.

Q. What are the issues in geriatric burn?

- Skin and wound healing: Prolonged healing time
- Early excision and grafting—risk to benefit ratio not clear
- With redundant tissue present in some body regions, scarring and contracture development are less frequent than in other adults
- Less acceptance of pressure garments
- Less cardiac reserve
- Less muscle mass
- Increased skin fragility.

POST MASTECTOMY LYMPHEDEMA

Summary

A 65-year-old house wife presented with gradual onset, slowly progressive swelling of right arm and fore arm with slight limitation of movement of right shoulder following her breast surgery and radiation therapy 3 months back. On examinations there is a right upper limb lymphedema with skin changes on right forearm. She is quite depressed and faces difficulty to perform ADL and special household works for last ten days.

P/D: Post mastectomy lymphedema.

Q. What are the differential diagnosis?
- Cellulitis
- DVT.

Q. What is the difference between lymphedema and venous edema?
- Venous edema: Swelling is pitting reversible when elevated. It mainly occurs in distal region generally associated with pain.
- Lymphedema: Swelling (apart from early stages) is nonpitting and non reversible when elevated and it occurs in whole limb and generally without pain.

Q. How will you classify lymphedema?
- Primary: Anomaly in lymphatic system
- Secondary: Filariasis, post radiation therapy
- High-output failure: Lymphangitis
- Normal output failure: Postmastectomy.

Q. What is the etiopathogenesis of lymphedema?
- Imbalance between lymph production and absorption
- Four major factor
  - Increased capillary hydrostatic pressure
  - Decreased plasma oncotic pressure
  - Increased capillary permeability
  - *Blockage of lymph return.*

Q. What are the causes of lymphedema after mastectomy?
1. Resection of lymph node
2. Radiotherapy
3. Chemotherapy (paclitaxel).

Q. Mention the clinical features of lymphedema?
1. May develop months to years later
2. Heaviness, tightness, numbness
3. Stiffness of joints.

Q. How will you take measurement?
1. Circumference: At different level, periodically measured.
2. Measurement of limb volume:
   - Water displacement limb emerged in water filled cylindrical container
   - Perometry: An infra-red optical electronic scanner and computer to calculate the volume of the body part.
3. ROM - Goniometry.

Q. What are the complications in lymphedema?
- Deformed limb
- Stewart treves syndrome (angiosarcoma)
- Elephantiasis.

Q. What is Peau d orange appearance?

Peau d orange describes anatomy with the appearance and dimpled texture like an orange peel, caused by lymphatic edema. However, the infiltrated skin is tethered by the sweat ducts in such a way that it cannot swell, leading to an appearance like orange skin.

Q. What are the stages of lymphedema?

Stage 0
- Latent, sub-clinical condition
- Swelling not evident despite impaired lymph transport.

Stage 1
- Completely and spontaneously reversible
- Soft, pitting edema.

Stage 2
- Spontaneously irreversible
- Tissues usually fibrotic
- Pitting requires strong pressure, or no pitting.

Stage 3 - *Elephantiasis*
- Irreversible
- No pitting, significant fibrosis
- Changes the skin.

Q. How will you manage this case?

Patient education and counselling
- Investigations:
  - Lymphography
  - USG doppler: To rule out axillary vein thrombosis
  - MRI/ CT: Entrapment neuropathy, metastasis.
- Medication:
  - Antidepressents
  - Skin Care

- Physiotherapy: CDT
  - Manual lymphatic drainage (MLD)
- Modalities: Faradism under pressure
- Intermittent pneumatic compression (IPC).

Q. What is full name of CDT?
Complete decongestive therapy.

Q. What are the components of CDT?
1. Manual lymph drainage.
2. Therapeutic exercise.
3. Multi-layer, short-stretch compression bandaging.
4. Skin care.
5. Education.
6. Elastic compression garments.

Q. Describe the phases of CDT?
- PHASE I:
  - Reductive phase
  - Primary goal is to decrease lymphoedema volume
  - Approximately 45 mins of MLD followed by compression bandage and exercise is done
  - Compressive bandage is left 21–24 hours/day
  - Optimally, CDT is performed daily (5 days/week) until the reduction of fluid volume has reached a plateau which can take 3–8 weeks.
- PHASE II: Started at the completion of Phase I CDT.
  - Compressive garments are used in day and bandages are in night
  - Remedial exercise daily
  - MLD as needed
  - A skin care regimen.

Q. What are the effects of CDT?
- Decreasec swelling
- Increase lymph drainage from the congested areas
- Reduce skin fibrosis and improve the skin condition
- Enhance patient's functional status
- Relieve discomfort and improve quality of life.

Q. What is MLD? How does it work?
- Manual lymph drainage is an essential part of CDT
- It works by increasing contractility of lymph vessels
- Through gentle and rhyhmic skin distension, congested lymph is directed through residual lymph vessel
- Treatment begins proximal, to "clear" proximal lymphotomes before moving to affected lymphatics
- Massage is directed towards the cleared lymphatics
- Pressure is very light (30–45 mm Hg)
- Strokes are rhythmic.

Q. How much pressure is given in faradism under pressure?
>30–32 mm of Hg.

Q. What is IPC?
Intermittent pneumatic compression.

Q. What are contraindications of IPC?
- Acute infection
- Severe arterial vascular disease
- Acute superficial or deep vein phlebitis (inflammation or clot)
- Recurrent cancer in the affected area
- Uncompensated CCF.

Q. What are the surgeries done in lymphadema?
- Excisional Operations, Including Debulking and Liposuction
- Tissue transfers
- Microsurgical lymphatic reconstruction.

Q. What are the indications of surgery?
- Not managed conservatively
- Cosmesis.

POST-POLIO RESIDUAL PARALYSIS (PPRP)

Summary

An 18-year-old young man presented with right lower limb weakness since childhood preceded by a febrile illness which last for a couple of days. He became suddenly sick followed by difficulty to walk.

On examination his gross power is 2/5 but his ankle power is 1/5 with genu recurvatum and high steppage gait for last few years. His tendo Achillis is tight and his right lower limb is shortened by four cm compared to his left lower limb. There is no sensory involvement.

P/D: PPRP of right lower limb.
D/D: Spina bifida.

Q. Why is it a case of PPRP?
- Asymmetric involvement
- LMN palsy
- No sensory involvement
- Preceding febrile illness.

Q. Which is the commonest muscle involved?
Quadriceps.

Q. Which is the most common completely paralyzed muscle?

Tibialis anterior.

Q. Which is the most common upper limb muscle to be involved?

Opponens pollicis.

Q. How to treat lower limb discrepancy?

Here shortening by 4 cm, correct 75% so need to correct 3cm.

First ½ inch (1.25 cm) by insole and rest by external heel and sole

Q. Difference between true and apparent shortening?

True shortening: The affected limb is physically shorter than the other leg. The cause may be above or below the trochanters. It is the measurement taken from the ASIS to the medial malleolar tip while both lower limbs are in identical positions and the pelvis is square.

Apparent shortening The amount of apparent shortening is the sum of the true shortening plus the shortening due to fixed deformity. It is the apparent shortening that matters to the patient. This measurement helps in assessing the extent of natural compensation developed for concealing the actual disparity at the hip joint especially by tilting the pelvis sidewards (fixed abduction and fixed adduction deformity) On many occasions this natural compensation improves cosmetic appearance.

Q. What is the rule of "2"?

2 days: Prodormal stage

2 weeks: Incubation period

2 months: Stage of acute illness

2 years: Stage of recovery

>2 years: Post polio residual paraparesis

20 years: Post polio syndrome.

Q. What is post polio syndrome (PPS)?

Long after the initial bout of poliomyelitis, some people suffer from further symptoms including new weakness, joint and muscle pain and fatigue.

Q. What are the living issues in PPRP?

There is no specific treatment for post-polio syndrome.

Symptoms may be controlled or improved if:

- Avoid physical overexertion or stress
- Keep comfortably warm and avoid exposure to cold temperatures
- Modify daily activities to conserve energy—for example, sit rather than stand at a workbench
- Use callipers, braces, walking sticks and electric scooters
- Ensure that all exercise is pain free and does not cause excessive tiredness
- Surgery can relieve a number of problems, such as:
  - A torn rotator cuff tendon in the shoulder—this can occur after years of using the arms to push up and out of wheelchairs
  - Foot deformities that can cause falls.

Q. Compare vaccinations with OPV and IPV?

Difference between OPV and IPV have been given in Table 3.14.

Table 3.14: Difference between OPV and IPV

OPV	*IPV*
Oral live attenuated vaccine	Inject able, inactive vaccine
Produced from sabin (attenuated) strains	Produced from wild polio virus strains
High systemic immunity	High systemic immunity
High mucosal immunity	Lower mucosal immunity
High efficacy	High efficacy
Contact immunity	No contact immunity
Herd immunity	Herd immunity
Risk of vapp (vaccine associated paralytic polio)	No risk of vapp
Risk of VDP (vaccine derived polio)	No risk of vdp
Contra indicated for immunosuppressant	Can be used
Easier to administer	Difficult (needs trained personnel)

Q. What is the mode of transmission of polio?

Feco-oral route.

Q. Eradication of polio from India? When was the last case of acute flaccid paralysis detected?

The last case of polio in the country was reported from Howrah district in West Bengal on January 13, 2011. On March 27, 2014 India was certified polio-free.

Q. What are the criteria's to notify AFP?

Any child under 15 years of age with AFP* or any person of any age with paralytic illness if polio is suspected.

Q. How will you manage this case?

- Counselling
- Pharmacological—supportive

- Nonpharmacological –
  - Exercise: Strengthening submaximal range, maintaining ROM
  - Modalities: TENS for pain
  - Orthosis: Shoe modification, AFO
- Surgery:
  - Hip flexion and abduction contracture—Ober release
  - Knee flexion contracture—Yount procedure
  - Equinus deformity—TA lengthening (only if quadriceps 3/5 or more)
  - Modified jones—Transfer of EHL to neck of 1st metatarsal.

PRESSURE SORE

Summary

A 42-year-old high-paraplegic wheelchair dependant male patient presented with an ulcer on his back for last fifteen days which was gradual in onset slowly progressive. He was also suffering from mild fever and wound discharge for last three days. That's why he has been readmitted for further care.

On examination there is 5cm × 3 cm wound with involvement of the muscles on his sacral area along with whitish discharge. There is no new neurodeficit apart from mild increase in spasticity.

P/D: Grade IV pressure sore in a paraplegic patient.

Q. Define pressure sore?

It is defined as injury to skin and/or underlying tissue usually over bony prominences due to prolonged pressure.

Q. What is the mechanism of pressure sore?

Pressure ulcers may be caused by inadequate blood supply and resulting reperfusion injury when blood re-enters tissue.

Q. How will you grade pressure sore?

See scales.

Q. What are the risk factors of pressure sore?

Extrinsic	Intrinsic
• Applied pressure	• Muscle atrophy
• Surface shear	• Impaired nutritional status
• Friction	• Anemia
• Local micro-environment	• Impaired vascular status
• Psychosocial	• Impaired mobility
	• Impaired sensation

Q. What is the minimum pressure needed to develop pressure sore?

>70 mm Hg.

Q. What are the common complications of pressure sore?

- Endocarditis
- Heterotopic bone formation
- Sinus tract or abscess
- Maggot infestation
- Perineal urethral fistula
- Septic arthritis
- Squamous cell carcinoma in the ulcer
- Contractures
- Increase in spasticity.

Q. How can you measure a pressure sore?

- Length
- Breadth
- Depth.

Q. How will you manage this case?

- Councelling and patient education
- Postural care in bed:
  - Pillows to maintain desired position
  - Bridging technique.
- Weight shifting while sitting(30 secs/15 to 30 mins)
- Change in position every 2 hours
- Prone position if tolerated
- In wheelchairs: Weight shifts, tilt in space, reclining wheelchair.

Investigations:

- Blood: Hb%, TC,DC, LFT, FBS
- Wound swab for C/S
- Urine RE/ME/CS
- X-ray to rule out osteomyelitis.

Pharmacological:

- Medicine: Antioxidants
- Wound care
- Antibiotics as per wound swab culture sensitivity report
- Anti inflammatory
- Anti-spasticity medicines.

Nonpharmacological:

- Proper mattress and overlays
- Exercise: Supportive

- Modalities: Ultra sound therapy (UST), Infra red (IR), electrical stimulation (ES)
- Hydrotherapy
- OT: Transfer techniques, postural care.

Q. How will a wheelchair bound patient shift his body weight to prevent pressure sore?
- Anterior shifts
- Lateral shifts
- Lifting
- Tilt in space wheelchair
- Reclining wheelchair.

Q. What are the different types of beds and mattresses?
- Air mattress (chance of dehydration)
- Water mattress.

Q. What are the new advances in treatment of pressure sore?
- Amniotic membrane
- Amniotic fluid injection (Still in research level).

Q. What is the role of stem cells?
It helps in healing and rapid recovery.

Q. What are the surgeries done in pressure sore?
1. Primary direct closure.
2. Skin grafting—
   - Split-thickness SG.
   - Full thickness SG.
3. Skin flaps.
4. Free flaps.
5. Musculocutaneous flaps and fasciocutaneous flaps.
6. Amputation and fillet procedures.

Q. What is the indication of surgery?
- Mainly required for stage III and IV.

Q. What are the prerequisites of surgery?
- Propрer nutrition
- No osteomyelitis
- Good support system
- Nonsmoker.

Q. What are the complications of surgery?
- Recurrence
- Dehiscence
- Seroma
- Hematoma
- Scarring
- Pressure on a new area with new site of ulcer
- Medical squeal
- Infection.

PROXIMAL MYOPATHY

Summary

A 40-year-old female patient presented with gradual onset difficulty to do over head activities for last six months without any pain. She was also complaining of difficulty to rise from ground and stair climbing for last three months. These features are gradually worsening. She does not have a history of alcoholism or any other drug intake. There is no history of weight loss, cachexia, lumps or bumps anywhere.

On examinations of proximal muscles of upper limbs power is 2/5 and lower limb is 3/5, sensory examination is within normal limits with normal jerks and flexor planter bilaterally.

Q. What are the differentials?
- Proximal myopathy
- Polymyalgia rheumatica.

Q. What are the classical features of PMR?
- Persistent pain
- Morning stiffness
- No weakness
- Raised ESR
- Good response to prednisolone
- Low-grade fever with weight loss.

Q. What are the different types of proximal myopathy?
- Hereditary myopathies
  - Muscular dystrophies.
- Dystrophinopathies
- Duchenne muscular dystrophy
- Becker muscular dystrophy
- Myotonic muscular dystrophies
- Facioscapulohumeral muscular dystrophy
- Limb-girdle muscular dystrophies
- Congenital muscular dystrophies
- Oculopharyngeal muscular dystrophy
- Emery–Dreifuss muscular dystrophy
- Congenital myopathies
  - Central core
  - Nemaline
  - Centronuclear
  - Multicore
  - Fiber-type disproportion
  - Reducing body
  - Fingerprint
  - Cytoplasmic body
  - Myofibrillar.

- Metabolic myopathies
  - Disorders of glycogenoses
  - Acid maltase deficiency (Pompe disease)
  - Myophosphorylase deficiency (McArdle's disease)
  - Disorders of lipid metabolism
  - Respiratory chain defects.
- Distal myopathies
  - Welander
  - Markesbery-Griggs-Udd
  - Nonaka
  - Miyoshi
  - Laing.
- Mitochondrial myopathies
  - Kearns–Sayre syndrome
  - Progressive external ophthalmoplegia
  - Mitochondrial encephalomyopathy, lactic acidosis, stroke
  - Myopathy and external ophthalmoplegia, neuropathy, gastrointestinal, encephalopathy
  - Leber's hereditary optic neuropathy
  - Leigh's syndrome
- Channelopathies
  - Myotonia congenita
  - Hyperkalemic periodic paralysis
  - Hypokalemic periodic paralysis
  - Paramyotonia congenital.
- Inflammatory myopathies
  - Polymyositis
  - Dermatomyositis
  - Inclusion body myositis.
- Toxic myopathies
  - Corticosteroid myopathies
  - Lipid-lowering agent myopathies
  - Alcohol-related myopathies
  - Myopathies related to other medications.
- Endocrine myopathies
  - Muscle disorders with glucocorticoid abnormalities
  - Myopathies with thyroid disease.
- Acquired myopathies
  - Myopathies with parathyroid disease
  - Pituitary dysfunction
  - Electrolyte disturbance.
- Infectious and granulomatous myopathies
  - Viral, bacterial, fungal, tuberculous, and parasitic myositis
  - Sarcoid myopathy.
- Myopathies associated with systemic disease
  - Critical illness myopathy
  - Electrolyte disturbances
  - Paraneoplastic.

Q. What is Gower's sign?

Gowers' sign is a medical *sign* that indicates weakness of the proximal muscles, namely those of the lower limb. The *sign* describes a patient that has to use their hands and arms to "walk" up their own body from a squatting position due to lack of hip and thigh muscle strength

Q. What is waddling gait?

Hip girdle muscles are responsible for keeping the pelvis level when walking. If there is weakness on one side, this will lead to a drop in the pelvis on the contralateral side of the pelvis while walking (Trendelenburg sign). With bilateral weakness, there will be dropping of the pelvis on both sides during walking leading to waddling. This gait is seen in patient with myopathies, such as muscular dystrophy.

Q. What is the management of this case?

- Counselling and education
- Investigations:
  - CBC,FBS, PPBS, TSH, K, Na, Ca, phosphate, CPK, Aldolase
  - EMG-NCS
  - Muscle biopsy
- Pharmacological
  - Supportive
  - Low-dose steroid
  - Medicine for complication like CHF, pneumonia.
- Nonpharmacological
  Physical therapy
  - Sub maximal strengthening
  - Avoid fatigue
  - Strengthening of the affected muscles
  - Stretching of the TA and Hamstrings
  - Electrical stimulation of the affected muscles.

Occupational therapy

- Balance training
- Gait training
- Wheelchair training.

Orthotic support

AFO only night time use (in BMD and DMD)

Note: Always stop any culprit drug, look for occult malignancy, if needed do initial malignancy screening.

PSORIATIC ARTHROPATHY

Summary

A 45-year-old female patient presented with bilateral symmetrical joint pain and swelling without any deformity. She is also suffering from symmetrical pain in other large joints with stiffness mainly in the morning.

On examination there is silvery scaly patches over her extensor surface of her elbow and knee. Her nail plates are thickened with hyperkeratosis and onycholysis. Her tender joint score is 16 and swollen joint count is 4.

P/D: Psoriatic arthriopathy

D/D: Rheumatoid arthritis

Q. What are the common sites of psoriatic lesion?
- Palms
- Soles
- Extensor surface of limbs
- Trunk
- Scalp.

Q. What is auspitz sign?

The Auspitz sign refers to the appearance of small bleeding points after successive layers of scale have been removed from the surface of psoriatic papules or plaques.

Q. What is Koebners phenomenon?

The Koebner phenomenon refers to skin lesions appearing on lines of trauma. The Koebner phenomenon may result from either a linear exposure or irritation.

Q. What is Nikolsky sign?

Nikolsky sign is a skin finding in which the top layers of the skin slip away from the lower layers when slightly rubbed.

Q. What are the etiologies of Koebners phenomenon?
- Psoriasis
- Pityriasis rubra pilaris
- Lichen planus
- Flat warts
- Lichen nitidus
- Vitiligo
- Lichen sclerosus
- Kaposi sarcoma
- Systemic lupus erythematosus
- Juvenile idiopathic arthritis
- Still disease.

Q. What is the classification criteria of Psoriatic arthropathy?

Caspars criteria ...see scales.

Q. What are the types of psoriatic arthritis?
- Monoarthritis
- Asymmetrical oligoarthritis
- Polyarthritis
- Spondyloarthropathy
- Arthritis mutilans.

Q. How will you manage this case?

Nonpharmacological management like RA apart from PUVA therapy for skin lesions.

Pharmacological management:
- Skin: Local ointment.
- Joint: NSAIDS.
- DMARDS: methotrexate.
- Biologics: Infiximab.

Q. Salient points on PUVA therapy?
- It stands for Psoralen + UVA (Ultraviolet A).
- UVA is relatively ineffective unless used with a light-sensitizing medication psoralen, which is administered topically or orally.
- Slows down excessive skin cell growth and can clear psoriasis symptoms for varying periods of time. Stable plaque psoriasis, guttate psoriasis, and psoriasis of the palms and soles are most responsive to PUVA treatment.
- The most common short-term side effects of PUVA are nausea, itching and redness of the skin.

RAYNAUD'S PHENOMENON

Summary

A young girl from middle class family presented with bluish discoloration of her fingers while lifting her both hands from cold water. She is also suffering from small joint pains without any swelling for last 6 months. There is history of gastric reflux after taking food along with constipation for last 6 months.

On examination there is skin thickening on face and both upper limb from fingers to her elbow along with mask-like facies. Her heart sounds are normal in auscultation and her breath sounds are normal without any crepitations and wheeze. She did not have any changes of her fingers or any red spots in her palm and sole.

P/D: Raynaud's phenomenon in a case of systemic sclerosis
D/D: Crest syndrome

Q. Why discoloration of hand occurs in Raynauds phenomenon?
- Pallor–Vasoconstriction
- Cyanosis–Depleted oxygen
- Rubor–Vasodilatation.

Q. What is Raynaud's phenomenon?
Raynaud's disease or Raynaud's phenomenon is excessively reduced blood flow in response to cold or emotional stress, causing discoloration of the fingers, toes, and occasionally other areas. This condition may also cause nails to become brittle with longitudinal ridges.

Q. What are the etiology of raynauds phenomenon?
Primary—Idiopathic (Raynauds disease)
Secondary—
- Connective tissue disorders:
  - Scleroderma
  - Systemic lupus erythematosus
  - Rheumatoid arthritis
  - Sjögren's syndrome
  - Dermatomyositis.
- **Obstructive disorders**:
  - Atherosclerosis
  - Buerger's disease
  - Takayasu's arteritis
  - Subclavian aneurysms
  - Thoracic outlet syndrome.
- **Drugs**:
  - Beta-blockers
  - Cytotoxic drugs—particularly chemotherapeutics and most especially bleomycin
  - Ciclosporin
  - Bromocriptine
  - Ergotamine.
- **Occupation**:
  - Jobs involving vibration, particularly drilling and prolonged use of a string trimmer (weed whacker), suffer from vibration white finger
  - Exposure to vinyl chloride, mercury
  - Exposure to the cold (e.g., by working as a frozen food packer).
- **Others**:
  - Physical trauma, such as that sustained in auto accidents or other traumatic events
  - Lyme disease
  - Hypothyroidism
  - Cryoglobulinemia
  - Malignancy
  - Reflex sympathetic dystrophy
  - Carpal tunnel syndrome
  - Erythromelalgia.

Q. What is CREST?
C—Calcinosis
R—Raynaud phenomenon
E—Esophgeal dysmobility
S—Sclerodactyly
T—Telangiectasia.

Q. What is scerodactyly?
Sclerodactyly is a localized thickening and tightness of the skin of the fingers or toes. Sclerodactyly often leads to ulceration of the skin of the distal digits and is commonly accompanied by atrophy of the underlying soft tissues.

Q. What is the difference between limited and diffuse scleroderma?
Difference between limited and diffuse scleroderma have been given in Table 3.15.

Table 3.15: Difference between limited and diffuse scleroderma

Presenting features	*Limited*	*Diffuse*
Raynauds phenomenon	Long duration	Short duration
Skin involvement	Distal to elbow and face	Proximal to elbow and trunk
Tendon friction rub	Absent	Present
Nailfold capillaries	Dilatation	Dilatation and loss
Autoantigen	Centromere	Topoisomerase 1
Pulmonary Hypertension	Absent	Present
Renal Involvement	Absent	Present

Q. What are the other features of scleroderma?
- Gastro—Dysphagia, reflux, hypomobility, Primary biliary sclerosis
- Musculoskeletal—Pain, swelling, stiffness, arthritis
- Pulmonary—Interstitial lung disease
- Cardiac—Pericarditis, effusion, heart failure, conduction block.
- Renal—Proteinuria, azotemia, hypertension, renal crisis.

Q. How will you manage Raynauds phenomenon?

- Avoid cold and stress
- Wear gloves, mitten and socks
- Avoid smoking and drugs like ergotamine, beta blockers
- Drugs—Nifedipine, ACE inhibitors, Prostacyclin analogues
- Antiplatelet—aspirin. Dipyridamole
- Intervention—Chemical sympathectomy
- Surgery—Surgical sympatectomy

Q. How will you manage this case?

- Patient counselling
- Investigation
  - Blood—Antibodies (Anti centromere, topoisomerase), LFT, urea, creatinine,
  - Endoscopy (for esophageal involvement)
  - ECHO (for pulmonary hypertension)
  - USG (for renal involvement, cortico medullary differentiation)
  - CXR, HRCT (for interstitial lung disease).
- Medical management
  - No definite treatment, symptomatic
  - Skin—local emollient (disease modifiers none is efficient)
  - Raynauds—already discussed
  - Pulmonary hypertension—Prostaglandin analogue, anticoagulant,Nifedipine, Bosentan
  - Renal - ACE inhibitor (Avoid high dose to prevent renal crisis)
  - Gastro - PPI, H2 blocker
- Nonpharmacological
  - Exercise—Maintain ROM, Isometric strengthening, deep breathing
  - Modalities—no role as per the current evidences.
  - OT - ADL training.

Q. Salient features of Raynaud's disease?

- Raynaud's disease refers to vasospasm that happens with cold or stress without any other related medical condition
- Affects more women than men
- Occurs more commonly in youth (between ages 5 and 35 years)
- May occur more frequently in members of the same family
- The best treatment is to avoid the cause of the attacks like:
  - Avoiding cold (using protective garments)
  - Avoiding abrupt changes in temperature
  - Avoiding smoking.

SCOLIOSIS

Summary

A 16-year-old girl presented with spinal deformity with convexity towards right of thoracolumbar spine for last five years, which was gradual in onset and slowly progressive. Recently she is having mild backache after coming back from school. On examinations there is right sided thoracolumbar scoliosis which is structural in nature without any trunk muscle wasting or weakness. There are no focal neuro deficit or bladder and bowel changes.

P/D: Right sided structural thoracolumbar scoliosis of adolescence.

Q. What is scoliosis?

The Scoliosis Research Society (SRS) has defined scoliosis as a medically significant frontal plane curve (scoliosis) as any curve which is greater or equal to 10 degrees, with or without a rotatory component.

Q. What is kyphosis?

It is the forward bending of spine. Normal thoracic kyphosis range from 20 to 40 degree.

Q. What are the etiology of scoliosis?

1. Idiopathic resolving

- Infantile (0–3 years old) < Resolving / Progressive
- Juvenile (4 years—puberty onset)
- Adolescent (puberty onset—epiphyseal closure)
- Adult (after epiphyseal closure)

2. Neuromuscular (Table 3.16).

Table 3.16: Neuropathic and myopathic causes of scoliosis

Neuropathic		Myopathic
Upper motor neuron	**Lower motor neuron**	Arthrogryposis
Cerebral palsy	Poliomyelitis	Muscular dystrophy
Spinocerebellar degeneration	Spinal muscular atrophy	Duchenne
Friedreich's	Amyotrophic lateral sclerosis	Limb girdle
Roussy–Levy	Charcot-Marie-Tooth	Fascioscapular
Spinocerebellar (olivopontine) ataxia	Myelomeningocele	Congenital hypotonia
Syringomyelia	Dysautonomia (Riley–Day)	Myotonia dystrophica
Spinal cord trauma or tumor	Others	

3. Congenital:

i. Failure to formation
- a. Wedge Vertebrae
- b. Hemi vertebrae

ii. Failure of segmentation
- a. Unilateral bar
- b. Bilateral bar
- c. Mixed

iii. Associated with neural tube defects:
- a. Myelomeningocele
- b. Meningocele
- c. Spinal dysraphism
- – Neurofibromatosis
- – Mesenchymal tissue disease
- – Marfan
- – Homocystinuria
- – Ehlers–Danlos
- – Osteogenesis imperfecta.

4. Acquired:

i. Traumatic: Fracture and/or dislocation without paralysis.

ii. Soft-tissue contractures:
- a. Postempyema
- b. Burns.

iii. Osteochondrodystrophies
- a. Achondroplasia
- b. Spondyloepiphyseal dysplasia
- c. Diastrophic dwarfism
- d. Mucopolysaccharidoses.

iv. Tumor
- a. Benign
- b. Malignant.

v. Rheumatic diseases

vi. Metabolic
- a. Rickets
- b. Juvenile osteoporosis.

vii. Related to lumbosacral dysfunction
- a. Spondylolysis
- b. Spondylolisthesis.

viii. Thoracogenic
- a. Postthoracoplasty
- b. Postthoracotomy.

ix. Hysterical

x. Functional
- a. Postural
- b. Due to leg length discrepancy
- c. Due to muscle spasm
- d. Other.

Q. What are the age of presentation of different types of scoliosis?
- Idiopathic: Infancy to adolescence
- Neuromuscular: Childhood to adolescence
- Bone or ligamentous dysfunction: Childhood
- Traumatic/posttraumatic: All ages
- Infectious or neoplastic: All ages
- Degenerative: Middle age to seniors.

Q. What are the different types of curve?
- Primary curve: Structural curve with wedging, angulation, rotation and not corrected spontaneously or by mechanical correction. Primary curve is usually greatest.
- Secondary curve: Non-structural curve, develops in response to primary curve
- Compensatory curve: Formed to balance primary one (1 or 2)
- Decompensated curve: Compensatory curve doesn't fully balance primary one
- Overcompensated curve: Compensatory curve more than primary curve.

Q. What is Adams forward bending test?
- Patient bends forward, spine horizontal to the floor, while holding palms together, arms extended and knee extended
- Examine from side and behind the patient
- Look for a "rib hump"
- Rib hump is a hallmark of a scoliotic curve greater than 10 degrees.

Q. What is scoliometer?
- Scoliometer measures trunk rotation
- Patient positioned as in forward bending above
  - – Place Scoliometer on midline, perpendicular to spine
  - – Position at Vertebral level of maximum rib prominence
  - – Scoliometer inclination <5 degrees typically warrants no further evaluation
  - – Inclination of 5-9 degrees suggest Scoliosis and warrants Scoliosis XRay (or 6 month recheck at minimum)
  - – Scoliometer inclination >10 degrees suggests severe Scoliosis and requires work-up
  - – Seven degrees by scoliometer correlates with 20 degree Cobb Angle on scoliosis X-Ray.

Q. What are the factors of curve progression?
- Gender
- Future growth potential
- Curve magnitude at time of diagnosis.

Q. Mention the hindrance in this case?
- Pain
- Cosmesis
- Curve progression.

Q. How will you manage the case?
- Patient councelling
- Goal setting
- Posture correction.

Investigations:
Routine blood
X-ray: D/L spine: to see Cobb's angle.
Rib vertebrae angle difference (Mehta's angle).
Rissers sign.
PFT.
NCV and EMG of trunk muscle.
MRI of L/S spine if Red flag signs present

Treatment:
Pharmacological: NSAIDS for pain.
Nonpharmacological:
Orthosis: Milwaukee (for apex above T8)
Boston brace (for apex below T8).
PT exercise: Scoliosis correcting exercise.
Modalities: Electrical stimulation—Cotrels stimulation.
Traction: Cotrels traction (no present evidence)
OT: Postural care.
Work station modification.
Surgery if needed

Q. What is apical vertebrae?
The vertebra which is displaced and rotated most. Its endplates are least tilted.

Q. How to measure Cobb angle?
- Choose the first and last vertebrae that tilt into the concavity of the curve
- Draw a line perpendicular to that vertebrae
- The angle created between these intersecting lines is the Cobb angle.

Q. What is Ressiers index?
- Based on ossification of iliac apophysis
- Graded from 0 (no ossification) to 5 (complete bony fusion).

Q. What is Mehta's angle and its implication?
- Line drawn perpendicular to apical thoracic vertebra end plate and line drawn down the center of concave side rib and convex side rib
- Concave - convex angle = RVAD (Mehta's angle)
- <20 degree: Curve likely to resolve (90%).

Q. What are the types of exercise and its role?
- Pelvic tilt:
  - Supine
  - Standing
  - Prone (cat and camel exercise).
- Active elongation of spine
- General stretching exercises can be performed in prone position by extending both arms and legs
- Stretching one side of the arm and ipsilateral leg will cause stretching of that side
- Crawling exercise
- Cotrel's EDF technique (elongation—derotation—flexion)
- Breathing exercise.

Benefits of exercise:
1. Improve posture.
2. Increase flexibility.
3. Increase strength.
4. Correct muscular imbalance.
5. Improve respiration.

*(**NB**: Cotrel—Surgery*
Traction
Exercise
Electrical stimulation)

Q. What are the different types of low-profile thermoplastic-moulded TLSO?
Different types of low-profile thermoplastic-moulded TLSO have been given in the Table 3.17.

Table 3.17: Different types of low-profile thermoplastic-moulded TLSO

Boston	*Miami*	*Lyonnaise*	*Rosenberger*	*Wilmington*
One piece	One piece	One piece	One piece	Same
Posterior opening	Posterior opening	Anterior opening	Anterior opening	Anterior opening
Cut out present	Cut out present	Cut out present	NO cut out	NO cut out
Xiphi Sternum (XS) to Symphisis Pubis(SP)	Shorter. Allows forward bending	XS to SP	Same. Corrective forces given in cast	SN to SP, Lateral upto Axilla. Corrective forces given in cast
Plastic band	Plastic band	Plastic band	Adjustable and floating	Absent
No plaster needed Moulded	Plaster required	Plaster required	Plaster required	Plaster required

Q. When is orthosis given?

- Adolescents idiopathic scoliosis
- Actively growing adolescents (Risser ≤ 2) with curves between 30–45°
- Very young patient (Risser=0 or premenarchal) with curve >25°
- If between 20–29° and Curve progression >5° every 4–6 months.

Q. Which orthosis is to be given?

Apex above T8—Milwaukee brace

Apex at T8 and below—low-profile thermoplastic moulded TLSO.

Q. What is Charleston brace?

It is a part-time brace used in night time. Applied after attaining corrected positioning.

Q. What are the evidences of ES and traction in scoliosis?

Previously it was used but presently no role as per current evidence.

Q. What is the role of pulmonary function test?

- In untreated cases: Curve angle
  - Achieves 70 degrees—Mild decrease in vital capacity
  - 90–100 degrees—dyspnea on effort
  - >100 degrees—Alveolar hyperventilation, pulmonary hypertension, right-sided heart failure.

Q. What are the indications of surgery?

- Failure of conservative management (>40°)
- In neuromascular case >35°
- Pain uncontrolled by nonoperative treatment
- Thoracic lordosis
- Significant cosmetic deformity.

Q. What are the types of surgery?

1. Posterior instrumentation
   A. Harrington rod.
   B. Sublaminar wire and cable.
   C. Cortel and Dubousset system.
2. Anterior Instrumentation.

Q. What are the postsurgery rehab plans?

- Early mobilization
  a. To prevent deconditioning.
  b. To prevent other secondary postoperative complication.
  c. Preventing secondary deformity.
  d. Providing adaptations to ADL.
  e. Avoiding strengthening exercise and ROM in operative region.
- Type and timing of brace depends upon surgical approach, instrumentation.

Following growth: 6 month bracing is needed

TASK SPECIFIC DYSTONIA

Summary

A 50-year-old male clerk is suffering from difficulty to write, finish his desk jobs for last one month. It started gradually but is worsening day-by-day. He is presently facing difficulty to write five lines at a stretch due to tightness in forearm and inability to hold pen properly.

On examination there is no motor or sensory deficit noted and reflexes are normal. He is having dystonia after he starts writing for sometimes.

P/D: Task-specific dystonia or writers cramp.

Q. What is dystonia?

Dystonia is a neurological movement disorder syndrome in which sustained or repetitive muscle contractions result in twisting and repetitive movements or abnormal fixed postures.

Q. What are the other abnormal movements?

- *Tremor*—It is the most common movement disorder. It is defined as "an involuntary rhythmical movement about an axis".
- *Tics*—These are stereotyped, repetitive, rapid coordinated movements. They caninvolve any body part but typically involve the head, neck, eyes or upper extremities.
- *Chorea*—From the Greek word "dance", chorea is characterized by involuntary, irregular, purposeless, asymmetrical, non-rhythmic movements.
- *Athetosis*—This means "without fixed position". The movements are purposeless, bizarre, complex and writhing.
- *Myoclonus*—These are sudden brief jerks, irregular or rhythmic, and may be focal, segmental or generalized.
- *Ballismus*—Means "to throw". These are dramatic, flinging, involuntary appendicular movements, more prominent in proximal than distal muscles. The movements are continuous and confluent.

Q. What is task-specific dystonia?

Task-specific dystonias are primary focal dystonias characterized by excessive muscle contractions producing abnormal postures during selective motor activities that often involve highly skilled, repetitive movements.

Q. What is the pathogenesis of task-specific dystonia?

- Reduced inhibition at different levels of the sensorimotor system
- Repeated movements resulting in abnormal sensorimotor integration.

Q. How will you manage the case?

Investigations:

- Routine blood
- Xray of cervical spine
- NCS of upper limb

Management:

Medicine: Trihexiphenidyl
Clonazepam
Botulinum toxin Type A injection

OT: Grip changes
ADL plus IDLs
Vocational councelling
Computer typing
Alternate training.

Q. Will this patient face problem in computer typing?

No, since the cramp is specific for writing.

Q. Which muscle is targeted in botulinum toxin injection?

- Flexor carpi ulnaris (FCU)
- Flexor digitorum superficialis (FDS)
- Extensor carpi radialis (ECR)
- Flexor policis longus (FPL).

Q. How frequently is it repeated?

Generally gives good result after single dose and lasts for years.

Q. Is there any other alternate treatment?

No.

TOPHACEOUS GOUT

Summary

A 35-year-old male patient presented with recurrent asymmetric joint pain along with febrile illness which subsided within few days. Initially he was only suffering from recurrent first MTP joint pain for last one year.

On examination there are multiple tophi on his helix of ear and on Achilis tendon. His musculoskeletal signs are absolutely normal clinically. There is no other abnormality noted in any other system.

P/D: Chronic tophaceous gout

D/D: Pseudo gout

Q. What is tophi?

A tophus is a deposit of uric acid crystals, in the form of monosodium urate crystals, in people with longstanding hyperuricemia.

Q. What are the common sites of deposits?

- Helix of ear
- Olecranon bursa
- Achillis tendon
- Ulnar aspect of forearm.

Q. Define the spectrum of gout?

- Asymptomatic hyperuricemia
- Recurrent acute gout
- Chronic tophaceous gout.

Q. What are the clinical features of gout?

- Commonest and earliest involvement—First MTP joint
- Arthritis
- Oligoarthritis—Asymmetrical and in lower limbs
- During acute attack:
  - Middle of night/early morning
  - Pain, swelling, redness
  - Fever
  - Stays for few days.
- Other changes:
  - Chronic arthritis
  - Dyslipidemia
  - Joint deformity
  - Secondary degenerative joint disease.
- Systemic changes:
  a. Renal.
     1. Stone, 2. Obstructive uropathy
  b. CVS: Conduction block due to deposition of tophi in conduction system.
  c. Ear: Deafness and tinnitus due to tophi deposition on foot plate of stapedeous.

Q. What are the precipitating factors of acute attack?

- Dehydration
- Sepsis
- Drug intake.

Q. What are the common associations of Gouty arthritis?

- Hypertension
- Diabetes
- Bronchial asthma
- Dyslipidemia—Type IV: Increased triglyceride, VLDL
- Hypothyroid/Hyperthyroid
- Obesity.

Q. Factors increasing serum UA?

- Drugs—Diuretics, pyrazinamide, nicotinic acidMyeloproliferative and lymphoproliferative disorder
- Chronic renal failure
- Alcoholism.

Q. How will you manage the case?

- Investigation:
  - Blood—Routine, uric acid, lipid profile, TSH, FBS
  - X-ray foot (to look for tophi)
  - Synovial fluid analysis—crystal study
  - ECG.
- Management:
  - Life style modification
    - Weight reduction
    - Increased fluid intake—3-4ltr/day
    - Diet: Avoid red meat, sea food
  - Pharmacological

    Acute attack:
    - NSAIDS—Etoricoxib, indomethacin (started as soon as possible)
    - Cholchicine—0.6mg thrice a day (until loose motion or tinnitus happens).

  Recurrence of attack—Start Hypouricemic drug

  Hypouricemic drugs:
  - Allopurinol: First choice. Starting dose: 300 mg/day (dose up to 800 mg/day—maximum) for 3 months then check level and adjust dose
  - If not responsive or intolerant: Febuxostat (initially 40mg/day, max dose 120 mg/day)
  - Proben acid : Indication : low exceretion of uric acid.

  Nonpharmacological:
  - Exercise—Maintaining ROM, Isometric strengthening
  - Occupational therapy—Joint protection, energy conservation technique
  - Orthosis—if any joint deformity.

Q. What are the indication of starting hypouricemic drugs?

- Recurrent classic attack of gout
- Clinical/Radiological tophi
- Renal uric acid stone
- Uric acid crystal in Synovial fluid analysis
- Secondary hyperuricemia
- When 24 hours urinary uric acid level is <8 mg/dL.

Q. How long should it be continued?

Life long.

Q. What is the target level of uric acid?

To keep uric acid level <6md/dL.

Q. What are the side effects of allopurinol?

- Agranulocytosis, bone marrow suppression
- Fever, sore throat, and headache with a severe blistering, peeling and red skin rash
- Nausea, upper stomach pain, itching, loss of appetite, weight loss, dark urine, clay-colored stools
- Hepatotoxicity
- Joint pain or flu symptoms
- Easy bruising, unusual bleeding, or purple or red pinpoint spots under the skin
- Severe tingling, numbness, pain, or muscle weakness.

Q. What is pseudogout?

Pseudogout is a form of arthritis that causes pain, stiffness, tenderness, redness, warmth, and swelling in some joints affecting one or several joints at once and commonly affects the knee or wrist. Less often, it can involve the hips, shoulders, elbows, finger joints, toes, or ankles. It may be commonly caused by deposition of calcium pyrophosphste crystal.

Q. What are the other crystal arthritis?

- Calcium appatite
- Calcium oxalate
- Calcium apatite
- Calcium pyrophosphate

TORTICOLLIS

Summary

A 15-year-old young girl presented with neck pain and muscle spasm for last two months. She is facing difficulty to turn to her left side due to twisting and turning of her head and neck to right side.She is not suffering from any cough and cold or difficulty in deglutition or any recent onset hoarseness of voice. She is not suffering from any fever, joint pain or tingling sensation in upper limbs

On examination she is having torticollis to her right side with muscle spasm in nape of neck . Her throat examination is normal. There is no other neurodeficit.

P/D: Torticollis.

Q. What is torticollis?

Torticollis, also known as wry neck is a dystonic condition defined by an abnormal, asymmetrical head or neck position.

Q. What are antecollis and retrocollis?

Retrocollis: Spasmodic torticollis in which the neck is drawn back.

Antecollis condition where the neck is bent forward and chin touches chest.

Q. What are the clinical features of torticollis?

- Chin rotated away from the affected side
- Ipsilateral lateral flexion
- Flattening of the contralateral occipital protuberance
- Pain on movement may be present
- Difficulty in swallowing may be seen
- Fever with lymphadenopathy may also be seen.

Q. What is the etiology of torticollis?

- Congenital torticollis
- Secondary torticollis
  - Congenital bone anomalies
  - Atlanto-axial rotatory displacement
  - Infection (lymphadenitis, retropharyngeal abscess, tonsillitis, discitis, tuberculosis)
  - Trauma
  - Juvenile rheumatoid arthritis
  - Posterior fossa tumors
  - Intraspinal tumors
  - Dystonia (benign paroxysmal torticollis)
  - Ocular dysfunction.

Q. How will you manage the case?

- **Investigation:**
  Blood: CBC, CRP, ESR, FBS, PPBS
  X-ray cervical spine
  MRI cervical spine and brain (features suggestive of mass)
- ENT examination
- **Treatment:**
  - Pharmacological—NSAIDS and muscle relaxant
  - Nonpharmacological-
    - Stretching exercise
    - ROM exercise
    - Traction
    - Modality—UST (after ruling out infection)
  - Surgery.

ULNAR CLAW HAND

Summary

A 14-year-old boy presented with difficulty in lateral hand grip in right hand due to wasting of hand muscles apart from thenar muscles. He is also complaining of loss sensation of medial one and half fingers of his affected hand. He had a previous history of fracture around the elbow region and deformity of elbow following immobilization. He didn't suffer from any patchy areas of sensory loss of his hand and forearm.

So, this is a case of right-sided Tardy ulnar nerve palsy.

Q. What are the differentials?

- Ulnar clawing due to Hansen disease
- Entrapment neuropathy at elbow.

Q. What are the muscles supplied by ulnar nerve?

- In forearm—Flexor carpi ulnaris, 3rd and 4th flexor digitorum profundus
- In hand—All intrinsic muscles except the 1st and 2nd lumbricals, opponens pollicis, Abductor pollicis brevis and flexor pollicis brevis (superficially).

Q. What is Froment's sign?

This test demonstrates an inability to hold a piece of paper by the thumb and index finger with pure thumb adduction (adductor pollicis weakness). The patient substitutes the median innervated flexor pollicis longus muscle, causing flexion of the interphalangeal joint.

Q. How would you differentiate between lesion above cubital fossa and wrist?

- Above the elbow—all ulnar innervated muscles affected
- Wrist—Flexor carpi ulnaris spared.

Q. What is ulnar paradox?

Higher the lesion, lesser is the clawing, since in higher lesion flexor digitorum profundus (FDP) is affected. FDP cause more clawing deformity since it opposes lumbricals.

Q. What are the other causes of ulnar clawing?

- Rheumatoid arthritis
- Hansen's disease
- Brachial plexus injury (Klumpke's paralysis)
- AHD (anterior horn cell disease)—PPRP, ALS (amyotrophic lateral sclerosis)
- Severe VIC (Volkman ischemic contracture).

Q. What is Tardy ulnar nerve palsy?

It is ulnar nerve palsy at elbow which occurs late (months to years) after a distal humerus fracture with resultant valgus deformity at elbow.

Q. How will you manage this patient?

Investigation

- X-ray elbow

- EMG-NCS
- FBS, ESR, CRP (to rule out vasculitis)
- Nerve and skin biopsy (thickened nerve and hypopigmented patch) for Hansen's disease.

Pharmacological
- Vitamin B12
- (Dapsone + Rifampicin) if Hansen's
- Management of vasculitis.

Nonpharmacological
- Exercise therapy
  - Maintaining ROM
  - Strengthening of the affected muscles.
- Modality
  - Electrical Stimulations to the affected muscles.
- Occupational therapy
  - Hand function training
  - ADL training.
- Orthosis
  - WHO (Wrist Hand Orthosis)—Interphalangeal joint extension with MCP flexion.
- Surgery.

Q. What are the surgeries?
- Decompression in situ
- Decompression with anterior transposition
- Medial epicondylectomy.

Q. What is ape thumb deformity?
It is the inability to abduct and oppose the thumb due to paralysis of the thenar muscles innervated by median nerve.

Q. What is pointing index?
Also called as the hand of benediction. Occurs as a result of median nerve damage at the elbow and seen when patient is asked to make a fist.
If the patient is asked to make a fist, they will be able to flex the little and ring fingers. The patient will not be able to flex the index and middle fingers. Thus, the patient displays a claw shape, where the little and ring fingers are flexed, the index and middle fingers extended.

Q. What is police man tip position?
Also called Porter's tip position. Caused by lesion at Erb's point. It is characterized by—
Adduction and internal rotation at shoulder, extension and pronation at elbow, and palm facing back and out.

VERTIGO

Summary

A 69-years-old female patient presented with sudden-onset severe vertigo since last fourty eight hours along with neck pain. She is feeling that everything around her is moving whenever she is trying to change her position. There is no history of earache, discharge, deafness, tinnitus, loss of consciousness, any weakness and numbness in the body.

On examination her pulse is 74/min, there is no postural hypotension and her neck range of motion is normal. DIX Hallipikes test is also negative. There is no objective signs of any neuro deficit, carotid bruit or murmur in heart on examination.

P/D: Vertibrobasilar insufficiency group of cervical spondylosis.

Q. What is vertigo?
True vertigo is described as a false sense of unidirectional movement related to one's surrounding. It is more a sense of spinning or rotation.

Q. What is dizziness?
Dizziness is a sense of a disturbed relationship between oneself and one's environment

Q. What are the types of vertigo?
- Vestibular system disorder
  - Peripheral
  - Central.
- Nonvestibular system disorder
  - Cardiovascular
  - Cervical
  - Unknown cause
  - Endocrine dysfunction
  - Drugs.

Q. What are the causes of vertigo?
Causes can aslso be divided into:
1. Postural:
   a. Postural hypotension
   b. Ear causes
   c. Cervical causes
   d. Carotid insufficiency.
2. Nonpostural:
   a. General causes
   b. CNS causes
   c. CVS causes

d. Metabolic causes
e. Idiopathic.

Q. What is the difference between central and peripheral vertigo?
Difference between central and peripheral vertigo has been discussed in Table 3.18.

Table 3.18: Difference between peripheral vertigo and central vertigo

	Peripheral vertigo	*Central vertigo*
Onset	Abrupt	Gradual
Frequency	Intermittent	Constant
Severity	Severe	Mild to moderate
Duration	Short	Long
Effect of change of position	More common	Less common
Nausea and vomiting	More common	Less common
Imbalance	Mild	Severe
Cochlear symptoms	Common	Uncommon

Q. How will you perfom Dix hallpikes test ?
- Patient sits upright, turn head 45 degrees to side being tested
- Patient keep eyes open and focused on examiner's eyes or forehead
- Then, supporting head, pt quickly lies supine (<2 s), allowing head to hyperextend 30 degrees past horizontal
- After 2–20 see latent period, onset of torsional upbeat or horizontal nystagmus denotes positive test
- Symptoms can last for 20–40 seconds
- Nystagmus will change direction when returning to upright.

Q. How will you manage the case?
Counselling and goal setting
Patient education
Investigations:
- Blood: Hb%, FBS, Na. K, LFT
- X-ray of cervical spine
- ENT examination and audiometry
- ECG and echo : If cardiac causes are suspected
- CT scan or MRI: if neuro deficit
- Doppler carotid: if bruit is present
- Special endocrinal investigations if clinical features are suggestive.

Pharmacological:
A. Vestibular Suppressants:
- Meclizine: 25 mg –50 mg BD
- Clonazepam: 0.5 mg OD
- Diazepam: 2–10 mg (1 dose given acutely PO/IM/IV)

B. Antiemetics:
- Prochlorperazine: 5–10 mg IM/PO 6–12 h
- Promethazine: 25 mg PO 6–8 h/ 12.5 mg IM 6–8 h
- Thiethylperazine: 10 mg PO tid/ 2 mL IM tid.

Nonpharmacological
- Head-eye coordination exercise
- Visual-ocular control exercise
- Adaptation/habituation exercise for motion-provoked symptoms
- Sensory substitution-promoting exercise
- Postural strategy practicing exercise
- General conditioning exercise
- Functional activity training

Orthosis: Cervical collar for cervicogenic vertigo.

Q. What are the special exercises for BPPV?
Canalith repositioning/restoration (Epley's) maneuver.
Brandt–Daroff exercise.

Q. What is the pathogenesis for BPPV?
Loose otolith in semicircular canals causing a false sense of motion.

Q. What is postural hypotension?
Orthostatic hypotension is defined as a decrease in systolic blood pressure of 20 mm Hg or a decrease in diastolic blood pressure of 10 mm Hg within minutes of standing when compared with blood pressure from the sitting or supine position.

Q. What is the etiology?
- Dehydration, fever, vomiting, not drinking enough fluids, severe diarrhea and strenuous exercise
- Heart problems—bradycardia, valvular disease and heart failure
- Endocrine problems—Thyroid conditions, Addison's disease, hypoglycemia
- Nervous system disorders—Parkinson's disease, pure autonomic failure, CVA, SCI
- After eating meals.

Q. How will you treat it?
- Stop the culprit drugs
- Oral salt intake
- Fludrocortisone
- Postural care
- Pressure garments.

WRIST DROP

Summary

A 50-year-old male patient is suffering from right-sided wrist drop since yesterday morning after a heavy drink

Q. What are the types of nerve injury?

Types of nerve injuries have been discussed in the Table 3.19.

Table 3.19: Types of nerve injuries

Characteristics	*Neurapraxia*	*Axonotmesis*	*Neurotmesis*
Etiology	Nerve compression injury	Nerve crush injury	Nerve transection injury
Description	Axon is intact Local myelin injury Conduction block	Axonal interruption Schwann cell intact Conduction failure	Axonal and connective tissue disruption Conduction failure
NCS	The signal is normal distal to the lesion and abnormal across it	Resembles neuropraxia for 4–5 days, until Wallerian deg occurs	Resembles axonotmesis, but does not demonstrate recovery

last night. Actually he spent his whole night on a chair and waking up with wrist drop since then.

On examination power of his wrist extensor and finger extensor is 0/5. He is quite depressed and anxious about his recovery because he lives alone in home.

So, this is a case of right-sided saturday night palsy.

Q. What is saturday night palsy?

Also called as Honeymooner's palsy caused by arm being positioned over a sharp ledge, such as a chair back or from a person's head resting on the humerus, leading to compression of radial nerve at spiral groove.

Q. What are the muscles supplied by radial nerve?

- **Arm**

  Innervation above the spiral groove:
  - Triceps brachii
  - Anconeus.

  Innervation below the spiral groove:
  - Brachioradialis (BR)
  - Extensor carpi radialis longus (ECR-L)
- **Elbow**

  Posterior interosseus nerve (PIN)
  - Extensor carpi radialis brevis (ECR-B)
  - Supinator
  - Extensor digitorum communis (EDC)
  - Extensor digiti minimi (EDM)
  - Extensor carpi ulnaris (ECU)
  - Abductor pollicis longus (APL)
  - Extensor pollicis longus (EPL)
  - Extensor pollicis brevis (EPB)
  - Extensor indicis proprius (EIP).

Q. What are the other causes of radial nerve injury?

- Fracture humerus
- Entrapment in healing callus after fracture humerus
- Tight tourniquet
- Entrapment at arcade of frohse (PIN)
- Elbow fracture
- Elbow synovitis
- Compression from soft-tissue mass
- Hansen's neuropathy (rarely).

Q. How will you differentiate radial nerve injury from PIN injury?

In PIN injury:

- Finger drop
- No sensory loss
- Supination and wrist extension preserved.

Q. What is the management?

- Counselling
- Pharmacological—Vit B12
- Exercise—ROM, strengthening exercise
- Modality—Electrical stimulation to affected muscle
- Orthosis—WHO- Cockup splint.

Q. What is the prognosis in this case?

Good since it is neuropraxia

Expected to recover in 3 weeks time.

Q. What is Jone's operation?

Original:

- PT to ECRL and ECRB—Wrist Extension
- FCU to EDC III-V—Finger Extension
- FCR to EIP, EDC II, and EPL—Thumb extension
- Modified:
- PT to ECRL and ECRB—Wrist extension
- FCU to EDC III-V—Finger extension
- FCR to EIP, EDC II, EPL—Thumb extension EPB and APL and abduction
- PT: Pronator teres
- ECRL: Extensor carpi radialis longus
- ECRB: Extensor carpi radialis bravis
- FCU: Flexor carpi ulnaris
- FCR: Flexor carpi radialis
- EPL: Extensor pollicis longus.

4

Chapter

Orthosis, Prosthesis, Mobility Aids and Wheelchair

ORTHOSIS

Q. What is an orthosis?

It is an external device applied to body parts to provide support or stabilization, improve function by restricting or assisting motion, correct flexible deformities, prevent progression of fixed deformities, or reduce pressure and pain by transferring load from one area to another.

SHOES

Q. What are the types of shoes?

1. BOOT: Extends proximal to ankle.
2. CLOG: Thick, wooden soled, backless, slip on.
3. OXFORD: Low cut shoes, fastened with laces.
4. MOCCASIN: Oldest form, made of single leather.
5. MULE: Backless shoe, slipper with low heel.
6. SANDAL: Shoe with upper having straps.
7. PUMP: Thin soled, slip on shoe.

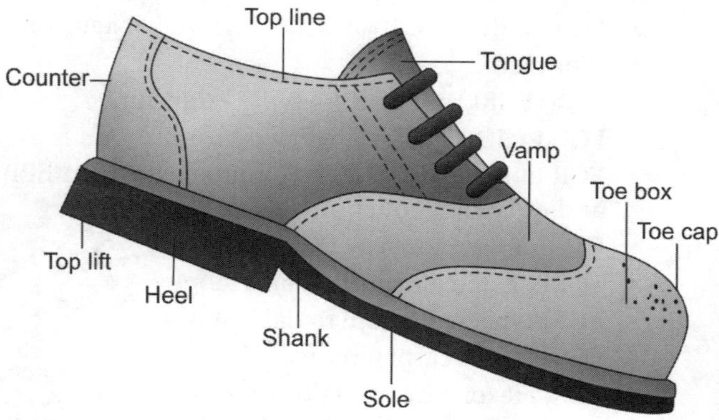

Figure 4.1: Parts of a shoe

Q. What are the functions of shoes?

1. **Protects** feet from trauma and uneven surfaces.
2. **Transfers** body weight to ground while walking hence relieves pain.
3. **Cosmetic** role.
4. **Supportive** to weak and sensitive foot.
5. Useful for **correction** of foot deformity.
6. **Foundation** for any lower limb orthosis.

Q. What is properly fitted shoe?

1. **Adequate** room for the foot to expand upon weight bearing.
2. Usually **1 cm** longer than the longest toe.
3. Widest part of shoe must correspond to foot's widest part.
4. It should be **snugly** fitted from heel to ball.
5. **Adequate** room for the foot to expand upon weight bearing.

Q. What are the parts of shoes (Fig. 4.1)?

Upper: Covers the dorsal part of foot.
Sole: Lies under the planter surface of foot.
Heel: Lies under the anatomic heel.
Tongue: Strip of leather under lace.
Throat: The base of tongue.
Lace stays: Contain eyelets for laces.

Q. What are the types of throat?

The type of throat are given in Table 4.1.

Table 4.1: Types of shoe throat

Blucher (Prussian general)	*Balmoral (English castle)*
Open lacing	Closed lacing
Wide opening for shoe insert	Narrow opening

Q. What are the external heel modifications?

- **Cushioned heel**: Wedge of compressible material inserted into heel to absorb shock at heel strike.
  Advantage:
  Reduces the knee flexion as there is more rapid ankle planter flexion.
  Indication: Patient wears orthosis with rigid ankle has anatomic ankle limitation
- **Heel flare**:
  Medially → Resists hind foot eversion
  Laterally → Resists hind foot inversion
- **External heel wedge**:
  Medially → Rotates hind foot into inversion
  Laterally → Rotates hind foot into eversion
- **Extended heel:**
  Projects anteriorly:
  In medial side: Thomas, orthopedic, S-shaped or keystone heel
  In lateral side: Reverse Thomas, reverse orthopedic heel
  Note: Thomas heel provides additional support to medial longitudinal arch
  Reverse Thomas →Support to lateral longitudinal arch
- **Heel elevation**: (Heel lift or shoe lift)
  Uses:
  - To compensate for fixed Pes Eqinus
  - Help reduce traction
  - Promote heeling of Achillis tendon.

  Note: Used to compensate for a leg length discrepancy of more than one cm (1/2 inch)

Q. What are the external sole modifications?

- **Rocker bar (Fig. 4.2):** Convex rigid strip placed across the sole just posterior to metatarsal heads.

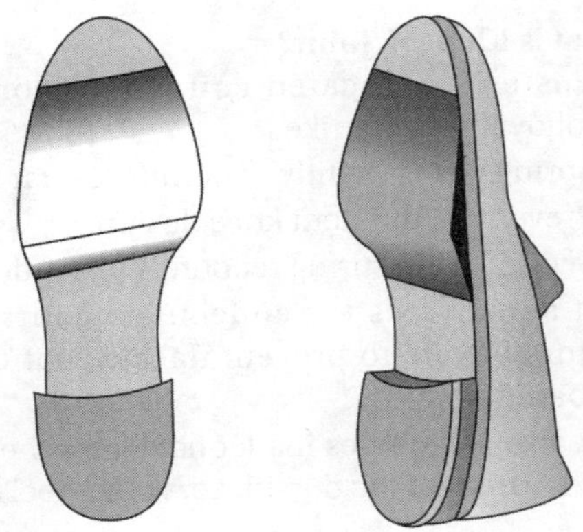

Figure 4.2: Rocker bar

  Use:
  - Shifts roll over point posterior to metatarsal head
  - Decreases pressure from metatarsal head to shaft
  - Decreases demand of planter fascia.
- **Metatarsal bar:** Flat strip of leather placed across the sole just posterior to metatarsal heads
  Advantage: During stance phase, transfers load from metatarsal head to shaft
  Example: Used in **metatarsalgia**

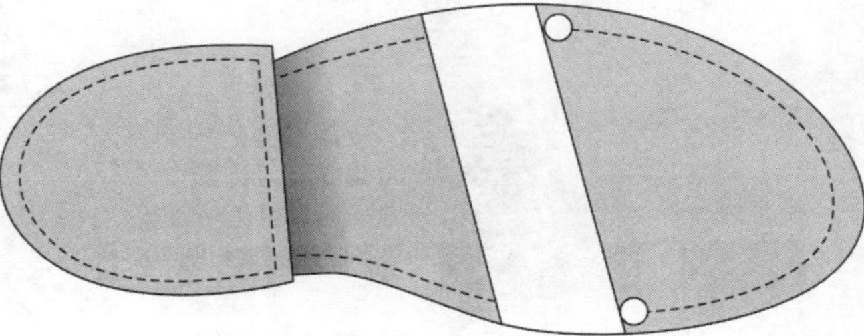

Figure 4.3: Metalarsal bar

- **Sole wedge:**
  Lateral wedge → Pronates forefoot
  Medial wedge → Supinates forefoot
- **Sole flare:**
  Medial flare → Resists eversion
  Lateral flare → Resists inversion
- **Steel bar:**
  - Inserted between inner and outer sole
  - Decrease motion of anterior sole.

  Used in metatarsal fracture

Q. What are the internal heel modifications?

- Heel excavation: Used in planter fasciitis
- Internal heel wedge: Used in inversion and eversion.

Q. What are the internal sole modifications?

- Internal sole excavation
- Metatarsal pad
- Scaphoid pad
- Toe crest.

Q. What is UCBL insert? (University of California Biomechanic Laboratory Inserts)

- Used to realign flexible flat foot, especially in runners
- Made of rigid plastic, custom fabricated over plaster mold of foot in maximum manual correction
- Has rigid medial, lateral and posterior walls
- Provides very effective longitudinal arch support.

LOWER LIMB ORTHOSIS

Conventional Ankle Foot Orthosis

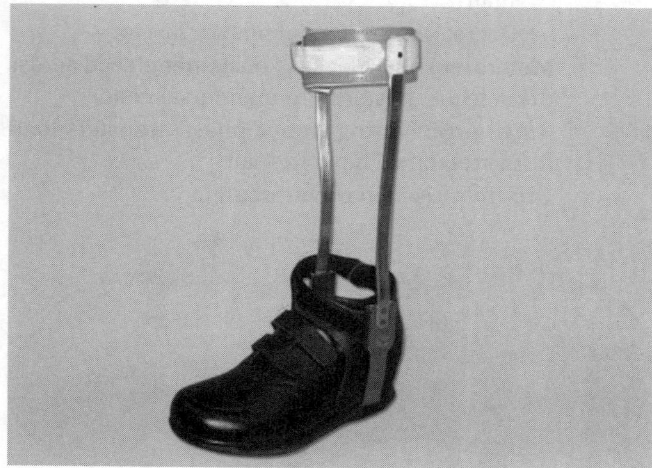

Figure 4.4: Conventional ankle foot orthosis

Q. What is this (Fig. 4.4)?

This is a leather metal ankle foot orthosis (AFO).

Q. What are the parts?

- Two metal uprights, calf band, ankle joint mechanism (anchored to shoe or foot attachment)
- Metal uprights attached to sturdy shoe by steel stirrup (solid or split) or caliper.

Q. What are the salient points?

- Mechanical ankle joints prevent mediolateral instability and either control or assist dorsiflexion or limit plantarflexion
- Ankle joints are:
  1. Free motion
  2. Ankle joint stop
     a. Plantar flexion
     b. Dorsiflexion
     c. Limited motion
  3. Ankle joint assist
     a. Dorsiflexion assist spring joint (klenzak)
     b. Spring wire dorsiflexion assist joint
     c. BICAAL joint
  4. Fixed ankle joint

Q. What are the advantages?

- Minimal contact design for fluctuating edema and for heat sensitive individuals
- For large and heavy wearer
- Satisfied previous wearer
- Prevent skin breakdown and skin irritation.

Q. What are the disadvantages?

- Heavy weight
- Poor cosmesis
- Metallic part gets rusted
- Produce sound when gets old.

Q. What are the indications?

- To improve gait and ensure safe ambulation
- To prevent or correct deformities
- Reduce hypertonicity
- To stabilize and reduce weight bearing in foot and ankle
- To reduce the energy cost of ambulation.

Q. What are the checkout points?

- Shell or calf band is comfortable
- Shell or upright conform to contour of the leg
- Fibular head sustains minimal or no pressure
- Mechanical ankle joint coincide with the anatomical ankle
- Varus or valgus correction strap supports foot
- Patellar tendon bearing brim reduces weight bearing on the heel.

Q. What are the different types and functions of ankle stops?

Ankle joint stops:

- Used in Achilles tendinitis to limit mediolateral foot motion
- Prevent instability caused by painful tendinitis

Plantar flexion stop:

- Used for patients with weak dorsiflexors and flexible pes equinus.

Dorsiflexion stop:

- Used by patients with weak plantar flexors
- Promotes knee extension.

Q. What is Klenzak joint?

- Posteriorly located coil spring compressed following heel strike
- Spring yields slightly to permit plantar flexion
- Prevent inadvertent knee flexion
- Swing phase, spring rebounds to aid dorsiflexion
- It substitutes for concentric contraction of dorsiflexors to prevent flaccid foot drop after toe-off
- It also substitutes inadequately for the eccentric activation of the dorsiflexors after heel strike.

Solid Ankle Foot Orthosis

Q. What is this (Fig. 4.5)?
This is solid ankle ankle foot orthosis (SAFO).

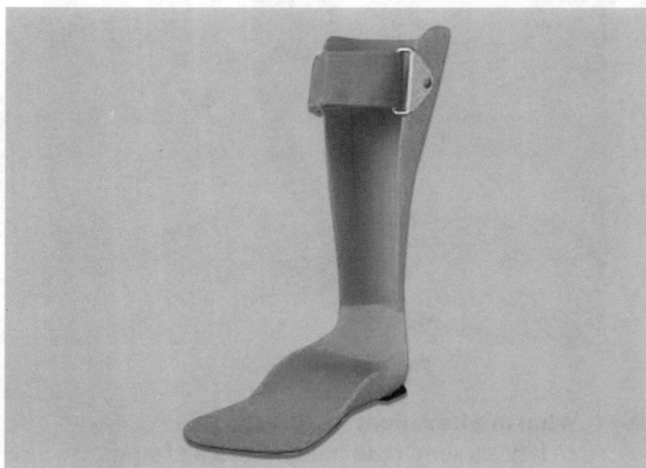

Figure 4.5: Solid ankle ankle foot orthosis (SAFO)

Q. What are the parts?
- Wider calf shell with trimlines anterior to malleoli.

Q. What are the salient points?
- Holds the foot in a fixed position resists all movements
- Provides maximum mediolateral stability
- Anterior band prevents knee buckling.

Q. What are the advantages?
- Good cosmesis
- Light weight.

Q. What are the disadvantages?
- Not for fluctuating edema and for heat sensitive individuals
- Not for large and heavy wearer
- Satisfied previous wearer of metal leather AFO do not like to change
- Skin breakdown and skin irritation.

Q. What are the indications?
- Structural collapse of foot ankle
- Pain with ankle movements
- Severe spasticity with clonus.

Q. What are the checkout points?
See conventional AFO.

Posterior Leaf Spring Orthosis

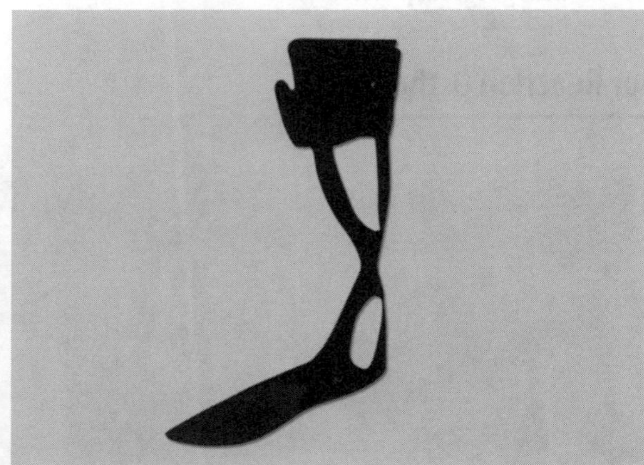

Figure 4.6: Posterior leaf spring (PLS) ankle foot orthosis

Q. What is this (Fig. 4.6)?
This is a posterior leaf spring (PLS) ankle foot orthosis (AFO).

Q. What are the parts?
- Consists of a shoe insert, narrow ankle with trimline behind malleoli and narrow calf shell
- No mechanical ankle joint.

Q. What are the salient points?
- Motion is provided by deformation and recoil of plastic.

Q. What are the advantages?
- Good cosmesis
- Light weight.

Q. What are the disadvantages?
- Does not provide ankle stability.

Q. What are the indications?
- Weakness of ankle dorsiflexors without significant plantar flexors weakness and adequate hip and knee strength.

Q. What are the checkout points?
Same as SAFO.

Q. How does PLS works?
- Early stance—narrow junction between calf shell and shoe insert bends backward slightly
- In swing phase, plastic recoils to lift foot into neutral position

- Resist plantar flexion at heel strike and during swing phase, preventing foot slapping and toe dragging, respectively.

Floor Reaction Orthosis

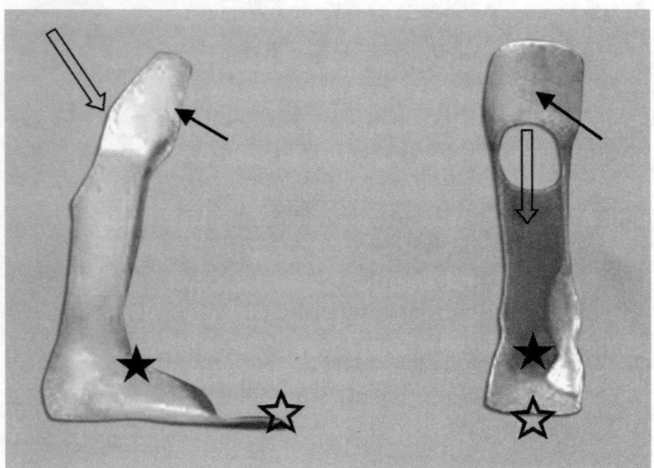

Figure 4.7: Floor reaction orthosis

Q. What is this?
This is a floor reaction orthosis (FRO) (Fig. 4.7).

Q. What are the parts?
- Consists of a shoe insert, narrow ankle with trimline behind malleoli and narrow calf shell
- No mechanical ankle joint.

Q. What are the salient points?
- Motion is provided by deformation and recoil of plastic.

Q. What are the advantages?
- Good cosmesis
- Light weight.

Q. What are the disadvantages?
- Does not provide ankle stability.

Q. What are the indications?
- For patients of quadriceps weakness without genu recurvatum.

Q. What are the contraindications?
- Genu recurvatum
- Knee contracture.

Q. What are the checkout points?
Same as SAFO.

Spiral AFO

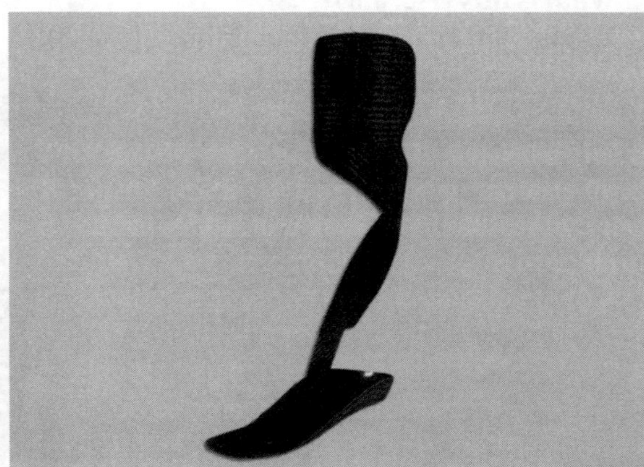

Figure 4.8: Spiral AFO

Q. What are its salient features?
- It has a semi rigid band in place of strap
- During midstance anterior band stabilizes the knee from buckling
- Ankle set at plantiflexion and molded anteriorly to just below the patella.

Q. What are advantages of spiral AFO?
- Lightweight and fastener free which makes it easy to don
- Must fit snugly and cannot be adjusted by the wearer.

Q. What are the indications and contraindications?
- *Indication*: Weak ankle dorsiflexors or plantar flexors with moderate mediolateral instability and weakness of knee extensors
- *Contraindications*: Edema, moderate-to-severe spasticity, severe mediolateral ankle instability.

Other Types of AFO

Q. What is hemispiral AFO?
- Makes only half a turn around the leg.

Q. What are the indications and contraindications of hemispiral AFO?
- *Indication*: Weakness of dorsiflexors and evertors with moderate to severe lateral instability or strong tendency to equinovarus, internal rotation of foot and moderate spasticity
- *Contraindications*: Severe spasticity with sustained clonus, valgus and fixed ankle deformity.

Q. What is hinged AFO?

- To enable ankle motion while maintaining more mediolateral control
- Ankle joints—plastic or metal
- Hinges can be designed to provide unrestricted motion or limited plantar and dorsiflexion with the use of stops.

Q. What is tone reducing orthosis?

- It is an AFO
- Broad foot plate to support foot, extending distally to toes and over foot medially and laterally to maintain neutral foot position
- Indicated for moderate spasticity with varus instability but whose deformities are not fixed.

Q. What is Vannini Rizzoli stabilizing boot?

- AFO with inner rigid calf shell continuous with footplate angled about 15° plantar flexion
- Used in SCI patients to achieve balance and ambulation.

Knee Ankle Foot Orthosis

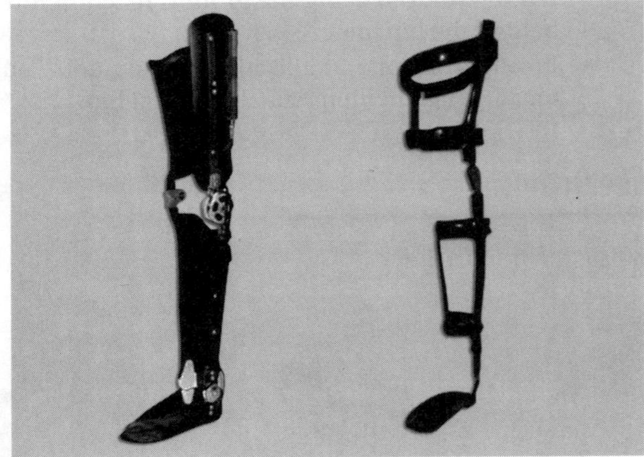

Figure 4.9: Knee ankle foot orthosis

Q. What is this?

- Long leg brace or above knee orthosis
- Also called as knee ankle foot orthosis (KAFO).

Q. What are the parts?

- Proximal thigh band/shell
- Thigh uprights
- Knee joints
- Two metal uprights, calf band, ankle joint mechanism (anchored to shoe or foot attachment)
- Metal uprights attached to sturdy shoe by steel stirrup (solid or split) or caliper.

Q. What are the types of knee joints?

A. Free motion knee joint
   1. Unlimited flexion with a stop to prevent hyperextension.
   2. Indicated in patiens with a tendency for genu recurvatum and mediolateral instability.

B. Offset knee joint
   1. Ground reaction force anterior to the orthotic knee joint.
   2. Allow knee to flex freely during swing phase.
   3. Step length is small.
   4. ***Careful steps while ascending ramps.***
   5. ***Should not be used in patients with knee or hip flexion contracture or with plantar flexion stop at ankle.***

C. Polycentric knee joint
   1. Double axis system to simulate flexion extension movement.
   2. Used in sports knee orthosis.

D. Stance control knee joint.

Q. What are the types of locks?

- Drop lock
  - Gives greatest stability
  - Has to be manually unlocked before sitting
  - Spring loaded retention button allows to unlock and prevents inadvertent locking
  - Some are provided with a spring loaded pull rod at thigh.
- Pawl lock with bail release
  - Consists of a pair of projections (pawl) that fit into recess when knee is extended
  - Unlocking—by moving the bail (semicircular lever attached posteriorly) upwards
  - Provides simultaneous locking and unlocking of both uprights
  - Disadvantage: Bulky bail and accidental release
- Adjustable knee joint locks
  - Provide stability in patients. with knee flexion contractures
  - Used in whom improvement is anticipated with gradual stretching
  - Types:
    - Fan
    - Serrated
    - Rachet
    - Dial lock.

Q. What are the advantages of knee lock?

- To prevent knee flexion during standing and walking
- Provide maximum knee stability.

Q. What are the disadvantages?
- Awkward gait
- Contraindicated in patients with knee flexion contracture.

Q. What are the advantages of conventional KAFO?
- Strong
- Most durable
- Easily adjusted.

Q. What are the disadvantages of conventional KAFO?
- Heavy
- Must be attached to shoe or shoe insert
- Less cosmetic
- Fewer contact points reduce control.

Q. What are the indications?
- When maximum strength and durability are needed
- For individuals with significant obesity
- For individuals with uncontrolled or fluctuating edema (e.g. congestive heart failure, dialysis).

Hybrid Knee Angle Foot Orthosis

Q. What is hybrid knee angle foot orthosis (KAFO)?
It is the combination of the metallic part as well as the plastic part.

Q. What are the advantages?
- The extended thigh shell provides greater support
- Helps control rotation
- Light weight
- Cosmesis.

Q. What are the disadvantages?
- Bulkiness in shape
- Skin breakdown over ischial tuberosity.

Q. What are the indications?
- Stabilize or support knee in quadriceps weakness or paralysis
- Control flexible genu valgum or varum
- Limit weight bearing of thigh, leg and foot.

Q. What are the checkout points?
See below.

Other KAFO

Q. What is supracondylar KAFO?
- Extends from the foot to the lower thigh
- Anterior proximal shell and foot segment—posteriorly directed force
- Calf band—anteriorly directed force
- *No knee joint is needed*
- Resists hyperextension force at the knee without hindering flexion
- In patients with knee extensor weakness the ankle foot component is set at a slight plantar flexion to produce an extensor moment at knee
- Disadvantages: Proximal shell protrudes above thigh—cannot be used bilaterally
- Contraindications—Fluctuating edema.

Q. What is Craig-Scott orthosis?
- *Intended for adults with paraplegia*
- Components:
  1. Bilateral uprights.
  2. Pawl lock with bail release.
  3. Posterior thigh band.
  4. Pretibial band.
  5. Distally plastic solid ankle or BiCAAL joint (with anterior and posterior adjustable pin stops).
  6. Longitudinal and transverse foot plate.
- Ankle joint is set at slight dorsiflexion (10°)
- To attain standing balance, patients hyperextend the hip joint to bring the ground reaction force behind the hip joint
- Provides orthotic stabilization at knee, ankle and foot and ligamentous stabilization at hip.

Knee Orthosis

Swedish Knee Cage

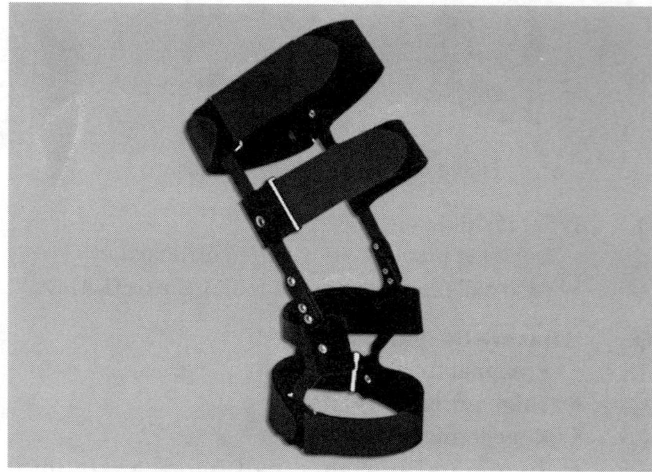

Figure 4.10: Swedish knee cage

Q. What is this?
This is Swedish knee cage.

Q. Why is it used?
- To control genu recurvatum
- Permits full knee flexion and prevents hyperextension
- Classic three-point orthotic system
- Helpful in early walking of hemiplegics.

Q. What is the disadvantage?
- Protrudes while sitting.

Q. What are the types of knee orthosis?
- Functional
- Rehabilitative
- Contracture reducing
- Prophylactic: Prevent injury but role is controversial
- Supportive.

Hip Knee Ankee Foot Orthosis

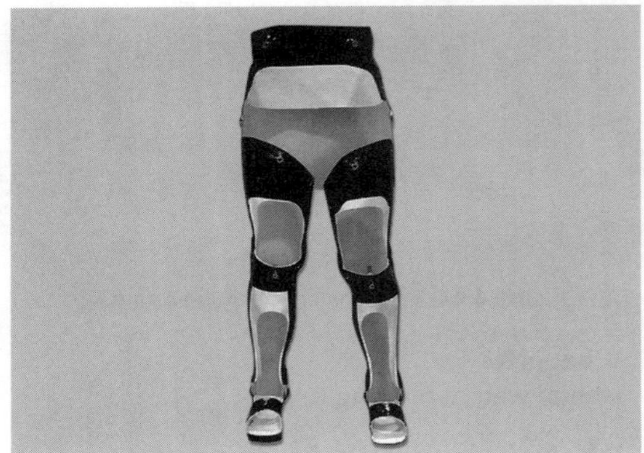

Figure 4.11: Hip knee ankle foot orthosis

Q. What is this?
This is a hip knee ankle foot orthosis (HKAFO).

Q. What are the parts?
- Consists of a pair of KAFOs with a pelvic band and bilateral hip joints.

Q. What are the salient points?
- It controls faulty hip abduction, adduction and rotation in paraplegics
- Hip joints are usually single axis with lock in extension or two position lock (at full hip extension and at 90° of flexion).

Q. What is the advantage?
- Hip joints are anterior and above greater trochanter so the patient can sit upright.

Q. What are the disadvantages?
- Adult patients mostly discard after 1 year of use due to tremendous energy expenditure and difficulty in donning
- When the hip joints are locked gait is restricted to swing to or swing through type.

Q. What are the indications?
- Most commonly prescribed for paraplegia, particularly pediatric patients with spina bifida
- Selectively recommended for adult SCI who tend to have abdominal control.

Q. What are the checkout points?
- Medial upright terminates below the perineum
- Lateral upright terminates below the greater trochanter.
- Knee and hip orthotic joint coincide with anatomical counterpart
- Distal thigh band and calf shell or band are equidistant
- Ischial bearing brim is comfortable
- Trunk components are comfortable.

Trunk Hip Knee AFO

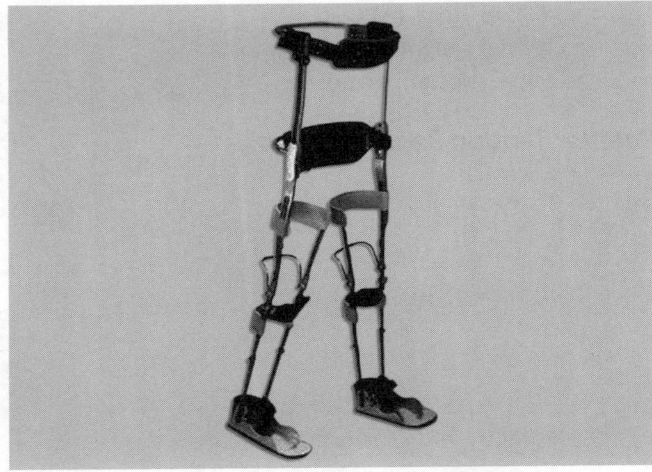

Figure 4.12: Trunk hip knee ankle foot orthosis

Q. What is trunk hip knee AFO?
- Incorporate a spinal orthosis with HKAFO to control trunk motion, maintain or modify spinal alignment and reduce loads on spine
- Heavy, cumbersome and very difficult to don
- Long-term usage minimal.

Reciprocal Gait Orthosis

Q. What is reciprocal gait orthosis (RGO)?

- Type of THKAFO—pair of KAFOs with solid ankle and locking knee joints, anterior leg and thigh straps, pelvic band unit with hip joint, uprights terminate in rigid dorsal band and anterior thoracic strap.

Q. What are the salient features of RGO?

- Hip joints are connected by two metal cables
- Knee joints stabilized by locks or posterior offsets or pretibial bands
- Feet are encased in a solid ankle AFO
- Hip joints are set to flex through a range of 25° or locked at 180°
- For sitting cables can be released for hip flexion
- As the patient extends one hip coupling mechanism induces hip flexion on opposite leg or vice-versa
- Using crutches the patient can perform slow four point gait.

Weight Releiving Orthosis

Q. What are the different weight relieving orthosis?

- PTB orthosis (AFO)
- Ischial weight bearing orthosis
- Patten bottom orthosis.

Patellar Tendon Bearing Orthosis

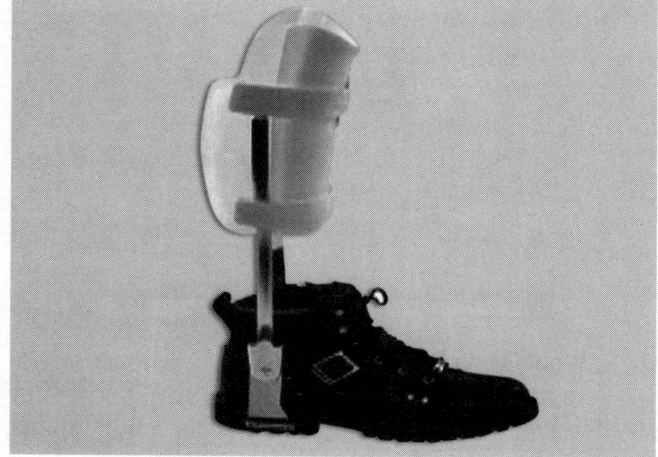

Figure 4.13: Patellar tendon bearing orthosis

Q. What is this?

It is PTB orthosis.

Q. What is PTB orthosis?

- Has plastic circumferential brim which supports substantial load on patellar ligament and tibial flare
- Load transmitted to shoe via metal uprights.

Q. What are the indications of PTB orthosis?

- Fracture fibula
- Foot gangrene.

Q. What are the contraindication of PTB orthosis?

Fracture patella.

Ischial Weight Bearing Orthosis

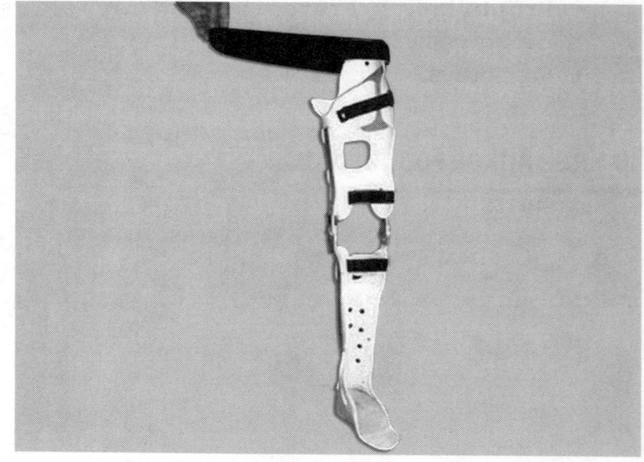

Figure 4.14: Ischial weight bearing orthosis

Q. What is it?

Ischial weight bearing KAFO.

Q. What is ischial weight bearing KAFO?

- Uses quadrilateral brim or ischial (Thomas) ring to transfer force from pelvis onto uprights of brace for partial unloading of leg
- Generally used with paralytic limbs
- Not as effective with larger or obese individuals.

Q. What is patten bottom orthosis?

- Uses uprights that terminate in floor pad distal to shoe
- Used with ischial weight bearing orthosis for complete unloading
- Shoe lift on opposite side.

Q. What is trilateral hip abduction orthosis?

- Less common approach
- KAFO: Triangular thigh cuff, locked knee joint and patten, hoof like platform at distal end, shoe placed laterally
- Used in early stages of TB hip.

SPINAL ORTHOSIS

Hard Cervical Collar

Q. What is this?

This is a hard cervical orthosis (Fig. 4.15).

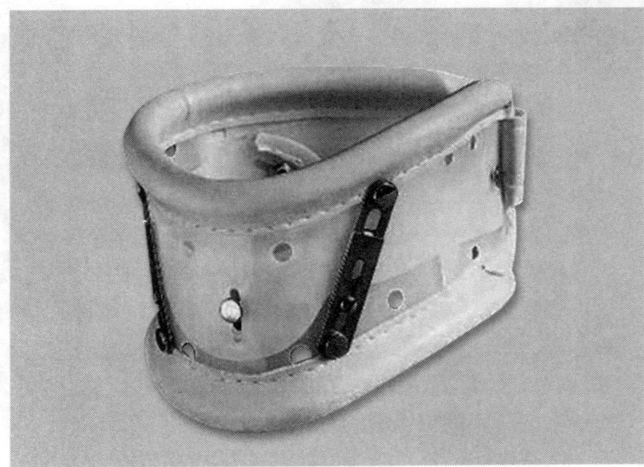

Figure 4.15: Hard cervical collar

Q. What are the different types of cervical orthosis?

- Soft cervical collar
- Hard cervical collar
  - Thomas
  - Philadelphia
  - Miami.

Q. What are the different types of cervicothoracic orthosis ?

- SOMI brace
- 4 Poster brace
- 3 Poster brace
- Yale brace.

Q. How much movement occurs using cervical orthosis?

The amount of movements that occur using cervical orthosis is given in Table 4.1.

Table 4.2: Extent of range of motion with cervical orthosis

	Flexion/ Extension	*Lateral flexion*	*Rotation*
Soft collar	74.2 %	92 %	83 %
Philadelphia	29 %	67 %	44 %
Miami	41 %	----	20 %
Minevera	46 %	----	14 %
SOMI	28 %	66 %	34 %
HALO	4 %	4 %	1 %

HALO Brace

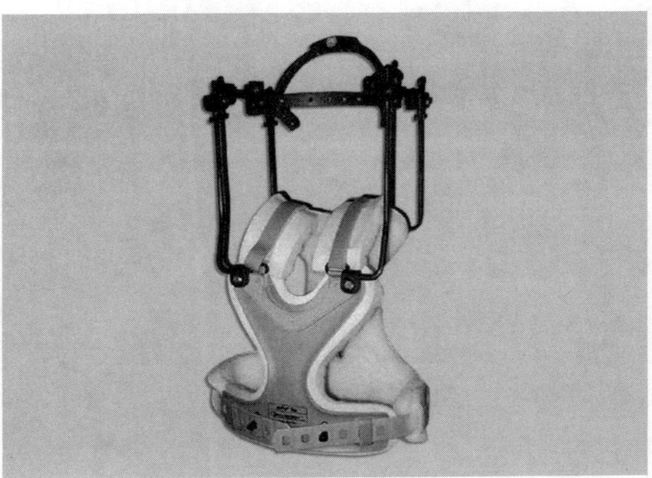

Figure 4.16: HALO brace

Q. What is this?

This is HALO brace.

Q. What is HALO Brace?

- It is a head cervicothoracic orthosis
- This orthosis provides maximum restriction in motion of all the cervical orthoses. It is the most stable orthosis, especially in the superior cervical spine segment
- A halo is used for approximately 3 months (10–12 weeks) to ensure healing of a fracture or of a spinal fusion
- Usually a cervical collar is indicated after the halo is removed, because the muscles and ligaments supporting the head become weak after disuse
- All pins on the halo ring should be checked to ensure tightness 24–48 hours after application.

Q. What are the indications of HALO brace?

- Unstable cervical fractures
- Postoperative management.

Q. What are the contraindications of HALO brace?

- Stable fractures whereless invasive management could be used
- Extremely soft skull might not tolerate the pin placement.

Q. What are the special considerations ?

- Skull density determines halo pin placement and the number of halo pins. While four pins are used on average, more can be necessary in soft skulls (osteoporotic, fractured or in an infant).

SOMI Brace

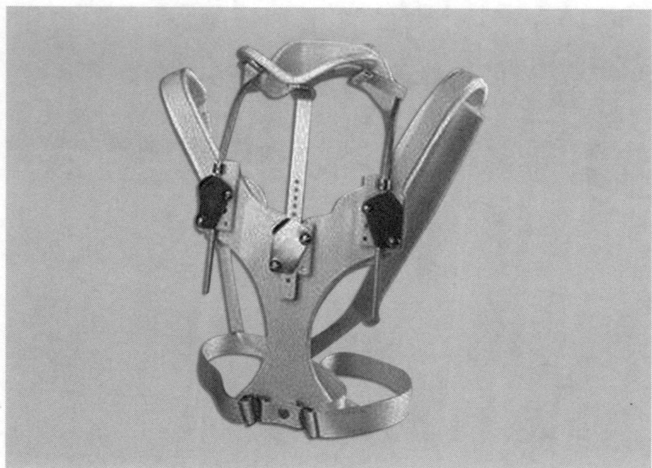

Figure 4.17: SOMI brace

Q. What is this?

This is a SOMI brace.

Q. What is SOMI?

- It is sternooccipitomandibular immobilizer
- Provides control of flexion, extension, and rotation of the cervical spine (F-E-R control)
- Pressure systems are used for control of motion, as well as to provide slight distraction for immobilization of the spine
- Donned while the patient is in the supine position
- Prefabricated, consisting of a cervical portion with removable chin piece and bars that curve over the shoulders
- Also has posts that fix the cervical portion to the sternal portion of the orthosis
- The anterior section supports the mandible and rests on the superior edge of the sternum, with the inferior anterior edge terminating at the level of the xiphoid
- The posterior aspect supports the head at the occipital level.

Q. What are the indications of SOMI?

- Cervical sprains, strains, stable fractures
- Protection and to limit mobility during the healing process in the postoperative patient.

Q. What are the contraindications of SOMI?

- Unstable fractures with ligament instability

Milwaukee Brace

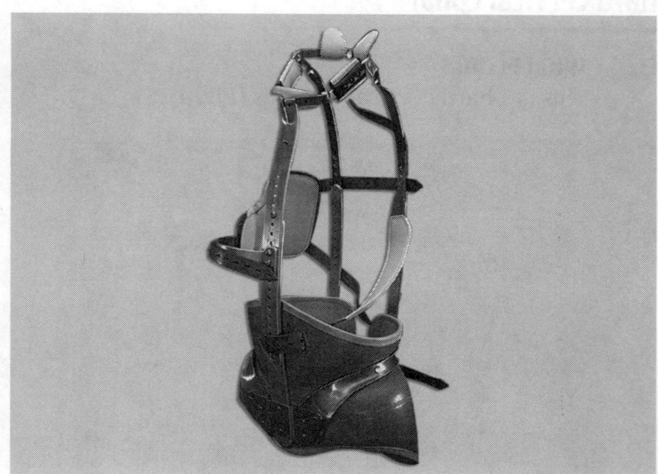

Figure 4.18: Milwaukee brace

Q. What is Milwaukee brace?

- It is a CTLSO
- Consists of a rigid plastic pelvic girdle connected to a neck ring over the upper thorax by 1 anterior, broad aluminum bar and 2 posterior paraspinal bars
- The cervical ring has mandibular and occipital bars, which rest 20–30 mm inferior to occiput and mandible
- Pads strapped to the bars apply a transverse load to the ribs and spine to correct scoliotic curvatures
- A good choice for patients who need correction in the higher thoracic region of the spine.

Q. How did the name Milwaukee come?

It has been first designed at Milwaukee.

Q. What are the indications of Milwaukee brace?

- Idiopathic or flexible congenital scoliosis with curves 25–40° if the curve apex is located superior to T8, the scoliosis shows signs of progression, and puberty has not finished
- Thoracic Scheuermann's disease kyphosis.

Q. What are the contraindications of Milwaukee brace?

- Lower thoracic and lumbar curves.

Q. What are the complications of Milwaukee brace?

- Jaw deformity
- Pain
- Skin breakdown
- Unsightly appearance
- Difficulty with mobility

- Difficulty with transfers
- Increased energy expenditure with ambulation.

Anterior Hyperextension Braces

Q. What are anterior hyperextension braces?
- The flexion control orthosis is also referred to as an anterior hyperextension brace, which functions to extend the thoracolumbar region
- It is prefabricated and lightweight
- Examples of this type of orthosis:
  - Jewett hyperextension orthosis
  - Cruciform anterior spinal hyperextension (CASH) braces.

Both use a three-point pressure system without any abdominal compression.

CASH Brace

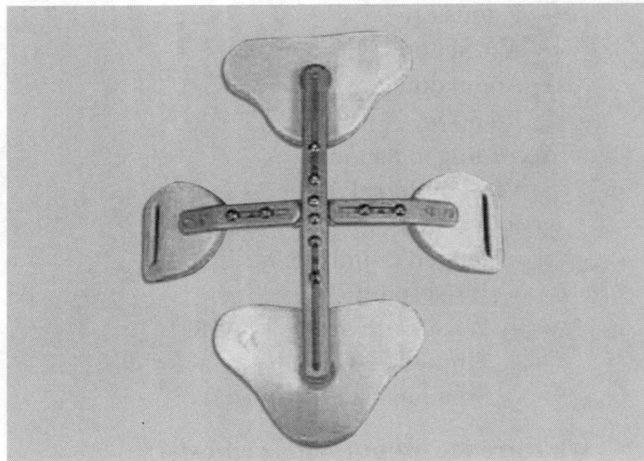

Figure 4.19: CASH brace

Q. What is this?
This is a CASH brace.

Q. What are the salient points of CASH brace?
- It is cruciate anterior hyperextension orthosis
- Biomechanics: Flexion control for the lower thoracic and lumbar regions
- Consists of posteriorly directed forces through a sternal and suprapubic pad, and an anteriorly directed force applied through a thoracolumbar pad attached to a strap that extends to the horizontal anterior bar
- When properly fitted, the sternal pad is one-half inch below the sternal notch, and the suprapubic pad is one-half inch above the symphysis pubis.

Q. What are the indications of CASH brace ?
- Mild compression fracture of the lower thoracic and thoracolumbar regions
- Osteoporotic fractures.

Q. What are the contraindications of CASH brace?
- Unstable fractures or burst fractures
- Spondylolisthesis.

Q. What are the special considerations?
- Excessive pressure on the sternum can result in poor compliance with wearing schedule
- Subclavicular pads may be added to help distribute this pressure.

Taylor and Knight Brace

Q. What is this?
This is a Taylor and Knight brace.

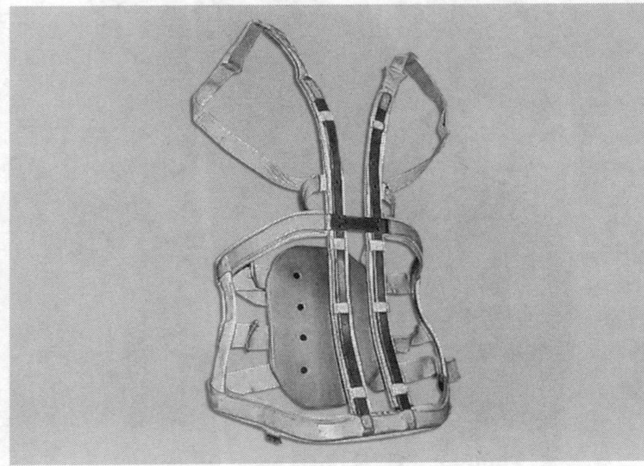

Figure 4.20: Taylor and Knight brace

Q. What are the salient points of Taylor and Knight brace?
- It is a thoraco lumbar sacral orthosis
- Biomechanics: Control of flexion, extension, and a minimal axial rotation via the three-point pressure systems for each direction of motion
- Design and fabrication: Posterior pelvic band extending past the midsagittal plane and across the sacral area. Two paraspinal uprights extend to the spine of the scapula. An apron front extends from the xiphoid to just above the pubic area
- Knight-Taylor has an additional thoracic band that extends from the uprights just below the inferior angle of the scapula to the midsagittal plane and a lateral upright on each side that connects the pelvic band and the thoracic band
- These bands provide additional lateral support and motion control to the trunk.

Q. What are the indications?
- Postsurgical support (for years) of traumatic fractures, spondylolisthesis, scoliosis, spinal stenosis, herniated disks and disk infections
- However, clinicians typically now prefer the custom-molded TLSO body jackets, because better control of position is obtained.

Q. What are the contraindications ?

- Unstable fractures that require maximum stabilization.

Q. What are the special considerations ?

- Pressure per square inch is higher because of the width of the bands and uprights.

LS Chair Back Orthosis

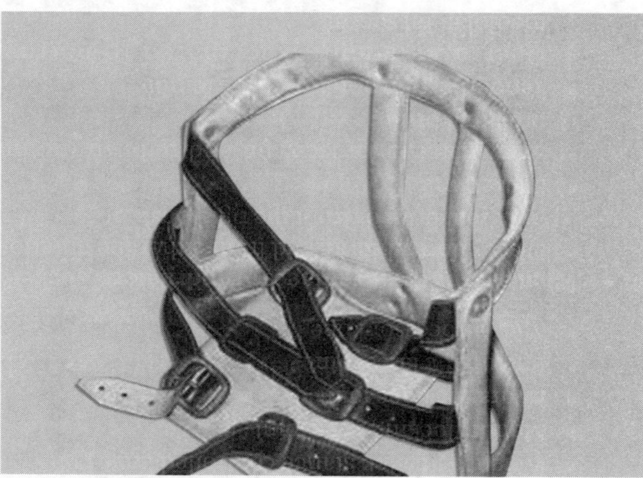

Figure 4.21: LS chair back orthosis

Q. What is this?

This is a lumbosacral chair back orthosis.

Q. What is LS chair back orthosis?

- It is a lumbosacral orthosis
- Biomechanics: It can limit flexion and extension. It also provides elevation of intraabdominal pressure
- Design and fabrication: This orthosis has a pelvic band that lies posteriorly and extends laterally to just anterior to the midsagittal line. Laterally, the ends fall midway between the iliac crest and the greater trochanter
- The superior edge of the thoracic band is at the level of T9–T10 or just distal to the inferior angle of the scapulae. The pelvic and thoracic bands are connected by two paraspinal uprights posteriorly
- Orthoses can be fabricated from a traditional aluminum frame covered in leather, or thermoplastic material molded into the same shape.

Q. What are the indications?

Degenerative disk disease, herniated disk, spondylolisthesis, and mechanical low back pain, postsurgical supports for lumbar laminectomies, fusions, diskectomies.

Q. What are the contraindications?

Unstable fractures, or conditions in the upper lumbar or thoracic area.

Q. What are the special considerations?

Adequate clearance of the paraspinal uprights is required to allow for some reduction of lumbar lordosis when the anterior apron is tightened and while sitting. Clearance on the lateral uprights over the iliac crests is also an area to be monitored.

UPPER LIMB ORTHOSIS

Q. How do you classify upper limb orthosis?

1. According to type:
   - Static
   - Dynamic.
2. According to function:
   - Flexion
   - Extension
   - Abduction
   - Adduction
   - Rotation.
3. According to region:
   - Volar or dorsal
   - Joints crossed
     - Finger/thumb splint
     - Wrist splint
     - Wrist hand orthosis (WHO)
     - Elbow (WHO)
     - Shoulder (Elbow- WHO).

Q. What are the uses of static orthosis?

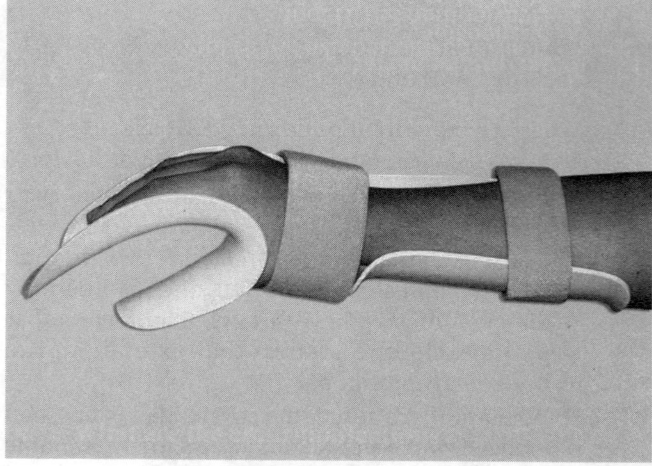

Figure 4.22: Static wrist hand orthosis

- Immobilize or support
- Help prevent deformity

- Prevent soft-tissue contracture
- Allow attachmentof assistive devices

Q. What are the uses of dynamic orthosis?

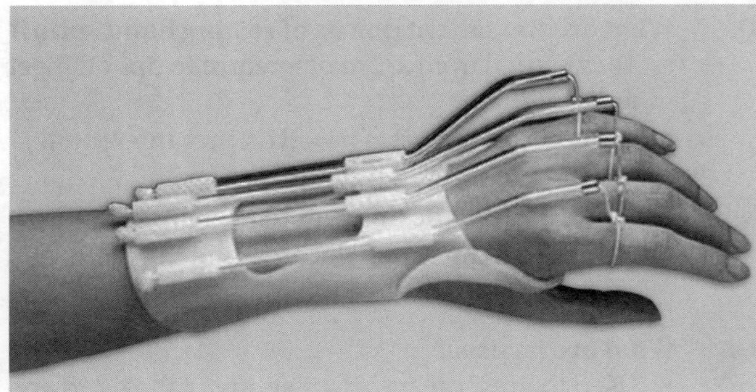

Figure 4.23: Dynamic wrist hand orthosis

- To substitute for loss of motor function
- To correct an existing deformity
- Aid in fracture alignment and wound healing.

Q. What are the different types of wrist hand and finger orthosis?

1. Assistive and substitutive:
   a. Positional
   b. Prehension
2. Protective:
   a. Digital stabilizers
   b. WHF stabilizers
   c. Tone reducing
3. Mobilization:
   a. Finger
   b. Thumb
   c. Wrist

Opponens Splint

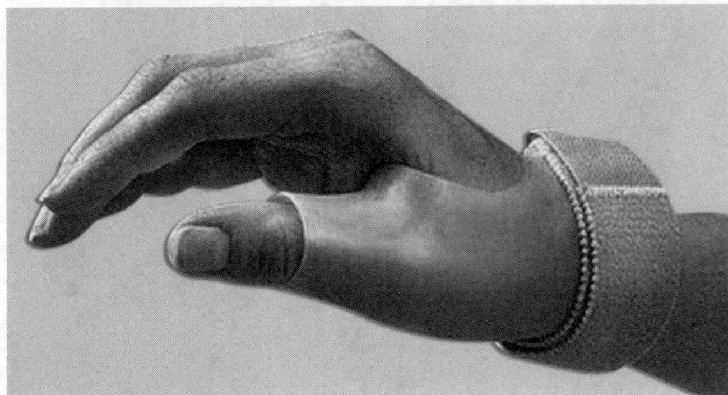

Figure 4.24: Short opponens splint

Q. What is this?

This is a short opponens splint.

Q. What is basic opponens splint?

- Also known as C-bar splints, short opponens splint
- Consist of a dorsal and palmar bar that encircle the mid palm with a thumb abduction bar and a thumb opponens bar on the 1st metacarpal.

Q. What is long opponens splint?

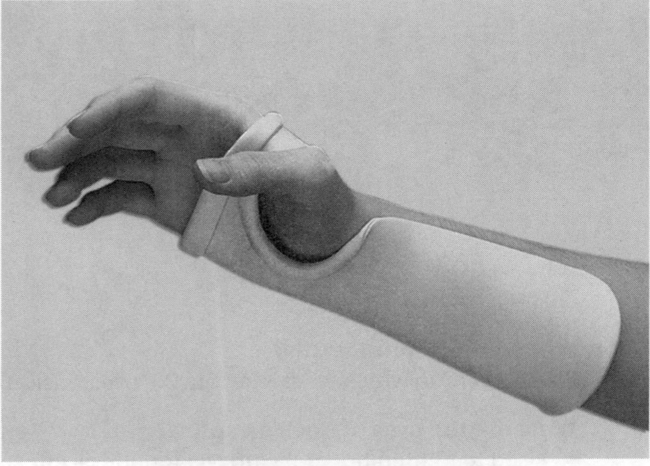

Figure 4.25: Long opponens splint

- Also known as thumb spica splint
- Additional forearm bar with proximal and distal crossbars for wrist control.

Q. What are the advantages of long opponens splint?

- Maintains wrist in extension
- Crossbars prevent ulnar or radial deviation in cases of RA.

Q. What are the indications of opponens splint?

1. Used to position the weak thumb in opposition to other fingers for three jaw chuck
   - SCI, stroke, TBI.
2. Immobilize thumb for tissue healing
   - Arthritis, fracture, dislocation, DQT, post surgical thumb.

Q. What is opponens orthosis with lumbrical bar?

- Hand based intrinsic plus splint, anti claw splint
- They prevent clawing by allowing MCP flexion, and preventing MCP hyperextension
- They also allow full extension at PIP and DIP
- Used in ulnar or combined median ulnar neuropathy, stroke, TBI.

Cock-up Splint

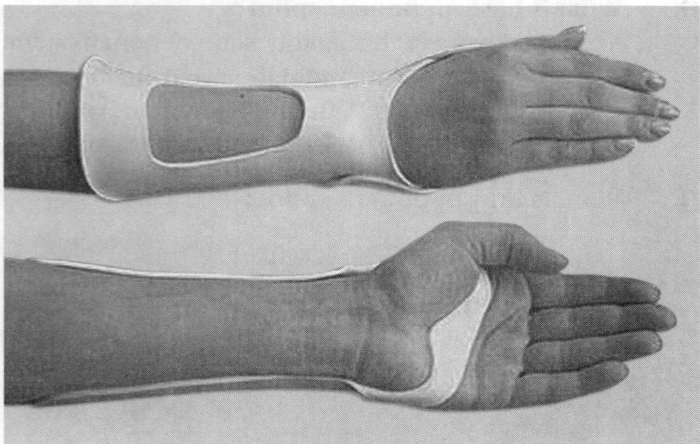

Figure 4.26: Cock-up splint

Q. What is this?
This is a cock-up splint.

Q. What type of splint is this?
Plastic WHO in which wrist is kept in 20° of extension.

Q. What are the uses of Cock up splint?
- Used to tighten finger flexors via tenodesis effect
- Prevent wrist flexion contracture in patients with radial neuropathy.

Q. What is dorsal cock-up splint?
- Stronger mechanical support of wrist and freeing up some of the palmar surface for sensory input.

Q. What are the advantages of it?
- Distributes pressure over the larger dorsal wrist surface area
- Better tolerated by edematous hand.

Wrist Hand Finger Stabilizer

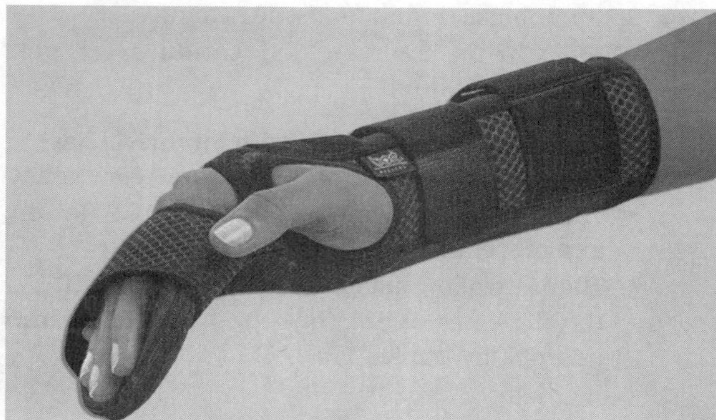

Figure 4.27: Wrist hand finger stabilizer

Q. What is it?
- It is wrist hand finger stabilizer
- Also known as resting hand splint, functional resting splints.

Q. What are the salient points of resting hand splint?
- They extend from 2/3rd of forearm to tips of finger and thumb
- Volar based or dorsal based or circumferential
- Wrist is held in slight extension
- MCP in 70–90° flexion and IP in slight flexion
- Designed to maintain the arches of the hand, and maintain the wrist in a functional position.

Q. What are its uses?
- Used to preserve the architecture of the hand and wrist on a patient with paralyzed musculature, reduce hypertonicity by abducting the fingers, to alleviate wrist or hand pain by immobilizing these tissues.

Miscellaneous

Q. What are epicondylar straps?
- Also known as forearm bands, proximal forearm arthosis
- Circumferentially applied to forearm distal to epicondyles without hindering elbow motion
- To reduce pain during activity in medial or lateral epicondylitis.

Balanced Forearm Orthosis

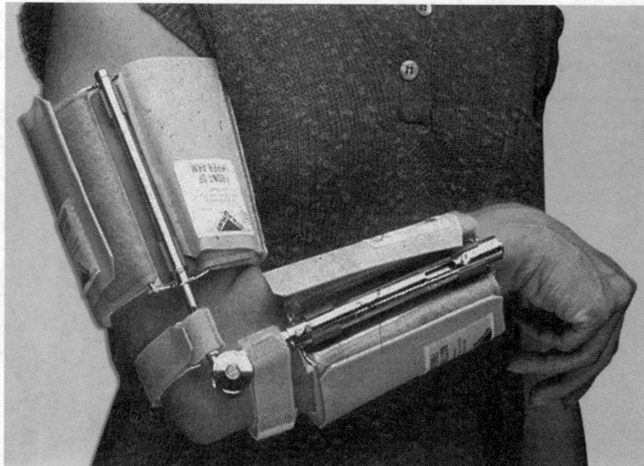

Figure 4.28: Balanced forearm orthosis

Q. What is this?
This is a balanced forearm orthosis (BFO).

Q. What are the salient points of BFO?
- It is a SEWHO (Shoulder elbow wrist hand orthosis)
- Also known as mobile arm support
- Consists of forearm trough attached by a hinge joint and consists of a mount which can be a WC, table, or onto a body jacket.

Q. What are the advantages of it?
Support the forearm against gravity and allow patients to move arm horizontally and flex the elbow to bring hand to mouth.

Q. Mention the uses of balanced forearm orthosis?
Used in patients of SCI, Polio, muscular dystrophy, brachial plexus injury.

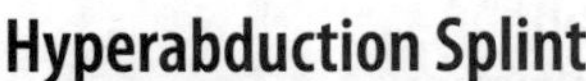

Hyperabduction Splint

Q. What is this?
This is a hyperabduction splint.

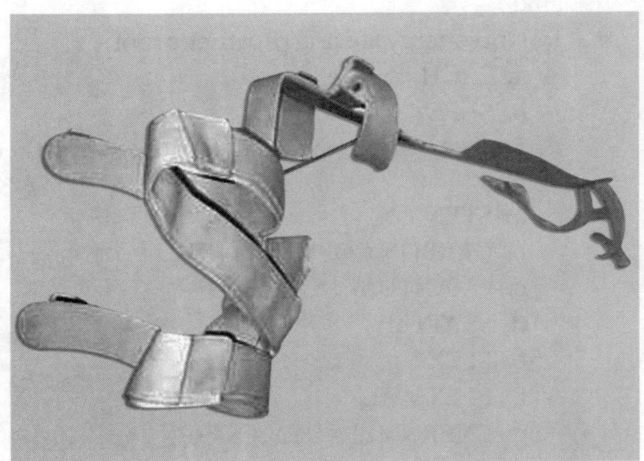

Figure 4.29: Hyperabduction splint

Q. What are its uses?
- Also called shoulder abduction stabilizer
- It supports the arm and shoulder
- Protect the shoulder from adduction contracture
- Example: Postrotator cuff surgery, brachial plexus injury, axillary contracture, etc.

PROSTHESIS

Lower Limb Prosthesis

Syme's Prosthesis

Q. What is this?
This is a Syme's prosthesis.

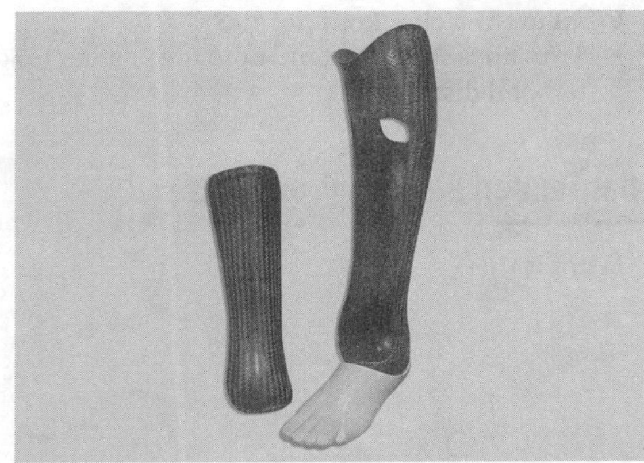

Figure 4.30: Syme's prosthesis

Q. What are the different types of Syme's prosthesis and their parts?
- Canadian Syme prosthesis: Plastic laminated socket attached to a modified SACH foot with a removable posterior wall
- Veterans administrative prosthetics center (VAPC) Syme prosthesis: Plastic laminated socket with a window on the medial aspect
- Flexible posterior build up Syme prosthesis: Non-fenestrated plastic laminated socket with a soft insert/expandable wall to allow passage of the malleoli.

Q. What are the characteristic points of an ideal Syme's prosthesis?
- Transmission of body loads
- Light enough to wear comfortably
- Lengthening of the limb to adjust for loss of the talus and oscalcis
- Distribution of the high forces developed in the ankle area
- Provision of shock absorption
- Cosmesis.

Q. What are the advantages?
- Medial opening type is more stronger design because of material in sagittal plane
- Stove pipe is the strongest.

Q. What are the disadvantages?
- Due to limited space available foot selection is limited to SACH foot and low-profile dynamic response foot
- They are directly bolted to the bottom of the socket.

Q. What are the indications?
Syme's amputation.

Q. What are the checkout points?
- Trim lines should extend upto the patellar tendon for load distribution.

Patellar Tendon Bearing Prosthesis

Q. What is this?

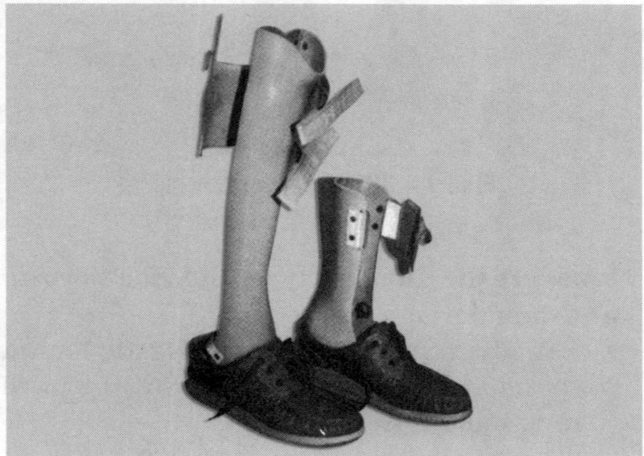

Figure 4.31: Patellar tendon bearing prosthesis

This is a patellar tendon bearing prosthesis with supracondylar cuff

Q. What are the parts?
- Supracondylar cuff
- PTB socket
- Exoskeletal shank
- Foot ankle assembly.

Q. What are the other suspension types?
- Fork strap with waist belt
- Joint and thigh corset
- Supracondylar cuff
- Sleeve
- Supracondylar brim
- Supracondylar suprapatellar brim
- Gel or elastomeric.

Q. What is PTB socket?
- Most commonly used
- Custom molded plastic socket
- Although the socket has total contact with the residual limb it concentrates force in pressure tolerant areas and relieves force in pressure sensitive areas
- The socket is aligned in slight flexion (5°) to:
  - Enhance loading on the patellar ligament
  - Prevent genu recurvatum
  - Resist the tendency of the residual limb to slide down
  - Facilitate contraction of quadriceps.
- Slight lateral tilt to reduce pressure on fibular head
- Total contact fit helps prevent edema, provides additional support, and probably provides greater sensory feedback.

Q. What are the pressure tolerant and pressure sensitive areas?
- **Pressure tolerant:** Patellar tendon, the pretibial and gastrocnemius musculature, the medial tibial flare and the fibular shaft.
- **Pressure sensitive:** The patella, hamstring tendons, fibular head, femoral epicondyles, tibial shaft, distal tibia and distal fibula.

Q. What are the other types of socket?
1. Plug fit.
2. Patellar tendon bearing (PTB).
3. Total surface bering (TSB).
4. Vaccum assisted socket system.

Q. What are the different types of foot ankle assembly?

a. **Non articulated:** No separation between foot and ankle
   - i. Non energy storing prosthetic foot:
     - a. SACH
     - b. SAFE
   - ii. Energy storing (dynamic response) prosthetic foot:
     - a. STEN
     - b. CARBON COPY II
     - c. QUANTUM
     - d. SEATTLE
     - e. FLEX
     - f. FLEX WALK
     - g. ENERGIZER (DYNA STEP)

b. **Articulated**
   - i. Single axis prosthetic foot
   - ii. Multiple axis prosthetic foot

Q. What is SACH foot?
- Introduced in 1956 by Foort and Radcliffe
- Most basic and widely used
- Rigid longitudinal keel surrounded by rubber
- No definitive ankle joint
- Posteroinferior compressible rubber heel wedge which simulates plantar flexion during early stance phase with heel wedge compressing upto ¾ to 1 inch.

Q. What is STEN Foot?
- Rigid polyurethane bolt block is attached to the shank
- Anterior part of the block terminates at a 45° making the keel more flexible
- Permits more inversion and eversion and adapts more readily to irregular surface

- Heel is cushioned like SACH foot
- Heavier than SACH foot.

Q. What is Jaipur foot?
- Developed by SMS medical college, Jaipur by Professor P K Sethi
- Provides barefoot ambulation.

Q. What is the difference between Jaipur foot and SACH foot?

The difference between Jaipur foot and SACH foot are given below in Table 4.3:

Table 4.3: Comparison between jaipur foot and SACH foot

	SACH	*Jaipur*
Flexibility	Less	More
Additional shoe	Essential	Not required
Wooden keel	Yes	No
Technology	Requires modern technology	Can be made by local products
Usable in muddy, uneven ground	Cannot be used	Can be used
Squatting/sitting cross legged	Not possible	Possible
Shape	Like a shoe	Like a foot

Above Knee Prosthesis (Transfemoral)

Q. What is this?

This is a transfemoral prosthesis.

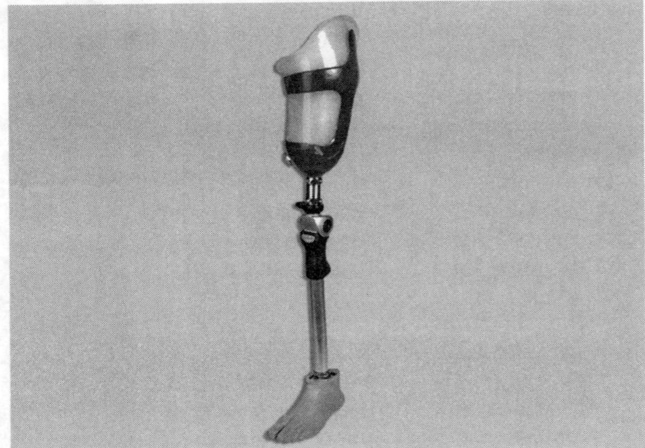

Figure 4.32: Above knee prosthesis (transfemoral)

Q. What are the parts?
- Suspension
- Socket
- Knee joint
- Shank
- Foot ankle assembly.

Q. What are the different types of suspension?
- Total elastic suspension
- Silesian belt
- Hip joint with pelvic band
- Suction suspension.

Q. What are the different types of socket?
- Quadrilateral design (ischial gluteal bearing)
- Ischial containment design.

Q. What are the different types of knee joint?
- Single axis knee joint
- Polycentric knee joint
- Weight activated stance controlled knee joint
- Manual locking knee joint
- Hydraulic knee joint
- Pneumatic knee joint
- Microprocessor knee.

Q. What are the disadvantages of qudrilateral socket?
- Discomfort while seated from either the anterior proximal brim or from the rigid posterior
- Socket wall
- Skin irritation at ischium and pubis from the proximal brim
- Tenderness on anterior distal femur
- Decreased stability compared to narrow mediolateral socket
- More lateral lurch when walking
- Poor cosmesis with gapping of lateral socket wall during stance
- Poor control of the residual femur allowing lateral shift of the socket.

Q. What are the advantages of ischial containment socket over quadrilateral socket?
- It stabilizes the relationship between the pelvis and proximal femur
- Narrow mediolateral design is intended to keep the femur in adduction
- Keeps the femur in adduction during the stance phase permits the hip abductors to be in a more stretched and efficient position
- More energy efficient ambulation at high speed
- More comfort in groin area compared to quad
- There is less lateral thrust of prosthesis at midstance
- Higher trimline results in better control of the short residual
- Able to accommodate smaller residual limb.
- There is greater medial-lateral control of the pelvis with this design.

Q. What are the disadvantages of ischial containment socket over quadrilateral socket?
- Difficult to fabricate
- More expensive
- More anterioposterior motion.

Q. What are the advantages and disadvantages of different types of knee joints?

Table 4.4: Advantages and disadvantages of different types of knee joints

	Advantages	*Disadvantages*
Constant friction knee (single axis with constant friction unit)		
• Friction mechanisms are devices used in swing control knee to dampen the pendular action of the prosthetic knee during swing phase, to decrease the incidence of high heel rise in early swing, and decrease terminal impact inlate swing • Single walking speed • May be used in kids • No stance control; a screw used to adjust the friction to determine how fast or slow the knee swings • K1 ambulator	• Inexpensive • Reliable	• Low stability (in early stance the single axis has the lowest zone of stability) • Fixed cadence • Too much friction prevents knee from flexing • Too little friction causes the knee to swing too easily; patient needs to vault
Stance control knee/safety knee/weight activated friction brake		
• Single axis knee with stance control • Stance control acts as a brake system • Indications: 1. Geriatrics 2. Short residual limb 3. General disability 4. Uneven surfaces 5. Amputees with weak hip extensors • K1 ambulator	• Improved knee stability	• Slightly increased weight • Increased cost • Increased maintenance • Must unload fully to flex Cannot use in bilateral AKA (knees will not bend with loading) → cannot bend both knees at the same time (patient cannot sit down) • Activities that require knee motion under weight-bearing, such as step-over-step stair descent, are incompatible with this knee
Polycentric knee joint		
• No stance control, but inherently stable • Short knee unit → can be used in knee disarticulation and long residual limb • K1 ambulator	• Excellent knee stability • Improved cosmesis in knee disarticulation and long residual limb patients	• Greater weight, cost, maintenance • Although durable, needs maintenance every 3–6 months
Manual locking knee		
• Knee of last resort used in: 1. Blind 2. Stroke patient with amputation • Commonly uses a spring-loaded pin that automatically locks the knee when the amputee stands or extends the knee • Knee is kept extended throughout the entire gait cycle to ↑ stability • K1 ambulator	Ultimate knee stability	• Abnormal gait • Awkward sitting • Cannot use in bilateral AKA because like the stance control knee, patients cannot sit. Knees lock on loading, therefore, cannot bend both knees at the same time to sit down
Constant friction knee (single axis with constant friction unit)		
1. Hydraulic 2. Pneumatic (air) • Cadence-responsive knee units through cadence dependent resistance • Allows for either swing phase, or swing and stance phase control • Indications: 1. For patients who vary cadence frequency 2. Active walkers 3. Ambulation in uneven terrain • K3 and K4 ambulators	• Variable cadence • Smoothest gait • Stable; will not lock unless at full extension • Pneumatic units are lighter but hydraulic units tolerate more weight (can support the heavier and more athletic amputee) • Can unlock for some activities (e.g. biking)	• Greatest weight • Increased cost • Increased maintenance

Q. What is the energy cost and speed of different amputations?

Table 4.5: Energy cost and speed of different amputations

Walking parameters	*Unilateral trans tibial*	*Bilateral trans tibial*	*Unilateral trans femoral*	*Bilateral trans femoral*	*Trans tibial and trans femoral*
% increase in energy expenditure/unit distance	23	41	99	186	118
% decrease in comfortable walking speed	20	20	51	60	56

UPPER LIMB PROSTHESIS

Below Elbow Prosthesis

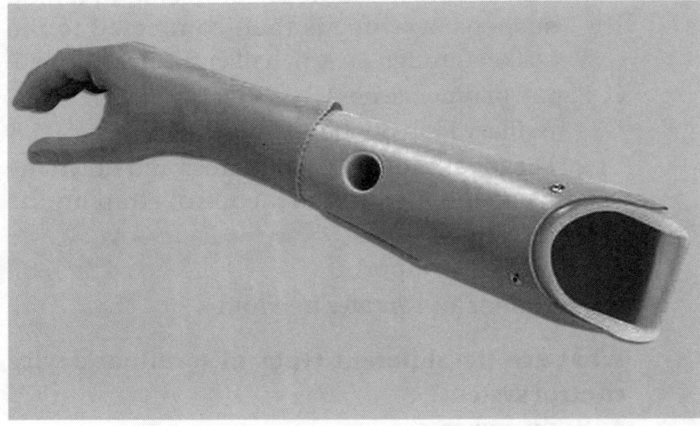

Figure 4.33: Below elbow prosthesis

Q. What is this?
This is a below elbow prosthesis.

Q. What are the parts?
1. A terminal device (TD).
2. A wrist unit.
3. Socket.
4. Elbow hinge.
5. Suspension and control system.

Q. What are the different terminal devices?
Passive
- No significant functional mechanism (though used for crawling, ball handling prosthesis for child)
- Do not provide grasp
- Should be relatively light weighted.
- Intended for cosmetic effect only.

Active
- Hooks, including prehensors—
- Artificial hands
  - Used to replace the grasp function of the hand
  - Unable to manipulate objects due to absence of sensory feedback.
  - Voluntary opening and voluntary closing types.

Q. What are the advantages of hooks?
- Basic grasp function
- Efficiency of use
- Ability to grasp small objects
- Durability
- Lower maintenance and repair costs
- Lighter weight
- Better ability of user to see what is being held.

Q. What are the advantages and disadvantages of prehensors?
Typical advantages: Do not look as threatening!!!
- Not as likely to scratch objects
- Not as likely to accidentally get caught on things.

Typical disadvantages: Not as good for picking up and working with small items
- Does not offer as much visual feedback because they are usually bulkier at the end
- Not as good for typing.

Q. What is voluntary opening hook?
- Curved and split hook in which sturdy rubber bands maintain the closed position
- Pinch force is determined by the number and type of rubber bands
- The amputee uses cable control powered by proximal muscles to open the hook fingers
- The rubber bands then act as a spring to close the hook
- In myoelectrically controlled hook, the electric motor turns in the opposite direction to close the hook
- External control generate increased force.

Q. What is voluntary closing hook?
- Maintained in an open position and has to be closed voluntarily by cable control or myoelectric control
- Better control of closing pressure
- Seldom used, because it is heavier and less durable than voluntary opening hooks.

Q. What are the advantages of hands?
- Provide palmar prehension by allowing the amputee to move the thumb, index and middle fingers through body power or myoelectric control
- More cosmetic, can be used for grasping a large or round object
- Less functional
- Bulkier and heavier.

Q. What is wrist unit?
- Metal devices used for attaching TDs to the anatomic wrist area at the distal end of the socket
- They position the TD into the best position for accomplishing a desired activity and also permit interchange of TD from hook to hand and vice versa
- The wrist unit provides orientation of the terminal device in space
- It can be positioned manually, by cable operation, or with external power.

Q. What are the types of wrist unit?

a. Wrist friction unit.
b. Quick disconnect/locking wrist unit.
c. Wrist flexion unit.
d. Wrist rotation unit.
e. Four function wrist unit.

Q. What is elbow hinge and its types?
- Connect the socket to a cuff or a pad on the upper arm and are important for suspension and stability.
- Three types:
  a. Flexible.
  b. Rigid.
  c. Residual limb activated locking types.

Q. What are the different types of socket design?

Self suspended socket design:

Less cumbersome and more popular than the harness suspended socket design. Here, harness is seldom used for suspension, it may still be used for control of TD.

Types:
- Suprastyloid suspension
- Sleeve suspension
- Supracondylar brim suspension
- Liner with locking pin suspension.

Harness suspended socket design:
- It uses a harnessing system to suspend the socket from the involved and uninvolved shoulder
- The harness is connected to an upper arm half cuff or triceps pad, which is then connected to the elbow hinge and socket.

Split socket:
- Total contact segment encasing the residual limb and connected by a hinge to a separate forearm shell to which the wrist unit and TD are attached
- It is used for very short residual limbs so that special elbow hinges (step-up or locking type) can be used.

Q. What are the different types of harness suspension?

These are used to suspend the prosthesis from the shoulder so that the socket is held firmly onto the residual limb and to transmit the force from shoulder and scapular motion via the cable system to operate the TD.

A. Figure of eight harness:
  - Is the most commonly used
  - It has an axilla loop worn on the sound side, which acts as a reaction point for transmission of body force to the TD
  - Anterior strap for support
  - Posterior strap for control.

B. Cross chest strap harness with shoulder saddle:
  - Consists of a shoulder saddle on the side of the amputed limb, which is connected to a chest strap looped around the opposite axilla
  - The shoulder saddle is connected to a loop suspensor, which is then connected to the socket through an arm half cuff or triceps pad.

C. Figure of nine harness:
  - Axillary loop on the sound side
  - Diagonal strap that runs across and down the back and attaches to a control strap on the prosthetic limb
  - No front support
  - Lighter and greater freedom.

Q. What are the different types of terminal device control system?

A. **Body powered**:
  - Use forces from the shoulder and scapula transmitted via harness and cable to operate the TD
  - The cable system used is the single control cable system.

B. **Electrically powered:**

  Controlled by switches or myoelectric signals and are powered with energy supplied from external batteries.
  - Myoelectric
  - Switch controlled.

Q. How does myoelectric controlled terminal device works?
- Uses surface electrodes placed on the muscles on the residual limb

- Myoelectric signals from the muscles are picked up by the surface electrodes
- Signals are amplified into volts to activate switch (myoswitch)
- Causes electricity to flow from a battery to an electric motor, thus activating the TD
- TD function can be controlled either in a constant manner or in proportion to the amplitude of the myoelectric signals.

Types of controller:

- Two site, two function myoelectric controller
- One site, two function myoelectric controller
- One site, one function myoelectric controller.

Q. What is switch controlled terminal device?

Uses either a push button electromechanical switch, which can be activated by a bony prominence, or a pull-switch which is incorporated in harness or cable.

Q. What is the advantage of body powered prosthesis?

- Lower initial cost
- Lighter
- Easier to repair
- Offer better tension feedback to the body.

Q. What are the advantages of myoelectric prosthesis?

- Do not require a harness or cable
- Looks like natural-appearing arm
- Battery powered, so motor strength and coordinated mobility not as important
- Newer batteries have reduced weight
- Provides strong grip force.

Q. What is the disadvantage of body powered prosthesis?

- Mechanical appearance
- Some people have difficulty using them
- Dependent on motor strength

Q. What is the disadvantage of myoelectric prosthesis?

- Higher initial cost
- Heavier
- Dependence on battery capacity and voltage
- Higher repair cost
- Dependence on battery life.

Above Elbow Prosthesis

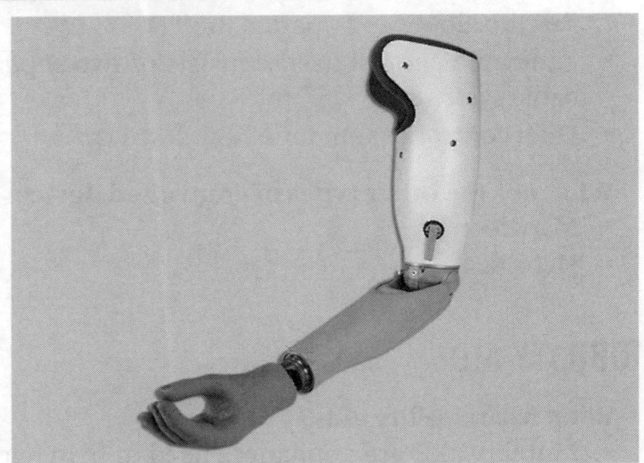

Figure 4.34: Above elbow prosthesis

Q. What is this?

This is a transhumeral prosthesis.

Q. What are the parts?

1. Terminal device.
2. Wrist unit.
3. Socket.

} See in BE prosthesis

4. Elbow units.
5. Harness and control system.

Q. What are the salient points of the elbow unit?

- Consist of hinge and cable systems, which can be locked to a position and maintain the prosthesis at various elbow flexion angle
- Uses internal elbow flexion locking system.

Q. What are the different types of suspension?

- Harness
- Suction
- Roll on liner
- Anatomically contoured.

Q. How the suspension and body powered control device works?

- Suspends the prosthesis from shoulders and transmits power from the shoulder to flex the prosthetic elbow, to lock and unlock the elbow unit, hence to operate the TD
- It uses a shoulder saddle with chest strap or figure of '8' harness

- Transmit forces from the shoulder and scapula via harness and cable to lock and unlock the elbow, flex the elbow and operate the TD
- The cable control used consists of two separate cable systems
- Dual control system for elbow and TD.

Q. What are the other types of controlled devices?
- Myoelectric
- Hybrid.

MOBILITY AIDS

Q. What are mobility aids?
- Mobility aids are appliances used to help people who have difficulty in walking
- They enable some of the body weight to be supported by the upper limbs
- Thus, building up stability and indirectly mobility
- As the condition improves the patient may progress through different types of aids
- Usually the stability of an aid is inversely related to the mobility it can achieve.

Q. What are the factors on which the selection of the mobility aid depends?
- Diagnosis and prognosis of the condition
- Strength of the upper and lower limbs
- Gait of the patient
- Stability of the patient
- Extent of improvement or deterioration of the patient
- Factors like motivation, age and acceptance
- Relief from weight bearing needed
- Coordination
- Vision and proprioception
- Architectural barriers.

Q. What are the function of mobility aids?
- To improve balance
- To give proprioception
- To decrease pain
- To reduce weight bearing
- To compensate for weak muscles
- To indicate the bystanders of the disability.

Q. What are the important points in prescription of mobility aids?
- The height of the appliance
- The location of the grip
- The rubber ferrule
- The material
- Its stability
- Whether used indoors or outdoors.

Q. What are the advantages of walking frame?
- Allows maximum stability
- Sense of security.

Q. What are the disadvantages of walking frame?
- Cannot be used safely on stairs
- Difficult to maneuver
- Limited to indoors
- Abnormal posture.

Q. How is a walking frame positioned with respect to patient?
- Placed 10–12" in front
- Elbow flexed 15°
- Handle at level of ulnar styloid.

Q. What are the different types of walking frame?
- Standard walking frame
- Gutter frame
- Rollator
- Reciprocal walking frame
- Stair climbing walker
- Reverse walker.

Q. What is so special about reverse walker?
- Facilitate extension posture
- Commonly used in spastic CP.

Q. How is a crutch different from a walker?

Crutches
- Two points of contact.
- Provide better stability than canes.
- Rubber tips.
- Padded hand grips.

NB: Should only be prescribed to patients with enough strength to extend the elbows and raise the body 1–2" off the floor.

Q. What are the different types of crutches?

A. Axillary crutches
   a. Standard axillary.
   b. Single upright.

B. Nonaxillary crutches
   a. Forearm (Lofstrand).
   b. Platform.
   c. Forearm crutches with closed cuff.
   d. Triceps.

Q. What are the advantages and disadvantages of axillary crutch?

Advantages:
- Provide better trunk support
- Short-term use by pts. with good balance and coordination
- Can free their hands.

Disadvantage:
- May cause crutch palsy.

Q. How is an axillary crutch measured?

Length measurement:
- Patient's height minus 16 inches
- 77 % of the patient's height
- Anterior axillary fold to a point 4–6" lateral to the anatomical heel (Supine)
- Anterior axillary fold to the heel plus 2"(Supine)
- Anterior axillary fold to a point 6" anterior and 2–4" lateral to the foot (Standing upright).

Hand bars:
- To give 15°–30° of elbow flexion with the wrist in maximum extension and the fingers forming a fist
- Distance from bottom of axillary piece to hand-bar equals the distance from patients olecranon to outstretched thumb.

Q. When are nonaxillary crutch used?
- Patients with good trunk balance and confidence in ambulation
- Long-term use.

Q. What are the important features of forehand (Lofstrand) crutch?
- Most popular non-axillary
- Padded handbar and forearm cuff with tubular aluminum
- Allow patient to free a hand
- The cuff should lie on the proximal third of the forearm, 4 cm from olecranon process.

Q. What are the disadvantages of canes?
- Single point of contact
- Less support than other gait aids.

Q. How is a cane measured?
- Patient upright, elbow 20°–30° degree flexed, highest point of the cane is at the level of the greater trochanter.

Q. What are the different types of cane?
- Regular (straight tip) cane
- Quad cane
- Walk-cane/Hemi-walker/side-stepper.

Q. In which side should a non axillary crutch/cane is given?
- It can be given in any side, but should be comfortable to the patient
- If given on the uninvolved side, we get normal gait pattern and a wide base of support
- If given on involved side, abnormal gait pattern is produced, e.g. right leg (involved side) and right hand goes simultaneously.

Q. What are the different types of crutch gait?

Point gait
- *Four point gait:* Sequence is right foot → left crutch → Left foot → right crutch. Very stable gait since 3 point of contact always on ground but slow
- *Three point gait:* Only 3 points of support in contact with floor
- *Two point gait:* Sequence is simultaneous advancement of right crutch and left foot followed by simultaneous advancement of left crutch and right foot
- *Tripod gait:* Sequence is right crutch then left crutch or both crutch simultaneously then drag lower limbs.

Swing gait
- *Swing to gait:* Both crutch are advanced simultaneously, arms pushed down and both lower limbs lifted and swing to the level of the crutches
- *Swing through gait:* Both crutch are advanced simultaneously, arms pushed down and both lower limbs lifted and swing beyond the level of crutches. It is the fastest gait but very energy demanding.

WHEELCHAIR

Q. What are the different types of wheelchair?
- Manual wheelchair
- Attendant-propelled wheelchair
- Powered wheelchair.

Q. What are the different parts of wheelchair?

A. Frame.
B. Propulsion unit.
C. Seat and backrest.
D. Hand grip.
E. Head rest.
F. Armrests.
G. Legrests.
H. Footplate.
I. Calf pads.
J. Safety system.

Q. What are the parts of propulsion unit?

1. Wheel.
2. Rear wheel axle.
3. Handrim.
4. Casters.
5. Tires.

Q. What are the different types of frame?

1. Folding (x-shaped) frame.
2. Rigid frame.

Q. What are the advantages and disadvantages of folding frame?

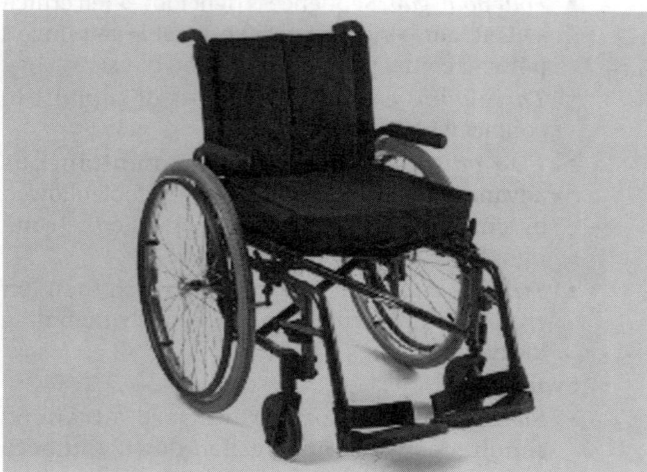

Figure 4.35: Folding frame wheelchair

Advantages:

- Easy to fold and transport
- Provides smoother ride than rigid frame.

Disadvantages:

- Less energy efficient
- May collapse when tilted sideways.

Q. What is rear wheel drive wheelchair?

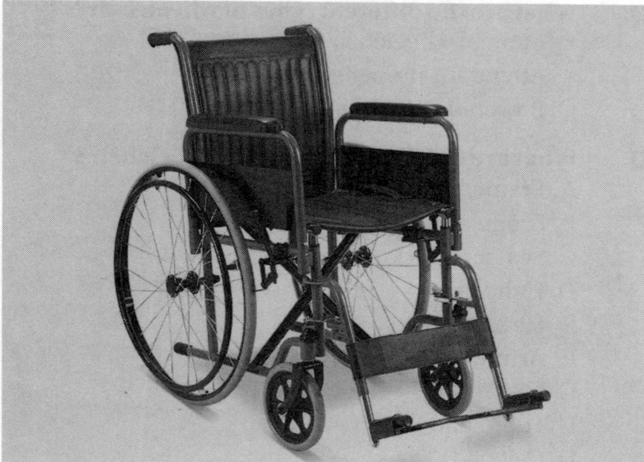

Figure 4.36: Rear wheel drive wheelchair

- Most common type of manual wheelchair
- Propelling wheels placed at the rear behind the casters
- Diameter of the wheel usually 24 inches
- Easy to maneuver than front wheel drive wheelchair.

Q. What is front wheel drive wheelchair?

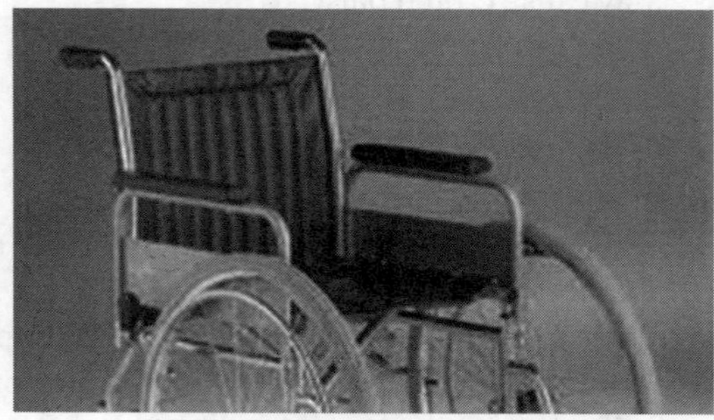

Figure 4.37: Front wheel drive wheelchair

- Propelling wheel placed in front of the casters
- Wheel diameter usually 26 inches
- Less risk of tipping backward
- Difficult to maneuver when used over curbs and particularly over stairs
- Generally used in indoors.

Q. What are the different types of wheel?

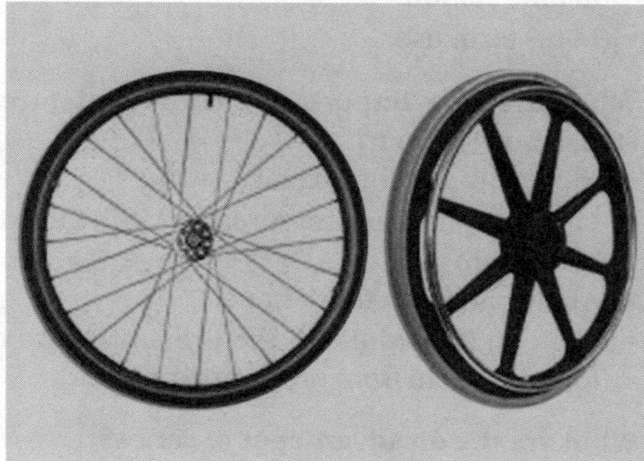

Figure 4.38: Spoked wheel and mag wheel

- **Mag wheel:**
  - Made of composite plastics or metal
  - Heavier than spoked wheel
  - More durable
  - Need less maintenance
  - Commonly used wheels in non sports wheelchair
  - Newer type of Mag wheels comprise high strength and lighter than spoked wheels, but they are more costly.
- **Spoked wheel:**
  - Lighter than Mag wheel
  - Less durable
  - Need greater maintenance
  - Less safe for elderly patients.

Q. What is camber?

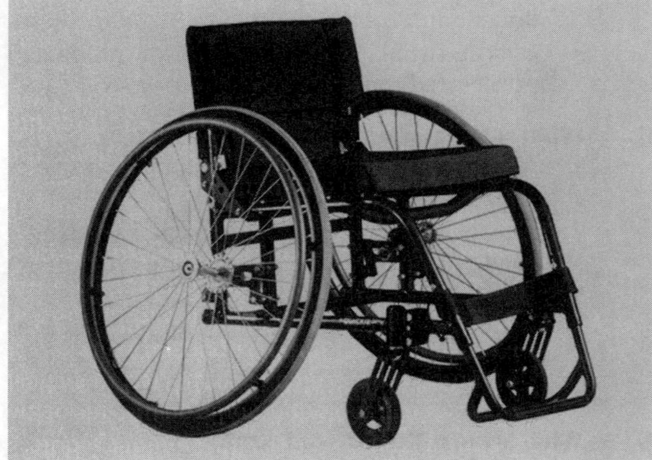

Figure 4.39: Wheelchair with increased camber

- It is the angle of rear wheel tilt
- Top is tilted inwards and bottom outward
- More the bottom of the wheel is moved outward, the greater camber and stability
- Reduces shoulder abduction
- Can be problematic while entering and exiting doors.

Q. How rear wheel axle position affects the wheelchair?

- Can be fixed or adjustable
- Axle placement can be adjusted either in the vertical direction or horizontal direction
- Posteriorly placed axle in respect to center of gravity increases wheelchair rear stability.
- Forward placement: Decreases stability but increases maneuverability and shortens turning radius.

Q. What is a hand rim? Types of hand rim?

- Used for self propulsion of the wheelchair
- Smaller in diameter than propelling wheel
- Attached slightly lateral to the propelling wheel
- Can be large, small, thick or knobby for better hand grip
- Large hand rim: Easier to propel, more arm strokes needed to cover given distance
- Athletes prefer smaller diameter rims to maximize the distance covered with each strokes
- Thicker the rim, easier the grip
- Knobby projections over rim may help to quadriplegics.

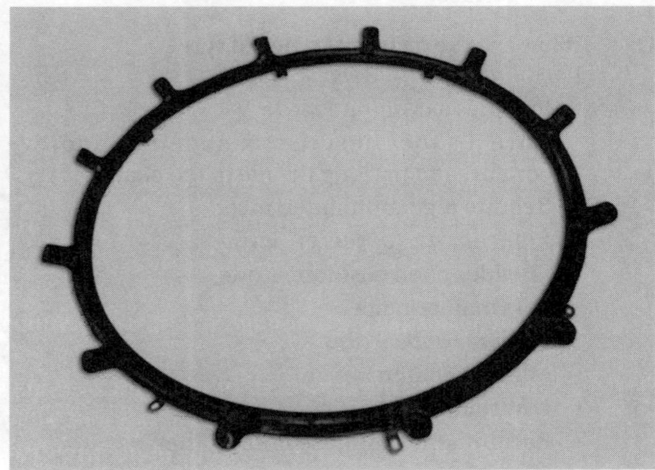

Figure 4.41: Knoby projections over hand rim

Q. What are casters?

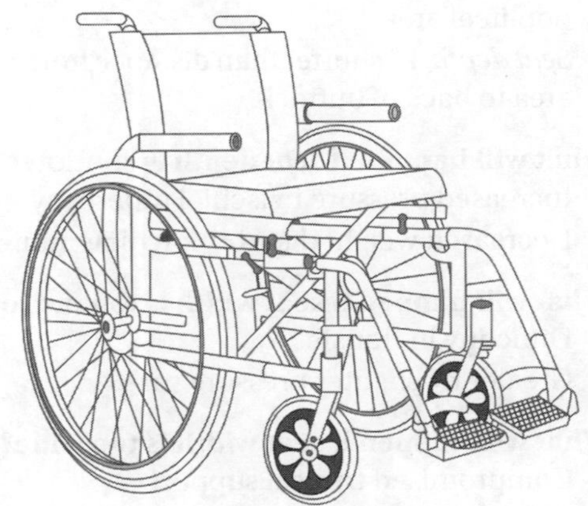

Figure 4.42: Casters

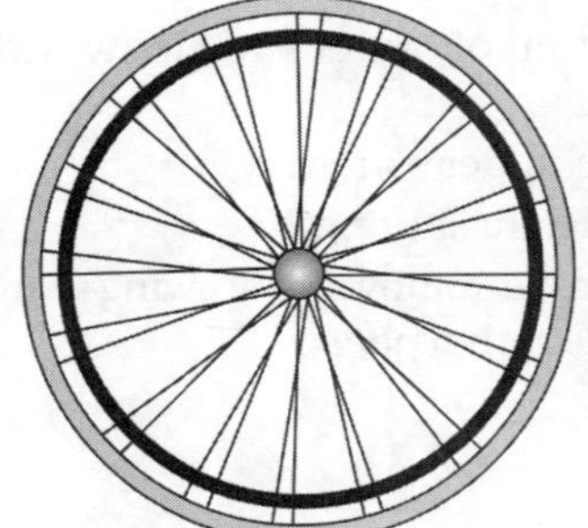
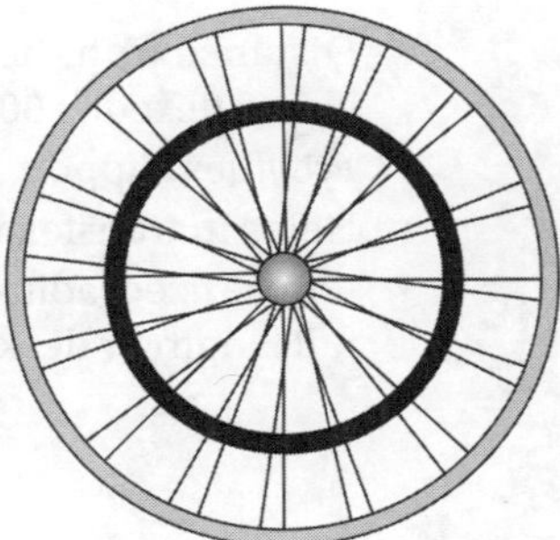
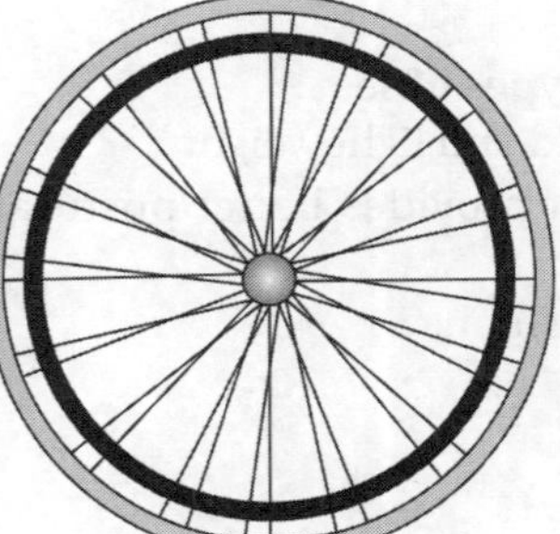
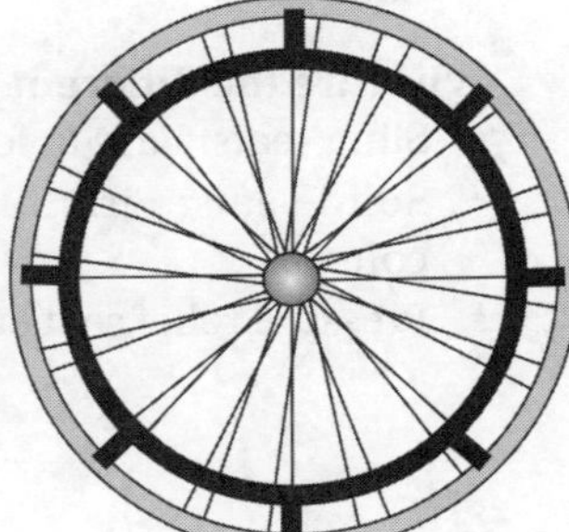

Figure 4.40: Different types of hand rims

- Small wheels in front of the rear wheel drive wheelchair or on the back of front wheel drive wheelchair
- Size:
  - Small (5 inch diameter) better for smooth surface
  - Large (8 inch diameter) better for rough surface.

Q. What are the different types of tyre?

Pneumatic (air-filled):
- Provides a cushioned ride
- Have a shock absorber function to improve comfort and prolong the life of the chair
- Require regular maintenance.

Semipneumatic (airless gel inserts):
- Provides good cushioned ride
- Less maintenance.

Solid (core rubber) tires:
- Minimal maintenance
- Low rolling resistance
- Recommended for use in smoother use.

Q. What are the measurement criteria for seat?
- *Seat width:* 1" wider than width of the widest part of buttock
- *Seat height:* 2" higher than distance from heel to popliteal area
- *Seat depth:* 2" shorter than distance from popliteal area to back of buttock.

Q. What will happen if seat depth is shallow?
- Increased pressure in ischial tuberosity
- Decreased weight distribution on femur.

Q. What will happen if seat width is too narrow?
- Difficulty in transfer
- Greater trochanter pressure sore.

Q. What will happen if seat width is too wide?
- Compromised truncal support.
- Difficult propulsion
- Scoliosis
- Back pain.

Q. What are the different types of seat?
- Sling seats: Easy to fold and light weight
- Solid seats: Firm but provides better postural control
- Pressure relief seat cushion.

Q. What is the disadvantages of sling seats?
- Promotes posterior tilt, hip internal rotation and adduction
- Collapsed trunk, head forward flexion, protracted and elevated shoulder.

Q. What is the measurement of backrest?
- 2" less than the distance from inferior angle of scapula to the sitting surface
- In a standard wheelchair the backrest height is usually 16–16.5" with 8° of backward tilt from the vertical
- Higher backrests give more support but less mobility
- Backrest width is similar to seat width.

Q. What is the utility of head rest?
- For posture and head alignment
- Adds comfort to the patient.

Q. What is hand grip?
- Used to push a wheelchair for attendant-propelled wheelchairs.

Q. What is arm rest? Its measurement and types?

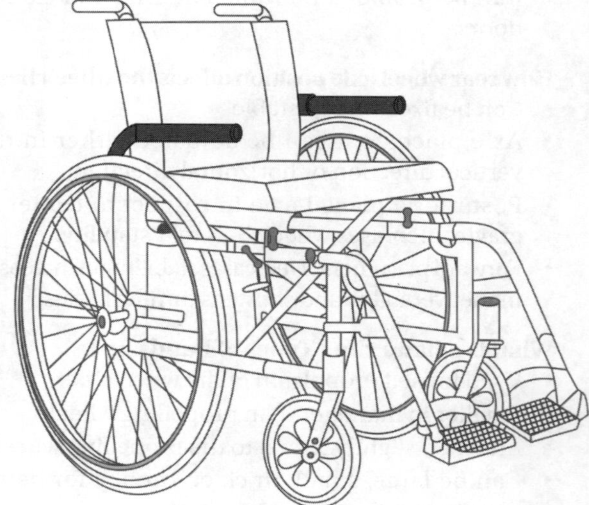

Figure 4.43: Arm rests

- Distance from bottom of buttock to elbow with elbow flexed at 90°
- Provides support to upper extremity
- Helps in transfer, weight shifting
- Can be fixed, adjustable, removable or swing away, full length or desk length type.

Q. What are leg rests?

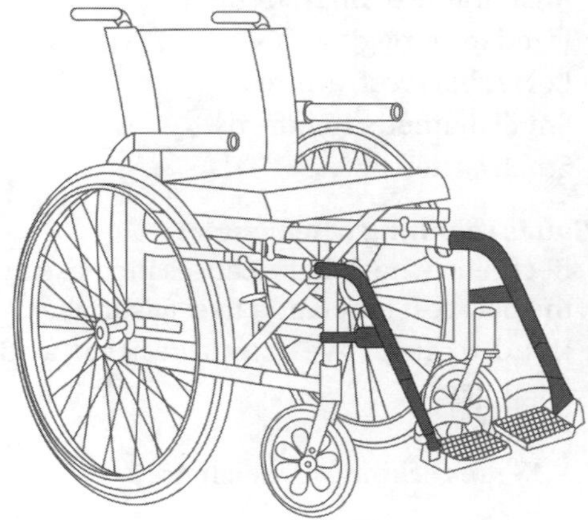

Figure 4.44: Leg rest

- Part of front rigging and support the legs
- Proper positioning of the lower extremity
- Can be removable, fixed or swing away type
- Elevating leg rests may helps in:
  - Reduction of LE dependent edema
  - Adds comfort when recline system are used.

Q. What is footplate?

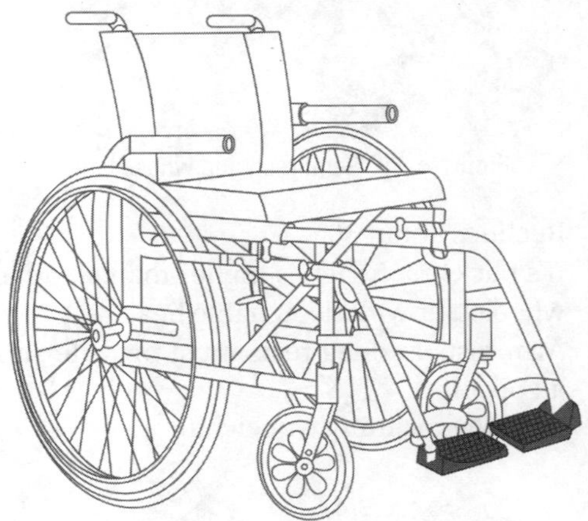

Figure 4.45: Footplate

- It supports the foot
- Can be fixed but most of the footplate generally swing up to allow the foot to reach the floor
- Can be equipped with heel loops or ankle straps
- The lowest point of the footplate should be at least 2 inches above the floor
- Keeps the ankle in neutral position.

Q. What are the calf pads?

- Attached to leg rest to provide support
- Supports the lower limb during elevation of the leg rests.

Q. What are the different safety systems in wheelchair?

- **Wheel locks (brakes)**

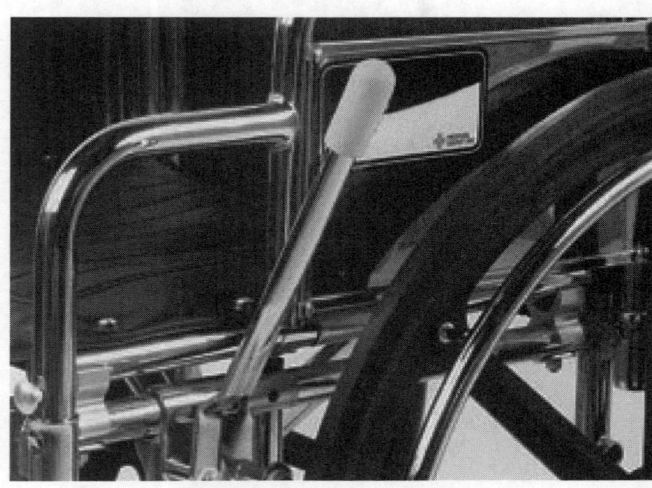

Figure 4.46: Wheel brakes

  - Fitted to side frame of the chair and work either "push-to-lock" or "pull-to-lock" mechanism
  - Installed to prevent unintended rolling.

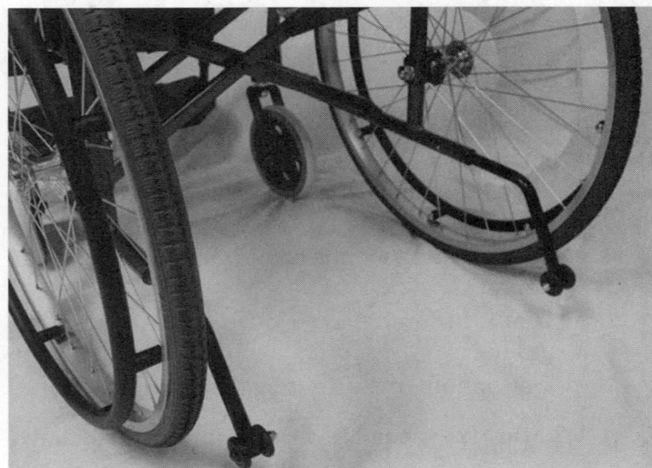

Figure 4.47: Antitippers

- **Antitipper**
  - Can be used on a wheelchair to prevent the chair from tipping backward
  - Attached to the rear of WC frame
  - Provides safety during wheelchair mobility.
- **Grade aids (hill holders)**
  - Spring loaded devices which prevent the wheelchair from rolling backwards
  - Selectively activated only when going uphill
  - Useful for patients with poor strength when propelling uphill.

Q. What is one arm drive wheelchair?

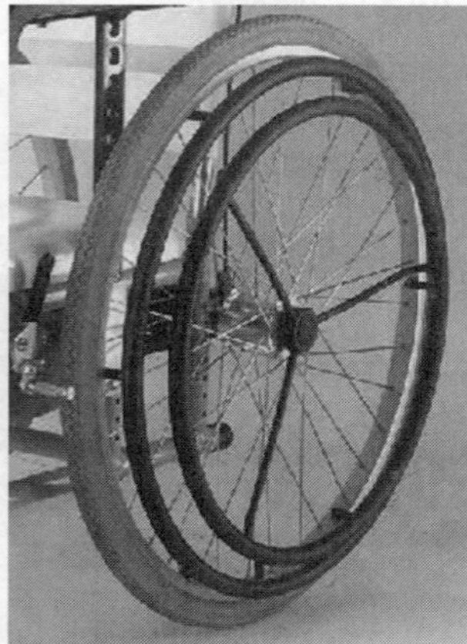

Figure 4.48: One arm drive wheelchair

- These are designed to be operated with one arm, either right or left
- Both handrims are typically mounted on one side
- The first handrim is the usual handrim connected with the wheel directly
- The second handrim is mounted outside the first and connected by an axle to the wheel
- The disadvantage is increased weight and width
- Used in hemiplegics, one arm amputee
- Propelling them requires a fairly high degree of strength and coordination.

Q. What are foot drive wheelchairs?

- These are practical alternatives to one arm drive wheelchairs
- Hemiplegics uses one handrim and one good foot to propel
- Seat is lowered 2 inch for the foot to reach the ground
- One or both of the front riggings is removed.

Q. What are the special features of sports wheelchair?

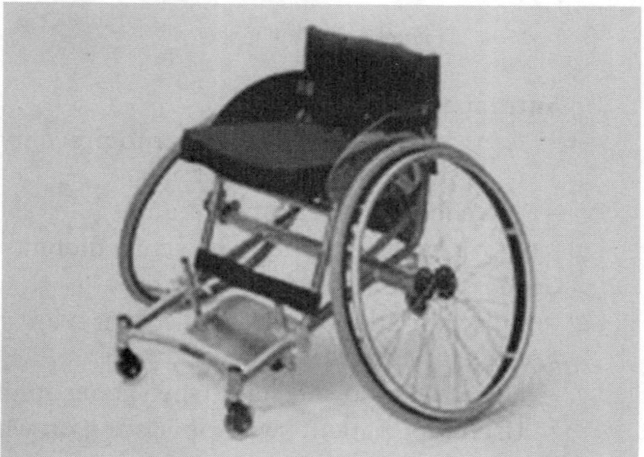

Figure 4.49: Sports wheelchair

- Light weight (15–20 lb)
- Rigid frame of high strength
- Fixed front riggings
- Lower backrest, armrest
- Small diameter handrims
- Small casters.

Q. What is reclining wheelchair?

- Reclining wheelchairs causes increase in angle of the backrest in relation to seat surface
- Used to improve trunk control and spinal alignment
- It can be:
  - Semi reclining wheelchair

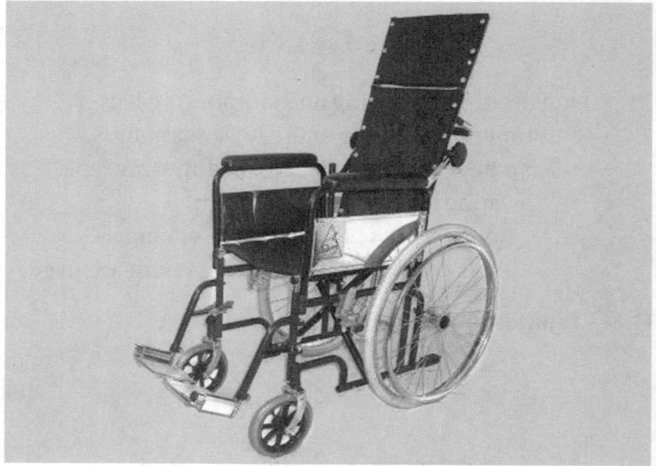

Figure 4.50: Semi reclining wheelchair

- Reclines about 30°
- It's back rest 5 inches higher than standard adult wheelchair with detachable head rest
- Arm rests and leg rests must provide support in all position.
  - Fully reclining wheelchair

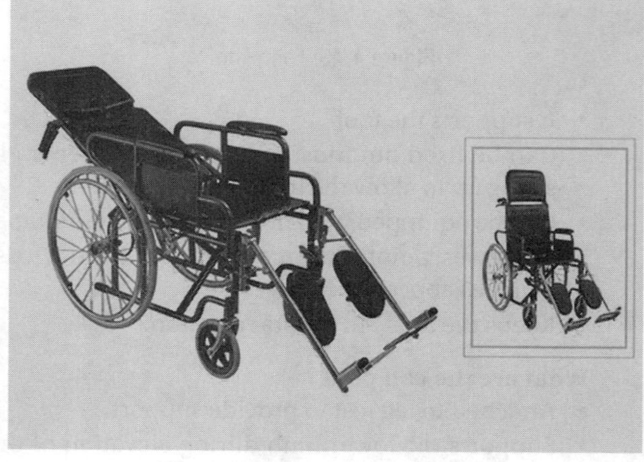

Figure 4.51: Reclining wheelchair

- Permits conversion from a wheelchair to a stretcher
- May be locked in any position
- It's back rest is 7 inches higher than standard adult wheelchair with detachable head rest
- Provides better relief of pressure from ischium and sacrum than semi reclining wheelchairs.

Q. What is tilt in space wheelchair?

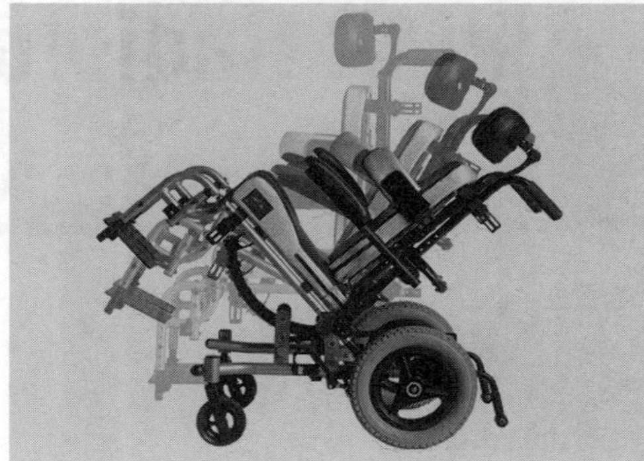

Figure 4.52: Tilt in space wheelchair

- Alternative to reclining wheelchairs
- Entire seat and back are tilted posteriorly as a single unit in the sagittal plane
- Angle between seat and backrest remains same in all position
- Advantage over reclining wheelchair is lack of shear stress during tilting movements
- Helps in better repositioning.

Q. What is the need for reclining and tilt in space mechanisms?

- To perform adequate weight shifts
- Minimizes skin breakdown
- Poor sitting balance
- Poor endurance
- Orthostatic hypotension
- Fluctuating respiratory status.

Q. What is power wheelchair?

See chapter in Paraplegia (SCI).

5 Chapter

PMR Radiology

X-RAY

Avascular Necrosis

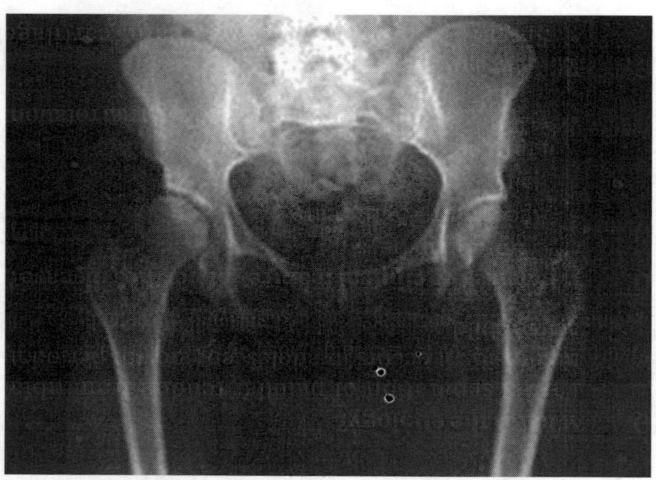

Figure 5.1: AP view of pelvis, both hip and upper part of femur, showing diffuse osteosclerosis of head along with osteolytic lesion in hip lateral part
(Early stage—Normal, Late—Head collapse Secondary OA hip)

Figure 5.1 is the AP view of pelvis, both hip and upper part of femur, showing diffuse osteosclerosis of head along with osteolytic lesion in hip lateral part. So, I think this is a X-ray of avascular necrosis of femur.

Q. What is AVN?

Necrosis of bone due to loss of vascularity secondary to dislocation of bones or due to fracture or disease.

Q. What are the causes of AVN?

- Idiopathic—commonest
- Sickle cell anemia
- End-stage renal disease on dialysis
- Perthes disease
- Slipped capital femoral epiphysis
- Dislocation
- Postpartum
- Steroid use
- Gaucher disease
- Infection
- Malignancy
- Radiation therapy
- Systemic lupus erythematosus (SLE).

Q. What are the investigations needed?

- Blood: CBC, ESR, CRP, ANF, if needed Sickling test
- X-ray
- CT scan
- MRI—for early diagnosis.

Q. What are the X-ray findings in AVN?

In early stage—normal

Classical—

- Sclerosis
- Flattening
- Crescent sign—subchondral radiolucent lines
- Collapse of cortex.

Q. What are the presentations?

- Progressive pain
- Limping
- Deformity and stiffness
- Antalgic gait
- Tenderness over bone
- Muscle wasting and weakness (75% are bilateral).

Q. How will you treat the cases?

- Analgesic for pain
- Bisphosphonate to prevent collapse
- Non/partial weight bearing

- Treatment of underlying cause
- ROM and strengthening of muscles
- Surgery
  - Realignment osteotomies
  - Decompression: Core decompression
  - Arthrodesis
  - Arthroplasty
  - Total hip replacement.

Q. What are the other AVN?

- *Kienbock's disease:* Idiopathic avascular necrosis of the lunate bone that leads to collapse and progressive carpal arthritis
- *Preiser disease:* Idiopathic osteonecrosis of scaphoid.

Perthes Disease

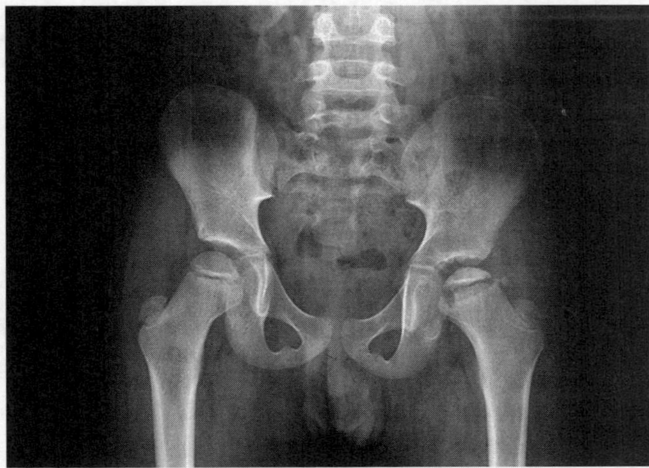

Figure 5.2: X-ray of pelvis, hip, upper part of femur of a young male showing collapse and sclerosis of epiphysis of femur head with increased hip space

Figure 5.2 is the X-ray of pelvis, hip, upper part of femur of a young male showing collapse and sclerosis of epiphysis of femur head with increased hip space. So, I think this is the X-ray plate of Perthes disease.

Q. What is Perthes disease?
It is the idiopathic osteonecrosis of capital femoral epiphysis.

Q. What is the etiology?
Mainly idiopathic due to vascular compromise.

Q. What is Osgood–Schlatter disease?
Inflammation at the tibial tuberosity due to overuse.

Q. What is the etiology?
Partial separation of patellar tendon from tibial tuberosity. It occurs in adolescent growth period in active child.

Q. What are the clinical features of perthes disease?

- Common in boys
- Age group—5–10 years
- Pain
- Limping
- Decreased ROM: Adduction and internal rotation.

Q. What are the stages of Perthes disease?

- *Stage1*: Ischemia and bone death, cartilage thickens
- *Stage 2*: Revascularization and repair
- *Stage 3*: Distortion and remodeling.

Q. What are the investigations needed?

- Bone scan
- MRI scan.

Q. How you will treat the case?

- Aim: To prevent head from malpositioning
- Head containment: By positioning, splinting, containment orthosis
- Pain by analgesic surgery:
  - Osteotomy-varous derotation osteotomy, salter osteotomy, chiari osteotomy.
  - 'Arthroplasty in severe cases

Q. Is there any specific treatment?
Usually self-limiting disease.

Ricket

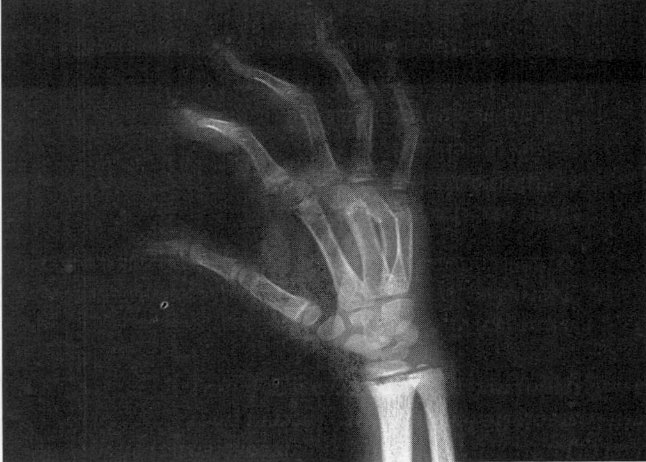

Figure 5.3: X-ray plate showing widening of epiphyseal spaces, fraying and cupping of metaphysis and splaying of metaphysis with rarefaction of diaphysis

Figure 5.3 is a X-ray plate of both wrist and hands showing widening of epiphyseal spaces (normal—2.4 mm), fraying and cupping of metaphysis and splaying of metaphysis with rarefaction of diaphysis.

I think this is the X-ray plate of rickets. (Early—delayed appearance of epiphysis; Bony deformity—knock knee, bow leg, coxa vera).

Q. What is rickets?

It is the disease of a growing child due to impaired mineralization of bone resulting in bony softening and deformity.

Q. What are the clinical features?

- Craniotabes
- Frontal bossing, delayed closure of anterior fontanelle
- Harrisson sulcus: Protruding of weakened ribs over lower chest
- Pigeon chest: Pulled sternum causing projection of ribs
- Funnel chest/pectus excavatum
- Richetic rosary: Costochondral junction deformity
- Hypotonic muscles: Pot belly
- Bow legs, knock knee.

Q. What are the investigations required?

- Blood for vitamin D_3, calcium, phosphate, alkaline phosphate, parathormone (PTH) level
- X-ray of hand and wrist, other areas
- Urine for bone metabolites.

Q. What are the types of rickets?

I. Nutritional rickets (Table 1)

II. Vitamin D dependent rickets—
   A. Type 1
   B. Type 2.

III. Vitamin D resistant rickets:
   A. Familial hypophosphatemic
   B. Pseudohypoparathyroidism
   C. Renal rickets

Q. How you treat the case?

- Vitamin D_3 supplementation—vitamin D (60k) once weekly for 3–4 weeks Or, 400 IU/day
- Exercise—muscle strengthening exercise.

Looser's Zone

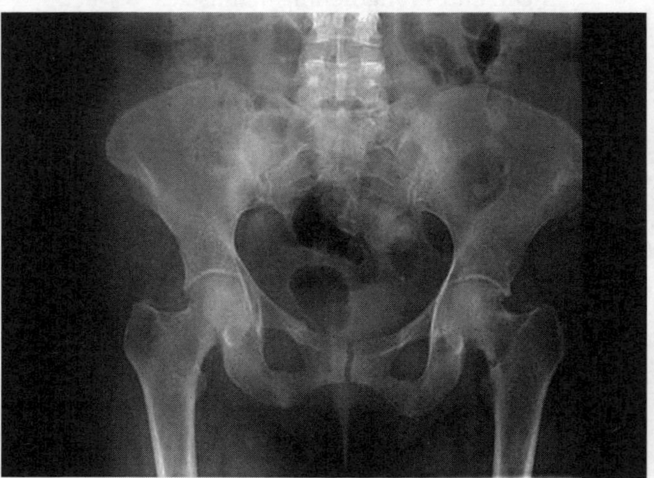

Figure 5.4: X-ray plate of pelvis, hip, upper part of femurs showing diffuse rarefaction of bones along with radiolucent zone occurring at the site of stress that is pubic rami, medial cortex of femur called loose zone, i.e. pseudofracture

Figure 5.4 is a X-ray plate of pelvis, hip, upper part of femurs showing diffuse rarefaction of bones along with radiolucent zone occurring at the site of stress that is pubic rami, medial cortex of femur called loose zone, i.e. pseudofracture. So, I think this is the X-ray showing looser zone due to osteomalacia.

Q. What are the common causes?

- Osteomalacia
- Fibrous dysplasia
- Hyperthyroidism
- Pagets disease of bone
- Renal osteodystrophy
- Familial hypophosphatemia.

Q. What are the common sites of Looser's zone?

- Ribs
- Pubic rami
- Proximal femur medially
- Lateral scapula
- Posterior proximal ulna.

Q. What is osteomalacia?

Disease of bone caused by demineralization and softening of bone after stoppage of bone growth.

Table 5.1: Types of rickets

Type	*Vitamin D3*	*1,25(OH)Vitamin D*	*Cal^{2+}*	*PO^{4-}*	*ALP*	*PTH*
Nutritional	Decreased	–	Decreased	Decreased	increased	–
Vitamin D dependent—Type1 Type2	– –	Decreased markedly Increased markedly	Decrease Decrease	Decreased Decreased	Increased Increased	Increased
Vitamin D resistant—Hypophosphatemic	–	–	Increased	Decreased	Decreased	--

Q. What are the clinical features?
- Difficulty rising from a chair
- Difficulty walking
- Low back pain, muscle weakness
- Weight loss, progressive deformities.

Q. What are the X-ray features of osteomalacia?
- Insufficiency fractures or pseudo fractures
- Protrusion acceptably
- Osteoporotic like features.

Q. What are the biomarker features?
- Decreased/normal calcium
- Decreased phosphate
- Increased alkaline phosphate
- Increased serum PTH.

Q. How you confirm it?
By bone biopsy.

Q. How you will manage the case?
- Weight relieving orthosis
- Exercise—Isometric strengthening exercise
- Vit D supplementation
- Calcium supplementation
- Treatment of underlying cause.

Cervical Rib

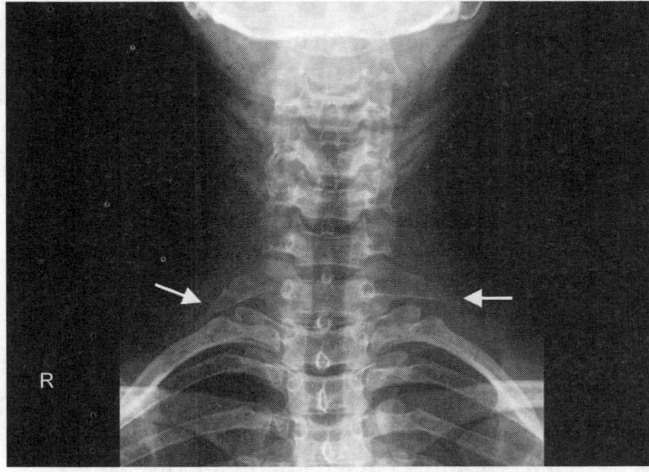

Figure 5.5: X-ray plate of cervical spine AP view showing extra rib originating from C7 vertebrae bilaterally

Figure 5.5 is a X-ray plate of cervical spine AP view showing extra rib originating from C7 vertebrae bilaterally.

Q. What may be the clinical features?
- May be asymptomatic
- Thoracic outlet syndrome.

Q. What are boundaries of thoracic outlet?
- Triangular-shaped space bound by anterior and middle scalene muscle with base by first rib.

Q. What are the structures passing through it?
- Subclavian artery
- Brachial plexus (subclavian vein passes anteriorly of the triangle).

Q. What are the clinical features of thoracic outlet syndrome?
- Often bilateral
- Vascular:

  Due to arterial involvement:
  - Pain
  - Fatigue
  - Limb ischemia
  - Limb necrosis
  - Decreased color and temperature.

  Due to venous involvement:
  - Pain
  - Bluish and swollen limb.
- Neurogenic—caused compression of lower trunk.
  - Pain and numbness
  - Intrinsic muscle weakness and atrophy
  - Decreased sensation
  - Difficulty in fine motor tasks.
- Manuevers
  - Elevation arm stress test/Roo's test:
    - Patient raises his or her hands above the head and clenches and releases the fist for 1–2 minutes
    - Appearance of the patient's typical symptoms with or without signs of vascular involvement should be considered as positive test.
  - Adson's test:
    - Locate the radial pulse
    - Arm to be held in extension, external rotation and slight abduction
    - Patient is asked to turn the head towards the test arm with extension of neck
    - In case of compression radial pulse will be diminished or absent.
  - Costoclavicular test:
    - Palpate radial pulse
    - Patient's shoulder has to be drawed down and back
    - In case of compression pulse will disappear.
  - Halstead maneuver:
    - Neck in hyperextension and rotated to opposite side
    - Give downward traction on the test upper limb

   - In case of positive test, there will be absence of radial pulse.
- Wright test (Hyperabduction test):
   - Arm is hyperabducted and overhead with elbow and arm in coronal plane
   - Patient's neck is rotated or extended
   - Decreased or absent radial pulse will be considered as positive test.
- Allen maneuver:
   - Shoulder in external rotation and horizontal abduction
   - Patient's head is away from the test side
   - Absent or decreased radial pulse considered as positive test

Q. Is there is any other investigations available to establish TOS?
- EMG NCS of both upper limbs
- Angiogram for arterial compression
- Computed tomography
- Phlebography for venous compression.

Q. Which investigation will you perform if patient is having TOS clinically and electrophysiologically but there is no cervical rib?
- Magnetic resonance imaging (MRI).

Q. How will you manage the case?
Pharmacological: For pain NSAIDs and muscle relaxant.
Nonpharmacological:
- Postural care—like avoidance of overhead activity
- Strengthening exercise—lower scapular stabiliser, upper limb muscle specially intrinsic muscle of hand
- Stretching of scalenes, pectorals, and trapezius muscle
- Relaxation technique
- Respiratory reeducation
- Modality—like TENS to relieve pain and for muscle relaxation.

Surgery—scalenotomy, removal of first rib.
Indication of surgery:
- Failure of conservative treatment
- Venous or arterial complication
- Nerve compression.

Osgood Schlatter Disease

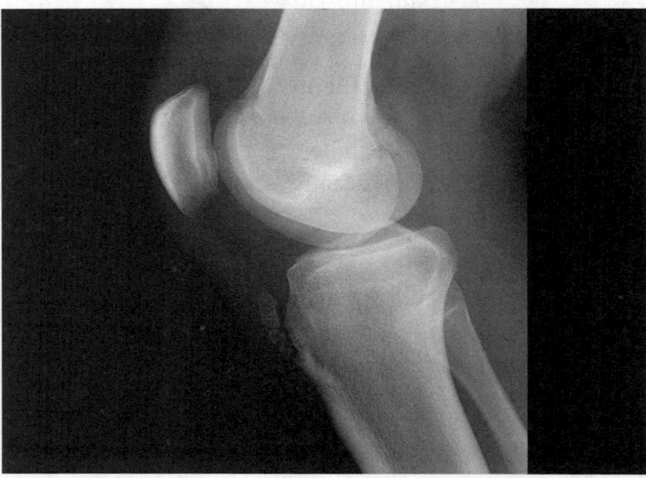

Figure 5.6: X-ray plate of lateral view of knee and upper part of tibia showing irregularities over tibial tubercle and fragmentation of part of it is just infront of tibial tuberosity

Figure 5.6 is a X-ray plate of lateral view of knee and upper part of tibia showing irregularities over tibial tubercle and fragmentation of part of it is just infront of tibial tuberosity. So, I think this patient is having Osgood Schlatter disease.

Q. What type of disease entity it is?
Osteochondritis.

Q. What are the age group involved?
Adolescent in growth spurt period.

Q. What are the clinical features?
- Seen in young adolescent child in growth spurt.
- Pain and tenderness at tibial tuberosity
- Bony overgrowth at tibial tuberosity.

Q. What are the exacerbating factors?
- Overactivity
- Direct contact.

Q. Is there any other investigation needed?
X-ray knee.

Q. What is Sinding Larsen Johansson disease?
Irregularity and fragmentation at the origin of patellar tendon in inferior pole of patella.

Q. What is the prognosis of the disease?
Symptoms resolve spontaneously after closing of growth plates.

Q. How you treat the case?
- Activity modification
- NSAIDs, ice for pain relief
- Strengthening exercise—gentle and progressive quadriceps strengthening
- Counselling and/or assurance of parents and family members.

Heterotropic Ossifications

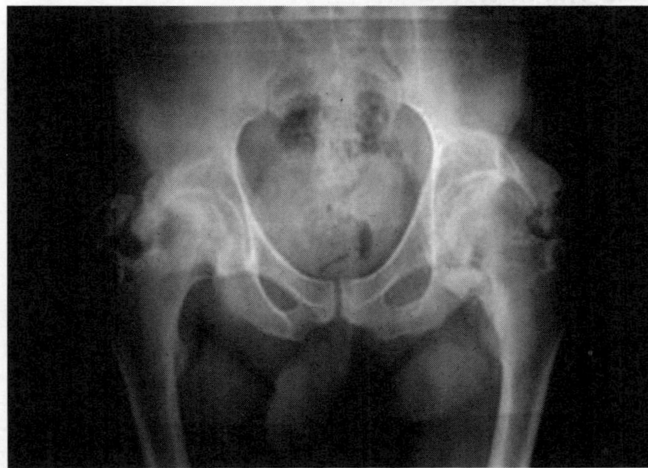

Figure 5.7: X-ray of hip and pelvis showing soft-tissue ossification in lateral aspect of hip joint isodense with other bony structures

Figure 5.7 is a X-ray of hip and pelvis showing soft-tissue ossification in lateral aspect of hip joint isodense with other bony structures. So, I think this patient is having heterotropic ossification (HO) around hip joint.
Differential diagnosis:
Myositis ossificans traumatica.

Q. What is HO?
This is formation of mature lamellar bone in abnormal areas usually in soft tissue surrounding a joint.

Q. Is it a true ossification? and why?
- No
- Because of lack of Haversian system in the bone.

Q. What is the pathogenesis of HO?
- Pathogenesis is not fully understood till now
- Possibly due to alteration in neuronal control over the differentiation of mesenchymal cells into osteogenic precursor cells
- Bone morphogenic protein is thought to play a role also
- Damage to the sympathetic tracts in the spinal cord may also promote HO by increasing the local vascularity and blood perfusion around the joint
- Forceful ROM of contracted limbs may cause microtrauma and bleeding, and lead to HO.

Q. What are the percentages of HO in SCI patient?
13–57%.

Q. What are the other risk factors?
- Older age
- Neurologically complete lesions
- Male gender
- Pressure ulcer
- DVT
- Spasticity
- Immobilization
- Fractures.

Q. What are common areas of involvement?
Hips (anteromedial aspect) > knees > shoulders > elbow.

Q. What are the common clinical features?
- May be asymptomatic
- Early clinical findings are increased temperature and soft-tissue swelling
- Pain
- Decreased range of motion of joints
- Joint erythema/joint effusion
- Low-grade fever
- In severe cases adjacent neurovascular structures may be compromised.

Q. What are the differential diagnoses?
- Thrombophebitis
- DVT
- Cellulitis
- Joint sepsis
- Fracture
- Hematoma.

Q. What are the biochemical parameters?
- Increased serum alkaline phosphatase
- Increased serum creatinine phosphokinase—more reliable
- Increased ESR and CRP for disease activity
- Urinary hydroxyproline and collagen metabolites—indicate presence of HO.

Q. What are the other investigations needed?
- Bone scan
- MRI for early diagnosis
- CT scan.

Q. How you will treat the case?
- ROM with gentle stretching
- Bisphosphonates:
  - Etidronate disodium × 6 months
    If CPK normal: 20 mg/kg/day × 3 months then 10 mg/kg/day × 3 months
    If CPK is elevated then 20 mg/kg/day × 6 months.
- NSAIDs: Indomethacin 75 mg/day × 6 weeks
- Radiation
- Surgery.

Q. What is the role of radiation therapy?
Radiation prevents further formation or recurrence of HO after surgery. It is used after 72 hours of surgery.

Q. What are the indications of surgery?
- Severely limited ROM that causes functional limitations
- Done after 12–18 months—after the ectopic bone matures
- HO compressing neurovascular structure.

Q. What is the surgical procedure done?
Wedge resection with pseudoarthrosis.

Q. How will the postoperative recurrence be reduced?
Prophylaxis by:
- Etidronate disodium 20 mg/kg/day × 2 wks then 10 mg/kg/day for 10 weeks
- Indomethacin 75 mg daily for 3 weeks within 5 weeks of injury
- Radiation therapy—single doses of 5–8 Gy are used within 72 hours of surgery

Salient points of myositis ossificans:
- *Pathogenesis*: Abnormal differentiation of fibroblast to bone forming cells leading to calcification of intramuscular hematoma
- *Myositis ossificans traumatica* when it occurs after trauma.

Clinical features:
- Pain, swelling and tenderness at the site of injury
- Stiffness
- Sometimes restricted ROM of joint
- Difficulty in weight bearing and antalgic gait in case of lower limb muscle and difficulty in daily activities by upper limb in case of upper limb muscle involvement.

Common sites:
- Thigh, arm (80%)
- Other site—Chest, itercostal space, gluteal region, erector spinae, etc.

Investigations:
- X-ray
- Bone scan and MRI scan for early cases

Management:
- Analgesic for pain
- Exercise—ROM and strengthening exercise
- Radiation prevent further bony formation
- Surgery in nonresponsive cases.

Radiologically differentiating points between MOT and HO:
- There is no such radiographic difference between two.
  - Myositis ossificans mostly found in large muscle
  - HO found associated with joints.

Total Hip Replacement

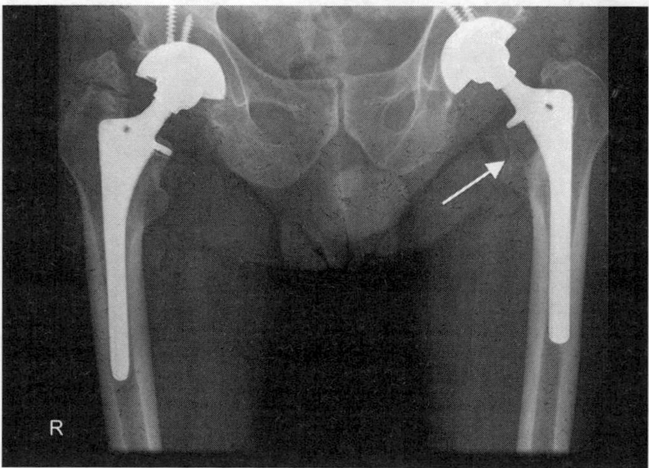

Figure 5.8: X-ray plate of pelvis and upper part of femur showing bilateral prosthetic hip joint without any subluxation

Figure 5.8 is the X-ray plate of pelvis and upper part of femur showing bilateral prosthetic hip joint without any subluxation. So, I think this patient is having bilateral total hip replacement (THR).

Q. What are the types of hip prosthesis?
I. Unipolar endoprosthesis.
II. Bipolar endoprosthesis.
III. True total hip replacement.

Q. What are the indications of THR?
Common disease requiring replacement:
- Osteoarthritis
- Rheumatoid arthritis
- Avascular necrosis (AVN)
- Post-traumatic degenerative joint disease
- Congenital hip disease
- Infectious diseases within the joint or adjacent bone.

In case of above disease patient requires replacement when there is:

- Severe pain
- Decreased ROM—rotation; abduction; flexion
- Contracture
- Disuse weakness
- Antalgic gait
- Decreased mobility—sit to stand, toilet
- Limited ADLs—dressing, bathing, household chores.

Q. What are the contraindications for THR?

- Active or recent joint infections
- Neurotrophic joints
- Inability of patient to take part in postoperative rehab plan
- Serious comorbid medical conditions
- Rapidly progressing or terminal cancer
- Gross malnutrition.

Q. What are the Do's and Don'ts after THR?

Dos:

- When sitting, sit with knees comfortably apart
- When lying on the uninvolved side, always have pillows between your knees
- Continue to use your elevated commode seat (usually around 6–10 weeks)
- Sit in a slightly reclined position-avoid leaning forward when sitting on the commode.

Dont's:

- Sitting in low chairs
- Lying on the involved side initially
- Cross legs while walking
- Bending past 80 degrees (e.g. touching your feet, pulling up pants, picking up off the floor)
- Raising knee higher than hip when in a chair
- Trying to get into a bathtub without a tub chair
- Prolonged sitting for longer than 1 hours before standing.

Q. What are the complications of THR?

- Anemia
- Pain
- Edema
- DVT
- Hematoma
- Infection
- Muscle weakness
- Restricted ROM
- Gait abnormality
- Contracture
- Hip dislocation fracture
- Trochanteric nonunion
- Limb length discrepancy.

Q. What are the preoperative counselling needed for THR?

- Counseling to clarify patients expectations
- Home exercise program:
  - Hip abductor and extensor strengthening
  - Quadriceps strengthening.
- ADL and transfer training (bed-wheelchair-toilet seat)
- Home visit for environmental modifications to aid in quick and safe discharge
- Basic use of gait aids.

Q. What will be the early rehabilitation program after THR?

Postoperative day 1:

- Bed rest with abduction pillow
- Wound monitoring
- IV and/or epidural analgesia
- Bedside exercise.

Postoperative day 2:

- Bedside transfer
- Bedside exercise
- Standing
- In room ambulation with walker
- Switch to oral analgesic
- Hip precaution.

Day 3 onwards:

- Exercise
- Ambulation training
- ADL training.

Q. What is the long-term outcome?

- Both short- and long-term prognosis is good
- Lasts for 10–15 years
- Depends upon:
  - Weight
  - Stress
  - Level of activity.

Q. What are the types of osteotomy?

I. Single innominate (Salter)
II. Acetabuloplasty (Pamberton)
III. Triple innominate (Steel)
IV. Shelf (Chiary)

Q. What are the indications of girdle stone osteotomy?

Excision arthroplasty of hip may be done in case of:

- Periprosthetic infection
- Recurrent dislocation
- Aseptic loosening
- Failed internal fixation of fracture neck femur.

Q. When it is done?

18 months to 6 years age.

Lytic Lesion

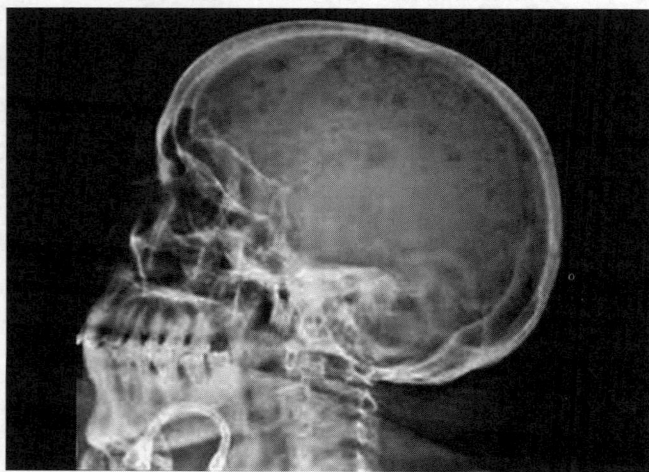

Figure 5.9: X-ray plate of skull of an elderly male showing multiple punched out lesion all over skull bones

Figure 5.9 is a X-ray plate of skull of an elderly male showing multiple punched out lesion all over skull bones. So, I think this patient is having multiple myeloma.

Q. What are the other common sites of lytic bone lesion?

- Ribs
- Pelvis
- Vertebrae
- Long bones.

Q. What is multiple myeloma?

- Malignant proliferation of plasma cells derived from a single clone.

Q. What are the common presentations of MM?

- Usually affect 6th–7th decade
- Male:female ratio is 2:1
- In early stage it may be asymptomatic
- Bone pain precipitated by movement
- Night pain
- Fracture
- Recurrent chest infection, UTI
- Anemia
- Weakness
- Neurological symptoms and signs
- Renal failure.

Q. What are the diagnostic criteria?

- M protein in serum and/or urine
- Bone marrow (clonal) plasma cells (10%) or plasmacytoma
- Myeloma-related organ or tissue impairment (end organ damage, including bone lesions):
- CRAB features:
  - **Calcium elevation** in the blood (serum calcium >10.5 mg/L or upper limit of normal)
  - **Renal insufficiency** (serum creatinine >2 mg/dL)
  - **Anemia** (hemoglobin <10 g/dL or 2 g <normal)
  - **Lytic bone lesions or osteoporosis.**
- **Updated definition of multiple myeloma:**
  The revised IMWG (International Myeloma Working Group) criteria will allow, in addition to the classic CRAB features, the following three markers as "myeloma defining events" (MDEs)
- **Bone marrow**: 60% or more clonal plasma cells
- **Serum**: Involved/uninvolved free light chain ratio of 100 or more, provided the absolute level of the involved free light chain is at least 100 mg/L
  [*Involved free light chain*—The one (either kappa or lambda) that is above the normal reference range; The uninvolved light chain—The one that typically is in, or below, the normal range]
- **MRI**: More than one focal lesion, at least 5 mm or greater in size.
  Any of the above is sufficient enough to diagnose multiple myeloma regardless of the presence or absence of symptoms or CRAB features.

Q. What are the systemic involvement and complications?

- **Neurological:**
  - Due to hypercalcemia—lethargy, weakness, depression, confusion
  - Due to hyperviscosity—headache, fatigue, shortness of breath, visual disturbances, ataxia, vertigo, retinopathy, coma
  - Cord compression
  - Radicular pain
  - Loss of bladder and bowel control
  - Carpal tunnel syndrome
  - Sensorimotor mono- or polyneuropathy.
- **Kidney:**
  - Renal failure: Hypercalcemia, glomerular deposits of amyloid, hyperuricemia, recurrent infections, frequent use of nonsteroidal anti-inflammatory agents for pain control, use of iodinated contrast dye for imaging, bisphosphonate use, and occasional infiltration of the kidney by myeloma cells.
- **Hematological:**
  - Microcytic hypochromic anemia
  - Megaloblastic anemia.
- **Bony involvement:**
  - Osteolytic lesion

- Pathologic fracture
- Vertebral wedge compression.

- **Infection:**
  - Recurrent chest infection
  - UTI.
- **Others:**
  - Thrombosis.

Q. What are the common biochemical features?

- Hypercalcemia
- Hyperuricemia
- Increased urea, creatinine
- Increased total protein, globulin, altered albumin/globulin ratio
- Normal alkaline phosphatase.

Q. What are the other radiological features?

- Fracture
- Vertebral wedge compression.

Q. What are the investigations to be done for this patient?

- Blood—routine blood, total protein, ESR, CRP, calcium, uric acid, urea, creatinine, IgM, IgG, LFT
- Serum immunoelectrophoresis
- Urine M protein, Ben Jones protein
- Bone marrow biopsy for plasmacytosis
- Imaging—MRI, bone scan.

Q. How will you stage the disease?

By any of these staging system:

1. **International staging system:** To predict survival.
   Stage I → beta2M <3.5, alb ≥3.5
   Stage II → beta2M <3.5, alb <3.5 *or* beta2M = 3.5–5.5
   Stage III → beta2M >5.5
2. **Durie–Salmon staging system:** No longer used because can not predict outcome.

Stage 1

- Hb>10 g/dL
- Serum calcium <3 mmol/L
- Normal bone X-ray or solitary lesion
- Low M component production.

Stage 2—Neither fitting stage 1 or 3

Stage 3—One or more of the following:

- Hb <8.5g/dL
- Serum calcium >3 mmol/L
- Advanced lytic bone lesion
- High M component production.

Q. What are the prognostic factors?

- Serum beta2M:
  - Levels <0.004 g/L—median survival of 43 months
  - Levels >0.004 g/L—median survival of only 12 months.
- Poor prognosis:
  - High labelling index, circulating plasma cells, performance status, and high levels of lactate dehydrogenase.
- Others:
  - Presence of cytogenetic abnormalities and hypodiploidy by karyotype, fluorescent in situ hybridization (FISH)—identified chromosome 17p deletion, and translocations t (4; 14), (14; 16), and t (14; 20).

Q. What are the causes of anemia in multiple myeloma?

- Replacement of normal marrow by expanding tumor cells
- Inhibition of hematopoiesis by factors made by the tumor
- Reduced production of erythropoietin by the kidney
- Effects of long-term therapy
- Mild hemolysis
- Megaloblastic anemia due to either folate or vitamin B_{12} deficiency.

Q. What are the options for treatment of MM?

- Treatment of choice is bone marrow transplantation
- Primary treatment of multiple myeloma is chemotherapy
- Symptomatic bone lesions usually respond rapidly to radiation treatment 40 Gy
- Standard treatment for newly diagnosed cases depends on whether the patient is a candidate for high-dose chemotherapy or with autologous stem-cell transplant
- Supportive care directed at the anticipated complications
- Patients with symptomatic and/or progressive myeloma require therapeutic intervention
  - 2 sorts of such therapy
    - Systemic therapy to control the progression of myeloma
    - Symptomatic supportive care to prevent serious morbidity from the complications of the disease.

Q. What is the drug of choice?

- Melphalan.

Q. What are the other medications?

- Glucorticoids, vincristine, doxorubicin, thalidomide.

Q. Role of radiotherapy in treatment?

- Symptomatic bony lesion responds rapidly by radiation.

Q. Common causes of death in MM?
- Progressive myeloma, renal failure
- Sepsis—pulmonary infection.

Q. What is the overall prognosis?
- Overall median survival is 5–6 years with subsets of patients surviving over 10 years.

Vertebral Wedging

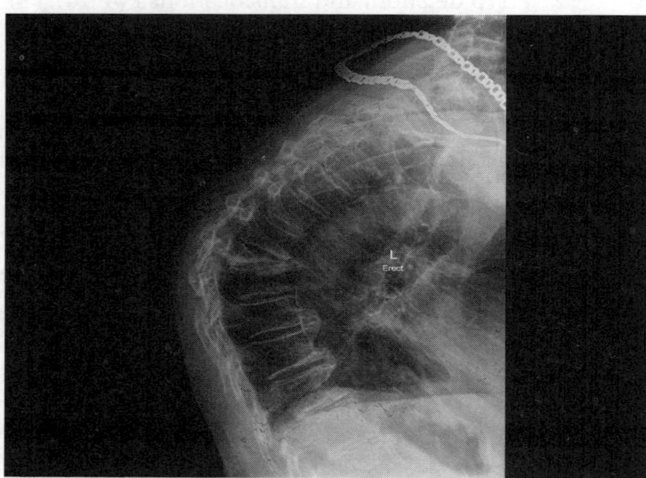

Figure 5.10: X-ray plate of dorsolumbar spine showing wedging of D12 vertebrae without any significant changes in disc spaces

Figure 5.10 is an X-ray plate of dorsolumbar spine showing wedging of D12 vertebrae without any significant changes in disc spaces. So, I think this is a case of vertebral wedging likely due to osteoporosis.

PD: Osteoporotic wedging

Differential Diagnosis
- Post-traumatic wedging
- Neoplastic wedging
- Metastatic wedging
- Infective (Carrie's spine) wedging.

Q. How will you investigate?
- Blood: For CBC, ESR, CRP
- Biochemical: Calcium, phosphate, alkaline phosphatase, uric acid, urea creatinine
- Chest X-ray for any lung lesion
- MRI dorsolumber spine to rule out infection, neoplasia, metastasis
- Lymph-node biopsy if lymphadenopathy present
- Bone marrow biopsy for plasmacytosis
- CT-guided FNAC from involved vertebrae for histopathological examination
- DEXA scan for osteoporosis.

Q. What are the indications of MRI?
- Extreme of ages:Back pain in children <18 years with considerable pain or onset >55 years
- Mild trauma in an aged patient
- Night pain
- Immunodeficiency: History of cancer, systemic steroids, drug abuse, human immunodeficiency virus infection
- Constitutional symptoms
- Persisting severe restriction of motion
- Intense pain or minimal motion
- Structural deformity
- Neurological involvement:
  - Difficulty with micturition
  - Loss of anal sphincter tone or fecal incontinence; saddle anesthesia
  - Widespread progressive motor weakness or gait disturbance.

Q. How you will manage the case?
- Postural care: Improve posture, transfers, and gait pattern to limit vertebral compression forces
- Pharmacology: Local NSAIDs, patch, muscle relaxant and oral analgesic
- Stabilisation of spine:
  - **Orthosis:** Thoracolumbar support, such as the CASH brace, lumbosacral corset, and thoracolumbosacral orthosis (TLSO) depend upon etiology and level of wedging
  - **Surgery:** Vertebroplasty, kyphoplasty.
- PT: strengthening exercise-> strengthening of paravertebral, abdominal, and gluteal muscles
- Modality: Dry heat for pain relief
- OT: To improve balance, flexibility, and posture and stress relieve
- Treatment of underlying cause.

Q. What is vertebroplasty?

It is a minimally invasive spinal procedure in which an acrylic bony cement is injected in a compressed vertebrae under fluoroscopic guidance or CT guidance in order to restore vertebral height.

Salient features of vertebroplasty:

Indications:

Pain due to vertebral compression associated with osteoporosis, tumor infiltration.

Contraindications:
- Infection
- Uncorrectable coagulopathy
- Neurological features—compressive myelopathy
- No middle column compromise.

Complications:
- Cement leak
- Cement pulmonary embolism
- Cord compression
- Hematoma, infection
- Probable adjacent vertebral fractures.

Vertebroplasty vs kyphoplasty (Table 5.2)

Table 5.2: Difference between vertebroplasty vs kyphoplasty

Vertebroplasty	*Kyphoplasty*
• Cheaper • Quicker	• Expensive • Takes longer time • Restoration of vertebral height questionable • Less adjacent fractures • Less cement leakage • Quality of life increased

Bamboo Spine

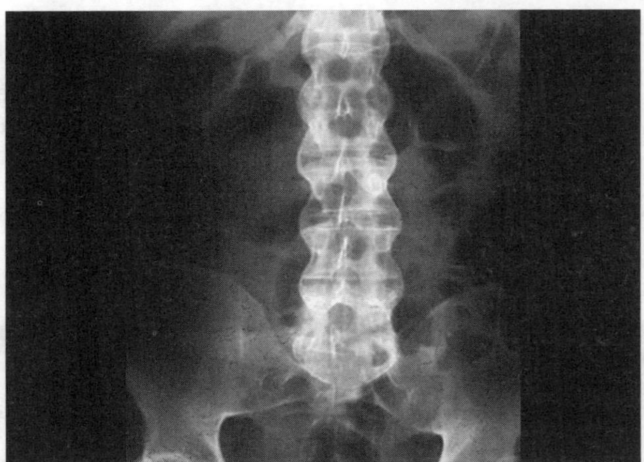

Figure 5.11: X-ray plate of AP view of LS spine and pelvis showing ligamentous calcification of anterior and lateral side of spine along with sclerosis of both SI joint typically looks like bamboo spine

Figure 5.11 is a X-ray plate of AP view of LS spine and pelvis showing ligamentous calcification of anterior and lateral side of spine along with sclerosis of both SI joint typically looks like bamboo spine. So, I think this patient is suffering from ankylosing spondylosis.

Q. What is bamboo spine?
It is a radiographic feature of AS which occurs due to vertebral fusion by marginal syndesmophytes.

Q. What is syndesmophyte?
Ossification of anterior portion annulus fibrosis of intervertebral disc.

Q. What are difference between syndesmophyte and osteophyte?
Osteophyte is bony spur occurs due to ossification of anterior longitudinal ligament, seen in degenerative changes and syndesmophyte is ossification of anterior annulus fibrosis, seen in AS.

Q. What is Romanus lesion?
It is a radiographic feature of AS characterized by sclerotic lesion on vertebral endplate usually at the junction of annulus fibrosis with vertebral endplate.

Q. What are the differences between radiological features of DISH and bamboo spine?
- In DISH there is flowing ossification of anterior longitudinal ligament, so characteristic features is flowing wax sign
- In bamboo spine there is vertebral body fusion by marginal osteophyte laterally and anteriorly.

Q. What are the hindrances of bamboo spine in rehabilitation point of view?
- Rigid spine with severely restricted spinal motion
- Increased chance of fracture
- Difficulty in ADL.

Q. Is there any indication of DEXA scan in this patient?
Yes: This patient is prone to osteoporosis, and easy pathological fracture. Hence, DEXA scan may be helpful for the patient.

Diffuse Idiopathic Skeletal Hyperostosis

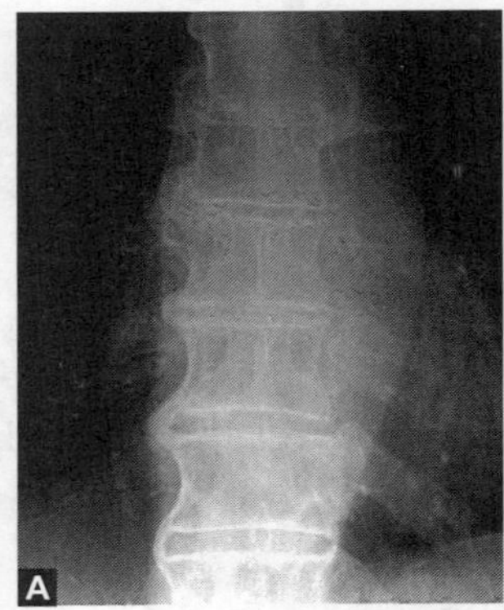

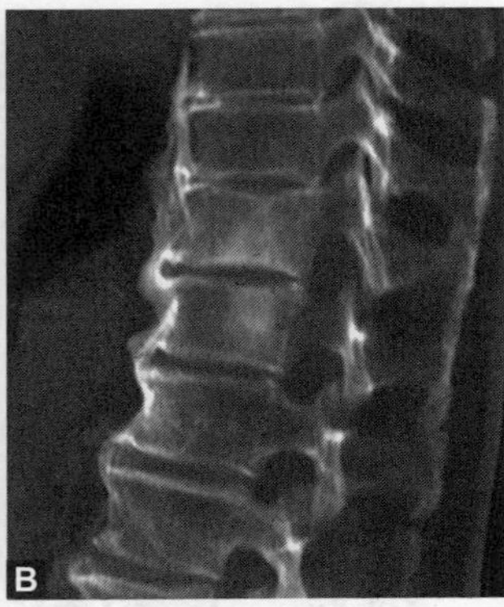

Figures 5.12A and B: X-ray of dorsolumbar spine showing marked calcification of ligaments along with flowing wax sign at dorsal spine

Figure 5.12 is a X-ray of dorsolumbar spine showing marked calcification of ligaments along with flowing wax sign at dorsal spine. So, I think this patient is suffering from diffuse idiopathic skeletal hyperostosis (DISH).

Q. What is DISH?
Presence of large flowing osteophyte at least 4 vertebrae, typically in thoracic spine (other vertebrae and peripheral joints may also be involved).

Q. What is flowing wax sign?

Appearance of sclerotic cortical thickening typically occurs in one side of bone and looks like melted wax from a bone.

Q. What are the diagnostic criteria of DISH?

- At least 4 contiguous vertebrae
- Preservation of IV disc and absence of extensive radiographic features of degenerative disc disease
- Absence of bony ankylosis and sacroilitis, intraarticular osseous fusion.

Q. What are the differential diagnoses?

- AS
- Fluoride exposure
- Paget's disease
- Osteopetrosis.

Q. What are the common clinical presentations?

- Most cases are asymptomatic
- Early morning stiffness
- Dorsolumbar pain
- Restricted spinal motion
- Joint pain
- Diminished chest expansion
- Complications:
  - Fracture
  - Neurological
  - Dysphagia, hoarseness, stridor
  - Myelopathy
  - Aspiration pneumonia
  - Sleep apnea
  - Atlantoaxial joint subluxation
  - Thoracic outlet syndrome.

Q. What are the areas involved?

- Thoracic
- Cervical
- Lumbar
- Peripheral joints (small and large)—not usually involved in OA
- Enthesis.

Q. What are the risk factors?

- Idiopathic
- Diabetes mellitus
- Obesity
- Hypertension
- Hyperinsulinemia
- Dyslipidemia
- Increased growth hormone/IGF-1
- Hyperuricemia
- Retinoids
- Genetics.

Q. How you will manage the case?

- Posture maintenance
- Weight reduction
- Diet low in fat and carbohydrate
- Pharmacological—analgesic, muscle relaxant for pain and stiffness—local or oral
- Treatment of underlying cause
- Treatment of complications
- Nonpharmacological:
  - PT
    - Strengthening of paravertebral, abdominal muscles
    - ROM exercise
    - Deep breathing.
  - OT
    - Relaxation technique
    - Joint protection.
- PO—depends upon symptoms and signs like soft insole for plantar fasciitis.

Q. What is the prognosis?

- Complete pathologic process requires 10 years
- Increased fracture risk
- It is associated with metabolic abnormalities (incidental finding of DISH should prompt careful evaluation of cardiovascular risk factor).

Q. What are the differentiating points between AS and DISH?

Difference between DISH and AS have been discussed in Table 5.3.

Table 5.3: Difference between DISH and AS

	DISH	*AS*
Age	Elderly—6th–7th decade	Middle aged—18–45 yrs
Nature of pain	Noninflammatory	Inflammatory
Site of pain	Usually dorsolumber	Usually lower back
Extra-articular features	Fracture, neurological complications, dysphagia, hoarseness of voice, stride, etc	Uveitis, conduction abnormality, ascending aortitis, apical fibrosis, fracture, etc
Biochemical	Increased IGF-1, growth hormone	In some patient elevated ALP
Inflammatory marker	Normal usually	Elevated ESR, CRP
HLAB27 linkage	Approximately 1/3 patient	60–80%
X-ray vertebrae	Flowing wax sign	Bamboo spine
Pharmalogical—Role of biologics	No	Yes, associated with peripheral arthritis

Chondrocalcinosis

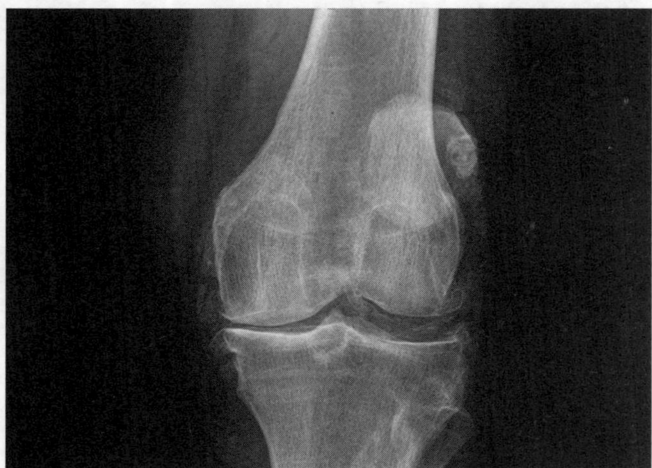

Figure 5.13: X-ray plate of knee joint AP view showing calcification of menisci in both medial and lateral joint space

Figure 5.13 is an X-ray plate of knee joint AP view showing calcification of menisci in both medial and lateral joint space. So, I think this patient is suffering from chondrocalcinosis.

Q. What is chondrocalcinosis?

Radiographic evidence of calcification in hyaline and/or fibrocartilage.

Q. What are the etiologies?

- Pseudogout
- Alkaptonuria
- Strong association with OA
- Aging
- Mechanical knee trauma/menisectomy
- Familial
- Hyperparathyroidism
- Renal failure on dialysis
- Hemochromatosis
- Gout
- Hypothyroidism
- Neuropathic disease
- Wilson's disease
- Articular amyloidosis.

Q. What is pseudogout?

Acute symptoms of joint inflammation or synovitis due to metabolic arthropathy caused by the deposition of calcium pyrophosphate dihydrate (CPPD) in and around joints, especially in hyaline and fibrocartilage of joints.

Q. What are the common joints involved in pseudogout?

- Knee
- Wrist, shoulder, elbow, hips and midtarsals
- Hand—2nd and 3rd metacarpophalangeal joints are most commonly affected.

Q. What are the salient features of pseudogout?

Clinical features

A. Acute pseudogout:

Most common cause of acute monoarthritis in elderly

- *Triggering factors:*
  - Direct trauma
  - Intercurrent illness
  - Any surgery.
- *Typical attack:*
  - Resembles gout
  - Rapidly developing
  - Severe pain, stiffness and swelling within 6–24 hours
  - Redness of joints.
- *Examination:*
  - Very tender joint
  - Loose pack position of joint
  - Marked synovitis
  - Large/tense effusion, warm, restricted movement and stress pain
  - Fever, confusion, ill looking.

B. Chronic pseudogout:

Most common in elderly female

Typical symptoms:

- Chronic pain
- Variable early morning stiffness
- Functional impairment
- Acute attacks may superimpose in chronic pain.

Examination:

- Features of osteoarthritis—bony swelling, crepitus, restriction of ROM
- Synovitis
- Wrist involvement—carpal tunnel syndrome
- Large/tense effusion, warm, restricted movement and stress pain.

- *Investigation:*
  - Synovial fluid examination—crystal study (negative birefrigent rhomboid-shaped crystal)
  - X-ray
  - Blood for calcium, alkaline phosphatase, magnesium, ferritin, LFTs.
- *Management:*
  - Aspiration of synovial fluid
  - Intraarticular steroid injection
  - NSAIDs and colchicine (avoid in very elderly patients)

- PT—early mobilization, strengthening exercise
- Home modification.

Q. What are the salient features of alkaptonuria?

- Autosomal recessive disorder affecting phenylalanine and tyrosine metabolism due to homgentisic acid dioxygenase (HGA) deficiency
- HGA accumulation causes ochronosis
- Blackening and destruction of cartilage and connective tissue (spine, hips, knees, shoulders, aortic valve)
- Clinical features:
  - Dark urine which become black after several hours
  - Arthritis
  - Blackening ear
  - Dark spot in eye.
- Investigations:
  - Urine analysis
    - After adding sodium or potassium hydroxide urine become dark
    - Fehling's test
    - Urine HGA (homogenticic acid).
- Treatment:
  - Prevention of ameliorating symptoms
  - Diet low in phenylalanine and tyrosine
  - Prevention of complication
  - PT—ROM and strengthening exercise
  - OT—relaxation, joint protection technique.

Spina Bifida

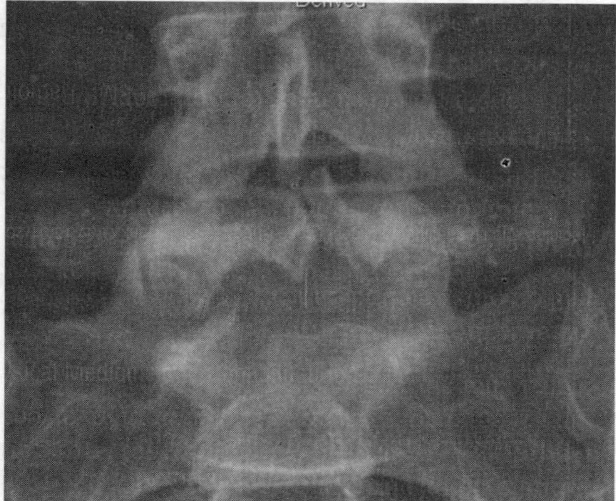

Figure 5.14: X-ray of LS spine AP view showing bifid spinous process of L5 vertebrae

Figure 5.14 is a X-ray of LS spine AP view showing bifid spinous process of L5 vertebrae. So, I think this patient is suffering from spina bifida occulta.

Q. What is spina bifida occulta?

- Just incomplete closure of the posterior elements of the spine without any protrusion of neurologic elements
- Spina bifida sometimes used nonspecifically to all patients with a spinal dysraphism or those with incomplete closure of the posterior neuropore.

Q. What are the types?

I. Open.
II. Closed.

Q. What is the commonest?

Open type.

Q. What are the clinical presentations of spina bifida occulta?

- May be asymptomatic
- Pain
- Swelling, dimple in skin, truft of hair
- Paralysis, loss of a sensation, hydrocephalus, seizures, blindness
- Complications—
  - Low fitness
  - Obesity
  - Pressure sores
  - Respiratory difficulties
  - Learning and perceptual difficulties
  - Difficulty in ADL.

Q. What are the other congenital anomalies associated with spina bifida?

- Anenchephaly
- Encephalocele
- Chiari malformation
- Meckel syndrome
- Dandy: Walker malformation due to arrest of cerebellar development prior to the 3rd month resulting in:
  - Agenesis/hypoplasia of cerebellar vermis
  - Cystic dilatation of 4th ventricle
  - Enlargement of posterior fossa.
- Congenital cardiac defects—ASD>VSD
- Facial defects—cleft lip, cleft palate
- GI tract anomaly
- Urinary tract anomaly—solitary kidney, malformed uterus.

Q. What is tethered cord syndrome?

In meningomyelocele the spinal cord can be fixed or tethered at one point causing traction and leading to progressive neurological, urological and orthopedic deficit.

Q. How will you manage spina bifida with tethered cord?

Prenatal: Folic acid supplementation, surgery

Postnatal: Surgery (24 hours after birth)

After surgery:

- PT/OT:
  - Group play is better
  - Upper body activities
  - Strength training
  - Aquatics
  - Flexibility—ROM exercise
  - Parachute activities
  - Wheelchair activities.
- PO:
  - Braces
  - Crutches
  - Wheelchairs
  - Other assistive device.
- Home modification.
- Counseling of family member and parents.
- Treatment of complications and associated anomaly.

Q. What are the complications?

- Pressure sore and skin irritations
- Latex allergy
- Bladder and bowel control problems
- Musculoskeletal deformities (scoliosis)
- Joint and extremity deformities—joint contractures, club foot, hip subluxations, diminished growth of non-weight bearing limbs
- Osteoporosis
- Tethered spinal cord syndrome.

Q. What are the risk factors of spina bifida?

- Multi-factorial inheritance
- Folic acid and vitamin B_{12} deficiencies
- Type 1 DM
- Maternal fever
- Mineral like zinc deficiency
- Viral infection
- Alcohol
- Medication—carbamazepine, valproic acid.

Q. What is spina bifida aparta?

Midline defect that communicates with the external environment.

Q. What is spina bifida cystica?

- Protrusion of sac filled with cerebrospinal fluid from the spinal column, also includes meningomyelocele and meningocele
- Meningocele:
  - Meninges protrude through the defect.
- Salient points on meningomyelocele:
  - Elements of the cord also protrude through the defect along with meninges, resulting in severe neural deficits
  - 1–2/1000 live birth
  - F:M—1.2:1
  - 85% occur in lumbosacral region
  - Most common neural tube defect.
- Clinical features:
  - Both meninges and spinal cord protrude from the defect
  - CSF leak
  - Paraplegia/Paraparesis
  - Meningitis
  - Neurogenic bowel or bladder
  - Hydrocephalus
  - Short stature, precocious puberty.
- Myelocele:
  - Part of spinal cord exposed in back with or without covering of meninges.

Spondylolysis/Spondylolisthesis

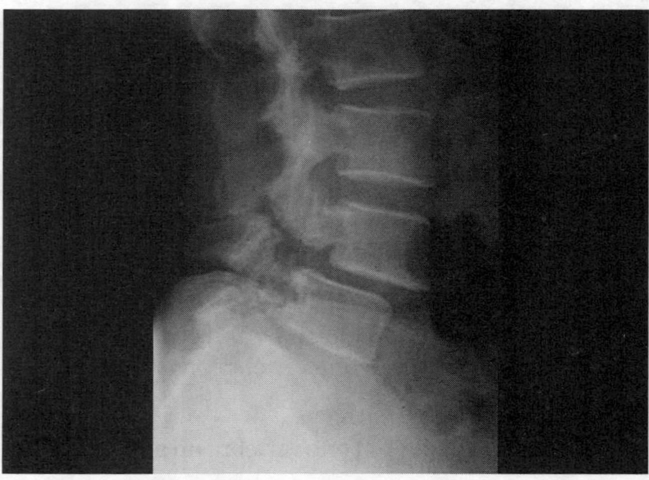

Figure 5.15: X-ray of LS spine lateral view showing break in pars interarticularis at L4–5 level with anterior displacement of L4 over L5

Figure 5.15 is a X-ray of LS spine lateral view showing break in pars interarticularis at L4-5 level with anterior displacement of L4 over L5. So, this patient is suffering from grade I anterior spondylolisthesis with spondylysis at L4–5 level.

Q. What is spondylysis?

Defect of the pars interarticularis or the isthmus between the superior and inferior articular facets.

Q. What are the etiologies?
- Acquired
- Injury
- Repetitive stress of spine
- Dysplasia.

Q. What are the grades?
By Tokushima classification:
- *Acute (early)*: Hairline defect
- *Progressive:* Moderately wide defect with round margins
- *Terminal (chronic):* Wide defect with sclerotic margins.

Q. What are the clinical features?
- Mechanical low back pain exacerbated by extension
- Local tenderness
- Hamstring tightness.

Q. Which X-ray view is best?
Oblique view.

Q. What are the other radiological tests?
- SPECT
- CT scan
- MRI.

Q. How will you manage the case?
- Relative rest—3 months
- Activity modification
- Immobilization—By LSO, not mandatory
- For pain—analgesic, muscle relaxant—local or oral
- PT—LS stabilization
  - Paraspinal, abdominal muscle strengthening
  - Aerobic conditioning.
- Surgery is rarely indicated.

Q. What is spondylolisthesis?
Anterior slippage of one vertebra on another.

Q. What is retrolisthesis?
Posterior slippage of one vertebra on another.

Q. What is laterallisthesis?
Lateral slippage of one vertebrae over another.

Q. What are the types?
I. **Isthmic spondylolisthesis**: Occurs as a result of a spondylolysis or stress fracture of the pars interarticularis.
II. **Dysplastic spondylolisthesis**: A congenital slip, caused by dysplasia of the facet joints, leading to an inability to resist shear stresses and forward slippage.
III. **Degenerative spondylolisthesis**:Long-standing intersegmental instability from degenerative facet or disc disease.
IV. **Traumatic spondylolisthesis**: Caused by acute fracture secondary to trauma.
V. **Pathologic spondylolisthesis**: Caused by decreased bony strength due to medical causes of generalized or local bone disease.
VI. **Postsurgical spondylolisthesis**: Caused by resulting instability from an extensive decompression surgery.

Q. What are the gradings?

Grade	percentage of slippage
1	<25
2	25–49
3	50–74
4	75–99
5	≥100 (spondyloptosis)

Q. Which X-ray view is best?
Ferguson coronal view.

Q. What is slip angle?
- Angle formed by intersection of a line drawn parallel to inferior or superior aspect of the L5 vertebrae and a line drawn perpendicular to posterior border of S1 vertebrae
- More than 55 degree indicates high probability and increased rate of progression.

Q. What are the clinical features?
- Asymptomatic
- Back pain or fatigue
- Muscle spasm, restricted spinal motion
- Radicular pain
- Step off sign
- Hamstring tightness
- Typical gait: Waddle with limited hip flexion, wide-based short stride
- Neurological involvement: Sensory disturbances, muscle weakness, bladder and bowel involvement
- Structural deformity: Hyperlordosis, lumbosacral kyphosis,scoliosis, spina bifida, flat buttock, etc.

Q. What are the risk factors for progression of curve?
- Younger age
- Female gender
- Dysplastic type
- Dome-shaped sacrum
- Slip >50%
- Slip angle >40–50% (N—<10%)

Q. What are the investigations?
- **X-ray:**
  - AP, lateral, flexion/extension, oblique
  - Reverse Napoleon hat sign: Severe slip of L5 through the sacrum
- **CT:** Best to pick up spondylolysis
- **MRI:** Best for neural element assessment

- **Technetium 99:** Most sensitive in acute fracture of pars articularis in child and young athlete.

Q. What is the treatment guidance?
- Patient education and assurance
- Relative rest
- Activity modification
- Immobilisation—By LSO (mandatory)
- For pain—analgesic like NSAIDs, muscle relaxant —local or oral; anticonvulsant-like gabapentine, pregabaline; tricyclic antidepressant like amitryptiline; opioids
- PT:
  - Exercise
    - LS stabilization
    - Paraspinal, abdominal muscle strengthening
    - Aerobic conditioning
    - Aquatic exercise
  - Modality—TENSE
  - Interventions—See chapter 10 page number 250.

Q. What are the indications of surgery?
- Grade 3 or more
- Persisting pain after appropriate rehabilitation program (9 months to 1 year)
- Persisting radiculopathy
- Progressive instability.

Q. What are the different types of surgery?
- Decompression (laminectomy) and stabilization surgery
- Fusion surgery.

Q. When intervention should be done?
See Chapter 10, page number 250.

Hemivertebrae

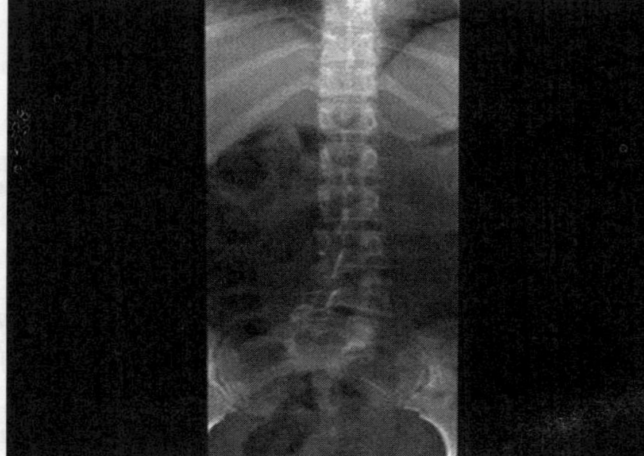

Figure 5.16: X-ray of lumbar spine showing absence of one side of L4 vertebrae with mild scoliosis

Figure 5.16 is the X-ray of lumbar spine showing absence of one side of L4 vertebrae with mild scoliosis. So, I think the patient is having hemivertebrae.

Q. What is hemivertebrae?
Congenital deformity resulting from defect in formation of vertebrae that will result in curvature.

Q. What are the centers of ossification?
- Primary:
  - One in center
  - One for each half of neural arch.
- Secondary:
  - Tip of spinous process
  - One in each tip of tranverse process
  - As ring epiphysis at the upper and lower surfaces of vertebral bodies.

Q. What are the congenital vertebral anomalies?
- Block vertebrae
- Hemivertebtrae
- Combination of both.

Q. What are the other anomalies associated with hemivertebrae?
- Genitourinary anomalies
- Cardiac anomalies
- Klippel–Feil syndrome
- Spondylothoracic dysplasia
- Absence rib
- Absence nerve root
- Sprengel's shoulder
- Hand and foot deformity.

Q. What are the common clinical presentations?
- Asymptomatic
- Scoliosis
- Pain.

Q. How you will manage the patient?
- Posture care
- Patient education and counselling
- Pain control—by NSAIDs, local/oral
- PT:
  - Scoliosis correcting exercise
  - Aerobic training
  - Deep breathing
  - Strengthening of paraspinal, abdominal, extremity muscle.
- OT:
  - Relaxation technique
  - Improvement and training of ADL.
- Bracing—in case of progressive scoliosis brace like Boston
- Surgery.

Q. What are the indications of surgery?

- Increasing curve in growing child
- Curve >40 degree before skeletal maturity
- In neuromuscular disease curve >35 degree
- Pain uncontrolled by nonoperative treatment
- Thoracic lordosis
- Significant cosmetic deformity.

Cobb's Angle

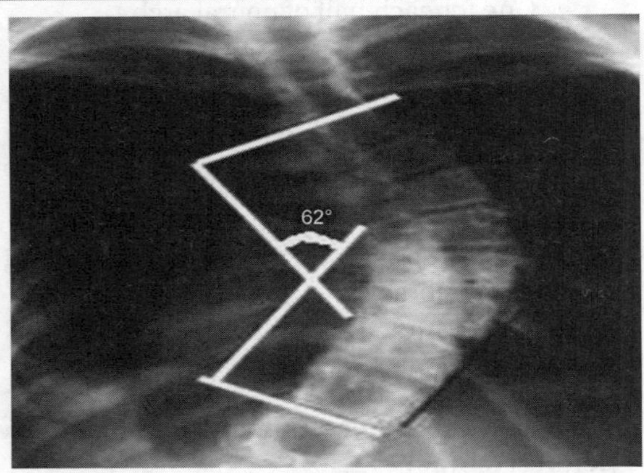

Figure 5.17: X-ray of dorsolumbar spine showing scoliosis of left-sided convexity with Cobb's angle 62 degree

Figure 5.17 is the X-ray of dorsolumbar spine showing scoliosis of left-sided convexity with Cobb's angle 62 degree. So, I think this patient is having scoliosis with Cobb's angle 62 degree with apical vertebrae D8.

Q. What is Cobb's angle?

- Choose the first and last vertebrae that tilt into the concavity of the curve
- Draw a line perpendicular to that vertebrae
- The angle created between these intersecting lines is the Cobb's angle.

Q. How you will measure?

See above.

Q. What are the implications of Cobb's angle in management strategy?

Implications of Cobb's angle in management have been discussed in Table 5.4.

Table 5.4: Implication of Cobb's angle in treatment

Cobb's angle	*Riser grade*	*X-ray /Refer*	*Treatment*
10–19	0–1	Every 6 months/no	Observe
10–19	2–4	Every 6 months/no	Observe
20–29	0–1	Every 6 months/yes	Brace after 25 degree
20–29	2–4	Every 6 months/yes	Observe/Brace
30–40	0–1	Refer	Brace
30–40	2–4	Refer	Brace
>40	0–4	Refer	Surgery

(For all other related question please see scoliosis, See Chapter 3 page number 112)

Caries Spine—X-ray

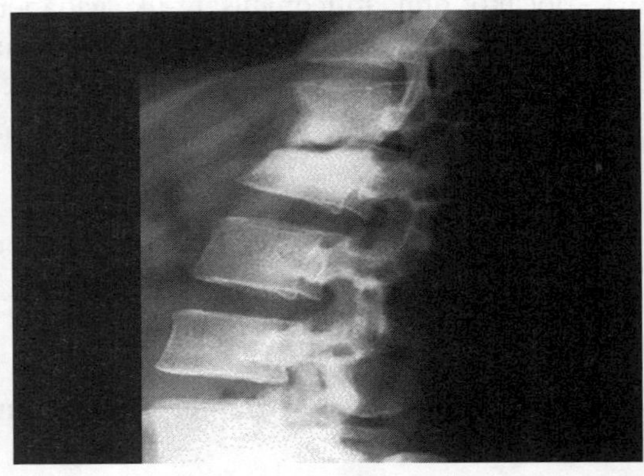

Figure 5.18: X-ray plate of dorsolumber spine showing reduced disc space of T12–L1 intervertebral disc with irregularity and sclerosis of adjacent vertebrae end plate and anterior wedging of L1 vertebrae

Figure 5.18 is a X-ray plate of dorsolumber spine showing reduced disc space of T12–L1 intervertebral disc with irregularity and sclerosis of adjacent vertebrae end plate and anterior wedging of L1 vertebrae. So, I think this patient is suffering from tuberculosis of spine.

Carries Spine—MRI Caries

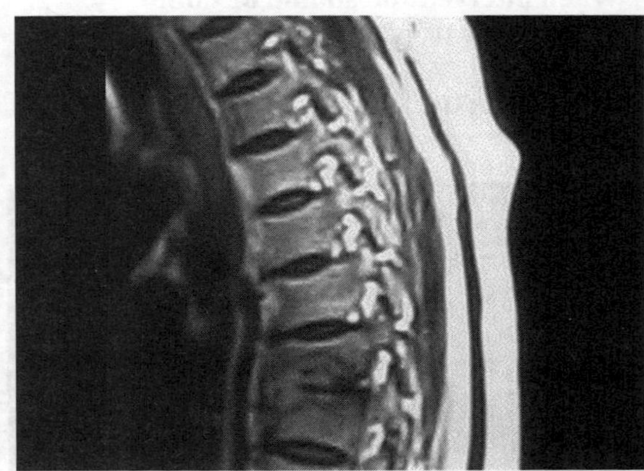

Figure 5.19: MRI of dorsolumbar spine in T2-weighted image showing hyperintense marrow with destruction of the intervertebral disc space and endplates of the adjacent vertebral bodies

Figure 5.19 is MRI of dorsolumbar spine in T2-weighted image showing hyperintense marrow with destruction of the intervertebral disc space and endplates of the

adjacent vertebral bodies. So, I think this is a MRI of carries spine.

Differential diagnosis

- Brucelosis
- Pyogenic infection
- Sarcoidosis
- Metastasis.

Mucopolysacharidosis

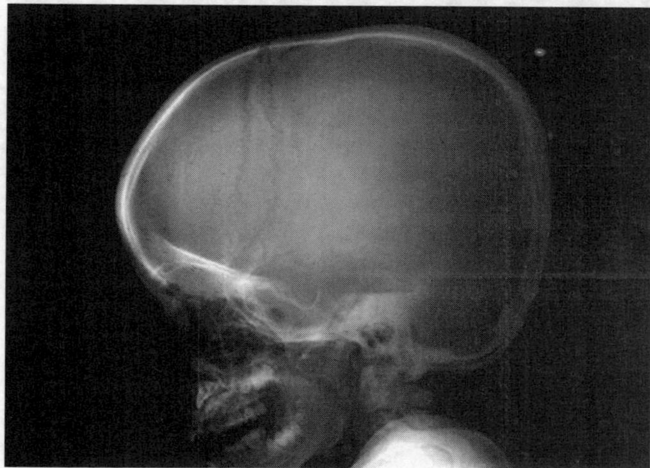

Figure 5.20: X-ray plate of skull showing J-shaped sella, thickened cortical bone, lack of pneumatization of mastoid and paranasal cavities

Figure 5.20 is a X-ray plate of skull showing J-shaped sella, thickened cortical bone, lack of pneumatization of mastoid and paranasal cavities. So, I think this is a x-ray of a patient of mucopolysacharidosis.

Other Area

- Spine X-ray
  - Central baking—Morquio disease
  - **Anteroinferior baking**—Hurler or other MPS
- Hand X-ray—**Bullet**-shaped metacarpals.

Q. What is mucopolysaccharidosis?

Deficiency of enzymes necessary to breakdown mucopolysaccharides (MPS) resulting in excessive accumulation of mucopolysaccharides in body tissues.

Q. What are the clinical features?

- Skeletal deformities (especially of the face)
- Mental retardation
- Decreased life expectancy.

Q. What are the different types?

- Hunter syndrome
- Hurler syndrome
- Scheie syndrome
- Sanfilippo syndrome
- Morquio disease
- Maroteaux–Lamy syndrome.

Complex Regional Pain Syndrome

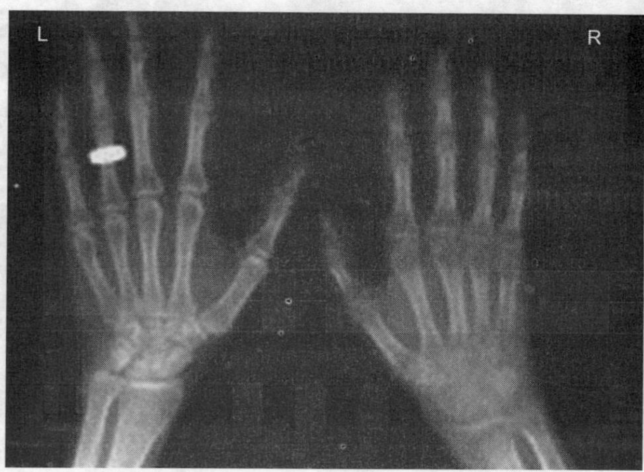

Figure 5.21: X-ray plate of both hand showing diffuse blotchy osteoporosis in right hand with malunited Colle's fracture in right wrist

Figure 5.21 is X-ray plate of both hand of middle-aged woman showing diffuse blotchy osteoporosis in right hand with malunited Colle's fracture in right wrist. So, I think this patient is suffering from complex regional pain syndrome (CRPS).

Q. What is CRPS?

Complex regional pain syndrome is a pain syndrome occurring most often in an extremity in association with abnormal autonomic nervous system activity and trophic changes.

Q. What is Colle's fracture?

Distal radius fracture with dorsal and radial displacement of wrist and hand without involvement of articular surface.

Q. What is the mode of injury?

Fall on outstretched hand.

Q. What are the complications of Colle's fracture?

- Malunion with dinner-fork deformity
- CRPS
- Carpal tunnel syndrome
- Extensor pollicis longus tendon tear
- Secondary OA changes.

Q. What is reverse Colle's fracture?

It is a fracture of distal radius with volar angulation of distal fractured fragment caused by fall onto flexed wrist.

See Chapter 3 Page no. 72 for further questions on CRPS.

Osteomyelitis

Chronic Osteomyelitis

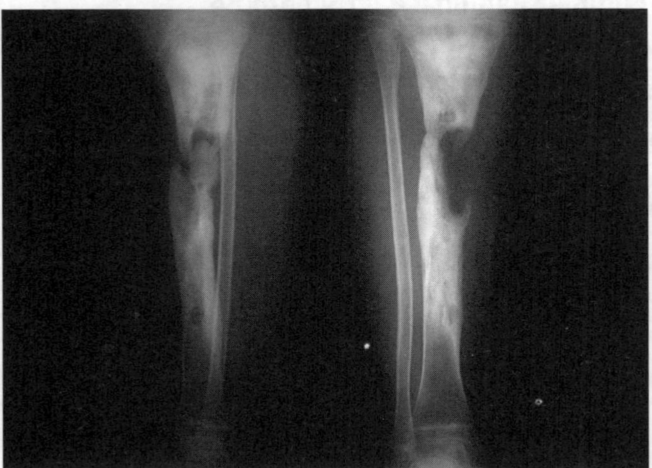

Figure 5.22: X-ray of right knee AP and lateral view showing destruction of bone both, periosteal reaction, new bone formation and peripheral sclerosis in upper and middle part of tibia

Figure 5.22 is a X-ray of right knee AP and lateral view showing destruction of bone both cortical and trabecular part, periosteal reaction, new bone formation and peripheral sclerosis in upper and middle part of tibia. So, this patient is having chronic osteomyelitis of right tibia.

Brodie's Abscess

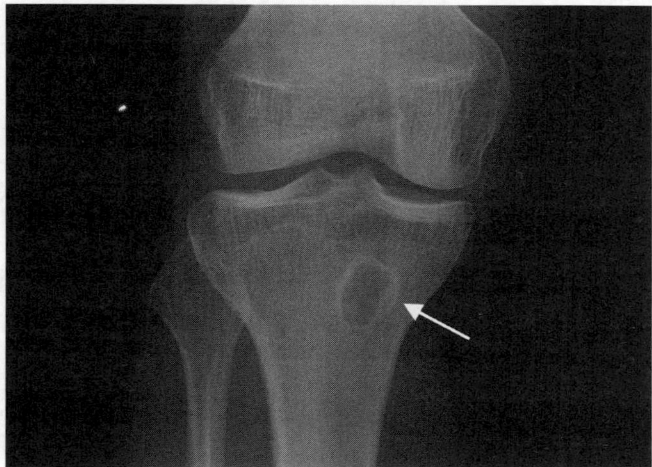

Figure 5.23: X-ray plate of knee and upper part of leg showing a circumscribed, oval cavity surrounded by a zone of sclerosis in upper tibia

Figure 5.23 is a X-ray plate of knee and upper part of leg showing a circumscribed, oval cavity surrounded by a zone of sclerosis in upper tibia. So, I think this is a X-ray of Brodie's abscess.

Brodie's abscess: Subacute pyogenic osteomyelitis manifested as intaosseous abscess.

See chapter 7 page number 213 for further questions on osteomyelitis.

BONE TUMORS

Giant Cell Tumor

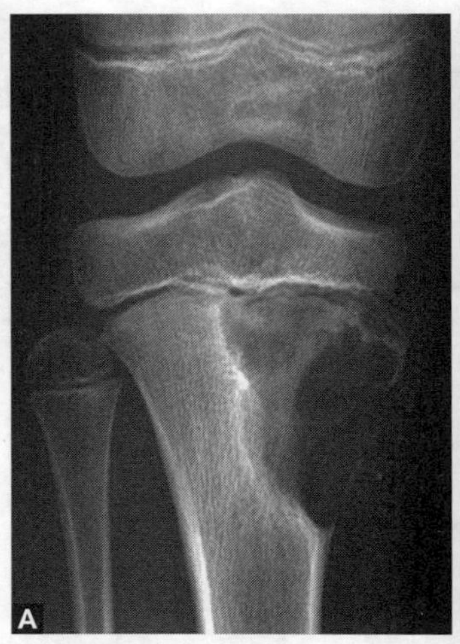

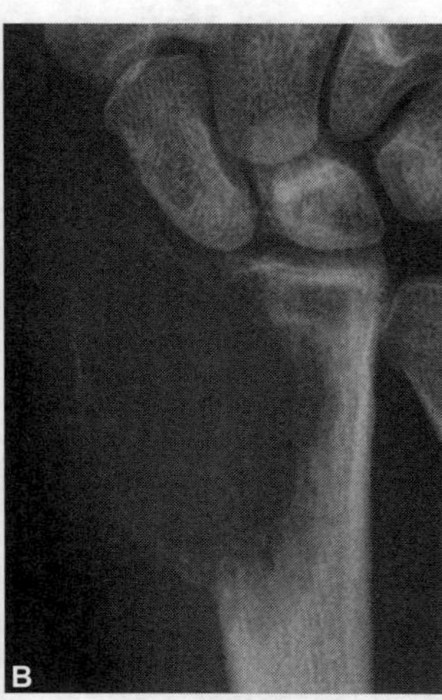

Figures 5.24A and B: X-ray plate of knee and wrist showing a well-defined lytic lesion in upper end of tibia and lower end of radius with closed growth plate and nonsclerotic margin resembles soap-bubble appearance

Figure 5.24 is a X-ray plate of knee and wrist showing a well-defined lytic lesion in upper end of tibia and lower end of radius with closed growth plate and nonsclerotic margin resembles soap-bubble appearance. So, I think this is a X-ray of giant cell tumor.

Q. What is the a of onset of giant cell tumor?
20–40 years.

Q. What are the common site of giant cell tumor?
- Around knee
- Lower end of radius.

Q. What are the common clinical features of GCT?
- Smooth swelling
- Pain
- Tenderness
- Egg-shell cracking sound
- Pathological fracture.

Q. Which investigations should be helpful?
- Routine blood investigations, ESR, CRP
- X-ray
- Bone scan
- CT scan
- MRI.

Q. What are the X-ray features of GCT?
- Solitary/Loculated lytic lesion
- Cortical expansion
- Soap-bubble appearance
- Sometimes sclerosis around the joint.

Q. What are the treatment options available?
- Excision of tumor
- Amputation
- Radiotherapy.

(Recurrence is the problem)

Osteosarcoma

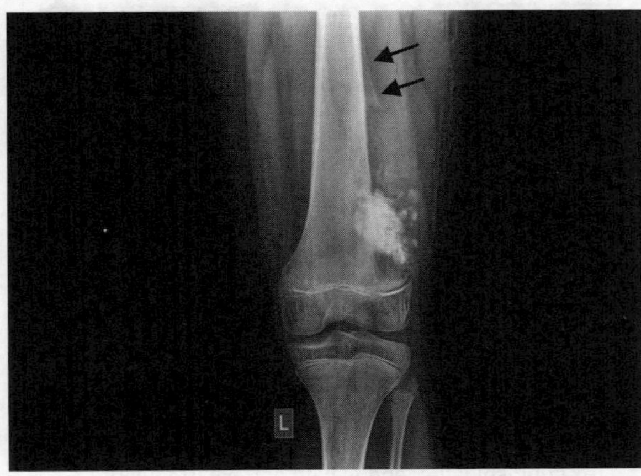

Figure 5.25: X-ray plate of knee showing destruction of cortex and medullary bone and new bone formation with irregular margin and Codman's triangle, appearing as sunray appearance

Figure 5.25 is X-ray plate of knee showing destruction of cortex and medullary bone and new bone formation with irregular margin and Codman's triangle, appearing as sunray appearance. So, I think this is a X-ray of osteosarcoma.

Q. What is the age of onset of osteosarcoma?
15–25 years.

Q. What are the common site of osteosarcoma?
- Lower end of femur—most common site
- Upper end of tibia
- Upper end of the humerus
- Any bone can be involved.

Q. What are the clinical presentation of osteosarcoma?
- Pain—increases with swelling
- Ill-defined swelling—warm and tender
- Often history of trauma
- Pathological fracture
- Limited ROM of adjacent joint
- Lymphadenopathy
- Symptoms due to compressed neurovascular structure.

Q. Which investigations will be helpful?
- X-ray
- Serum ALP—increased but no diagnostic value
- Bone biopsy
- Bone scan
- CT scan
- MRI scan.

Q. What are the X-ray features of osteosarcoma?
- Irregular destruction of metaphysis
- Erosion of cortex
- New bone formation
- Periosteal reaction
- Codman's triangle: Triangular area at the ends of tumor formed by subperiosteal new bone at the tumor host cortex junction
- Sun-ray appearance.

Q. What are treatment options available?
Depend upon extent of involvement of affected bone and spread of tumor:
- Amputation surgery
- Limb saving surgery
- Chemotherapy: High-dose methotrexate, citrovorum factor, cisplatin
- Immunotherapy
- Radiotherapy for local recurrence
- Follow-up every 6–8 weeks.

Q. What is secondary osteosarcoma?
Development of osteosarcoma over premalignant lesions called secondary osteosarcoma.
Premalignant disease causing osteosarcoma:
- Postradiation
- Paget's disease
- Diaphysial aclasis
- Enchondromatosis.

Simple Bone Cyst

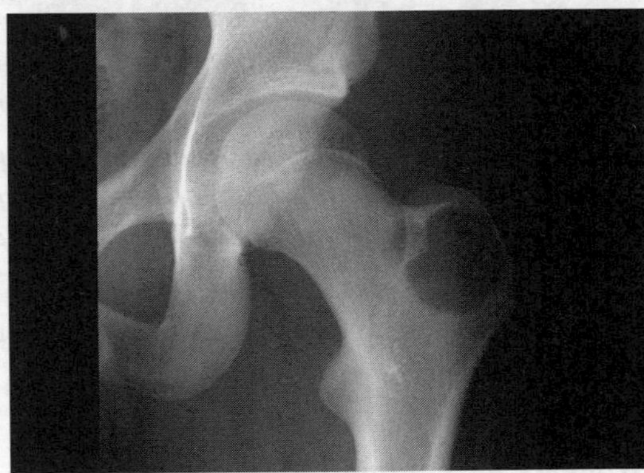

Figure 5.26: X-ray of left pelvis showing a well-defined, lobulated radiolucent cavity in upper end of femur, width is less than width of epiphyseal plate

Figure 5.26 is a X-ray of left pelvis showing a well-defined, lobulated radiolucent cavity in upper end of femur, width is less than width of epiphyseal plate. So, I think this is a X-ray of simple bone cyst.

Q. What is the age of presentation of simple bone cyst?
Children and adolescent.

Q. What are the common site?
- Upper end of humerus—commonest
- End of long bones.

Q. What are the clinical features of simple bone cyst?
- Asymptomatic
- Accidental findings in X-ray
- Little pain
- Pathological fractures.

Q. What are the treatment options available?
- Spontaneous healing
- Steroid injection
- Curettage
- Bone grafting.

Aneurysmal Bone Cyst

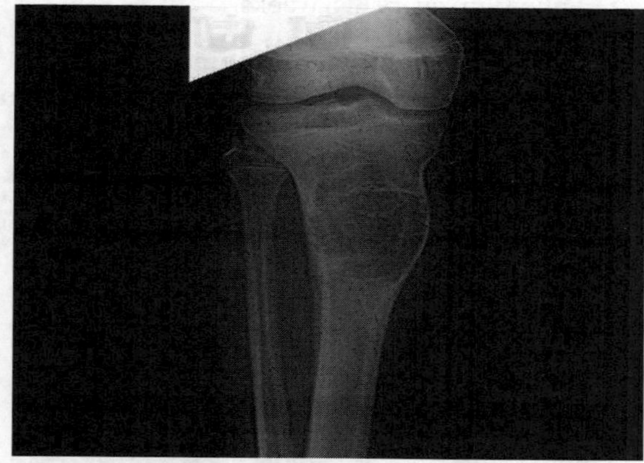

Figure 5.27: X-ray plate of knee showing well-defined, eccentric lytic lesion with overlying cortical expansion in upper end of tibia

Figure 5.27 is a X-ray plate of knee showing well-defined, eccentric lytic lesion with overlying cortical expansion in upper end of tibia. So, I think this is a X-ray plate of aneurismal bone cyst.

Q. What is the age of presentation of aneurismal bone cyst?
10–40 years.

Q. What are the common site?
Usually end of long bones.

Q. What are the clinical presentation of aneurismal bone cyst?
- Gradually increasing swelling
- Little pain
- Pathological fracture.

Q. How you will treat the patient?
Curettage and bone grafting.

USG: SHOULDER

Supraspinatus Tendinitis

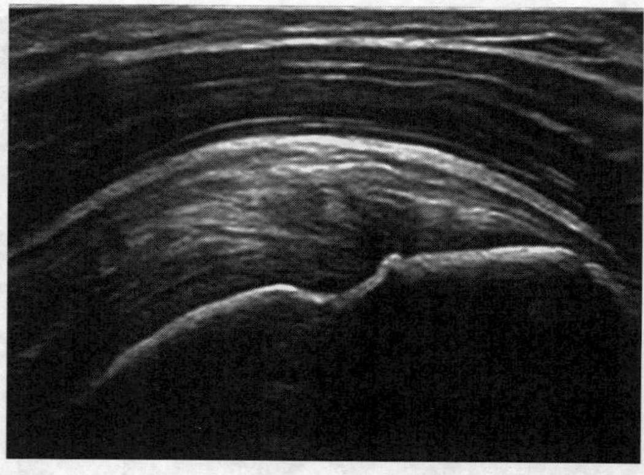

Figure 5.28: USG of shoulder joint showing tendinosis of supraspinatus tendon with cortical irregularity

Figure 5.28 is a USG of shoulder joint showing tendinosis of supraspinatus tendon with cortical irregularity.

Q. What is supraspinatus tendinitis?
Inflammation, pain and tenderness of supraspinatus tendon.

Q. What are the clinical features?
- Most commonly involved rotator calf tendinopathy
- More occassionaly presented with impingement syndrome
- Soulder stiffness and pain often radiating to upper lateral arm
- Symptoms increased by overhead activity, sleeping on affected side
- Shoulder ROM often painful specially abduction
- Difficulty in overhead activity due to pain
- Jobe's test:
  - Arm abducted in the plane of the scapula
  - Thumb pointing down
  - Resist elevation of the arm.

Q. What are the investigations needed?
- X-ray to rule out occult fracture
- USG of shoulder
- MRI of shoulder.

Q. How will you treat the patient?

- Pain: NSAIDs
- Ice compression
- Corticosteroid injection
- Modality: UST sometimes used
- Exercise:
  - Shoulder ROM ex
  - Strengthening of shoulder girdle muscle.
- Surgery: Subacromial decompression (open or arthroscopic) if impingement present.

(It may be advised after failure of conservative management after 3–6 months)

Supraspinatus Tear

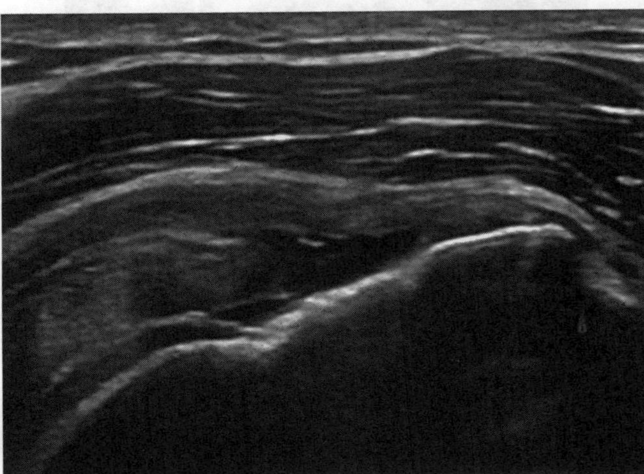

Figure 5.29: USG of shoulder joint showing full-thickness supraspinatus tear with thickened bursae

Figure 5.29 is USG of shoulder joint showing full-thickness supraspinatus tear with thickened bursae.

Q. What are the causes of supraspinatus year?

- Intrinsic factors:
  - Vascular supply (hypervascularity with tendonitis)
  - Degenerative changes: Age-related change in proteoglycan and collagen content in symptomatic tendons.
- Extrinsic factors:
  - Impingement
    - Acromial spurs (Type III acromion)
    - Coracoacromial ligament
    - AC joint osteophytes
    - Repetitive use causing tensile overload, muscle fatigue and microtrauma
    - Glenohumeral instability accentuates abnormal loading or internal impingement.

Q. What are the investigations needed?

- X-ray
- USG
- MRI.

Q. What are the clinical features?

- Almost similar to supraspinatus tendinitis
- Pain
- Tenderness
- Weakness of muscle
- Painful ROM
- Drop arm sign:
  - Abducts the patient's shoulder 90 degrees
  - The patient is then asked to slowly lower the arm back to the side
  - Pain and an inability to slowly lower the arm to the side indicate supraspinatus tear.

Q. What are the type of injury?

- Partial
  - <50%
- Complete.

Q. How will you treat the case?

- Pain: NSAIDs
- Ice compression
- Exercise:
  - Posterior capsular stretching
  - ROM exercise
  - Isometric strengthening supraspinatus—isotonic
  - Strengthening of shoulder girdle exercise
  - Propioceptive technique.
- Surgery: Repair of muscle.

Q. What are the indications of surgery?

- Failure of conservative treatment after 3–12 months
- Acute injury causing full-thickness tear
- Progressive weakness.

Q. What are the contraindications of surgery?

- Asymptomatic tear
- Chronic massive irreparable tears
- Unwilling or unable to participate in post-op rehabilitation
- PAS stage 2 or 3.

Bicipital Tendinitis

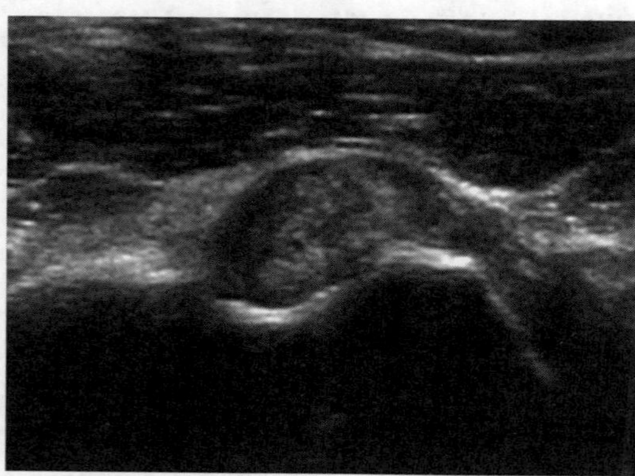

Figure 5.30: USG of shoulder joint showing thickened hypervascularized biceps tendinosis

Figure 5.30 is USG of shoulder joint showing thickened hypervascularized biceps tendinosis.

Q. What is biceps tendinopathy?
Inflammation, pain and tenderness of biceps tendon.

Q. What are the clinical features?
- Pain, tenderness of tendon or muscle
- Often radiating up to elbow
- Tenderness in bicipital groove
- Speed test:
  - Shoulder is forward flexed to 90 degrees
  - Elbow fully extended and the palm facing up
  - Applies a downward force against the patient's active resistance
  - Pain in the region of the bicipital groove—bicipital tendonitis.

Q. What are the investigations required?
- X-ray
- USG.

Q. How you will treat the case?
- Ice or heat compression
- Exercise:
  - Isometric strengthening—isotonic
  - Stretching exercise
  - ROM exercise.
- Local corticosteroid injection.

Q. What is the advantage and disadvantages of USG?
Advantages:
- Realatively inexpensive
- Readily available
- No radiation
- No contrast
- Dynamic evaluation possible
- Guided intervention possible.

Disadvanges:
- Less sensitive
- Cannot accurately diagnosed labral pathology.

See Chapter 3 page number 63 for further questions on adhesive capsulitis.

CT SCAN

Brain

Intracranial Hemorrhage

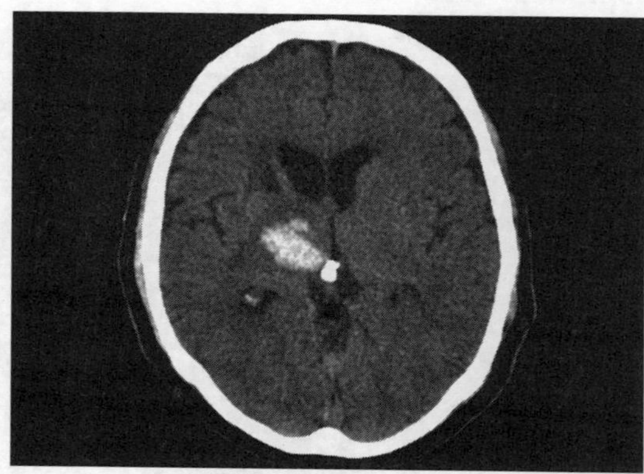

Figure 5.31: CT scan of brain in transverse section showing a hyperdense region in right basal ganglia

Figure 5.31 is a CT scan of brain in transverse section showing a hyperdense region in right basal ganglia. So, this is a CT scan of a patient with right basal ganglia hemorrhage without ventricular extension.

Infarct

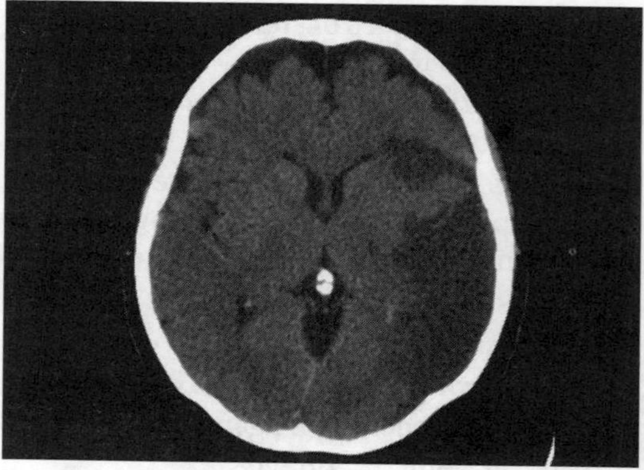

Figure 5.32: CT scan of brain in transverse section showing a cortical hypodense region with peripheral parenchymal swelling and loss of gray and white matter differentiation in middle cerebral artery territory

Figure 5.32 is a CT scan of brain in transverse section showing a cortical hypodense region with peripheral parenchymal swelling and loss of gray and white matter differentiation in middle cerebral artery territory. So, this is a CT scan of a patient with left-sided MCA territory infarct.

See Chapter 2 page number 6 for further questions on stroke.

MRI

Knee

ACL Injury

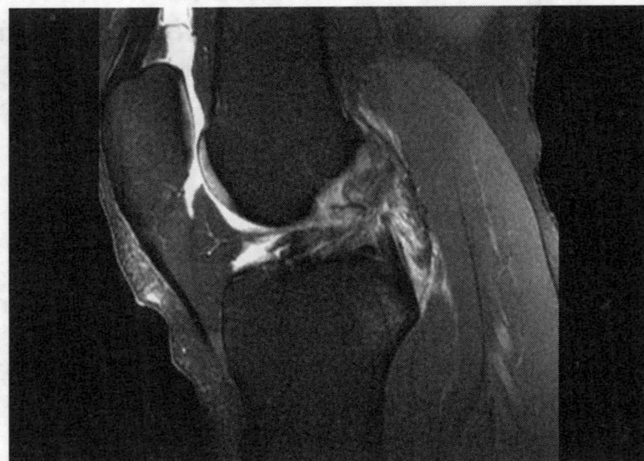

Figure 33: T2-weighted sequence MRI of right knee showing not only no visualization of ACL but also replacement of ligament by extensive edema fluid sequence in intercondyler notch

Figure 5.33 is a T2-weighted sequence MRI of right knee showing not only no visualization of ACL but also replacement of ligament by extensive edema fluid sequence in intercondyler notch. So, I think this is a MRI of acute ACL injury.

Q. What are the types of ACL injury?

- *Grade I*: Mild injury, only microscopic tears, do not affect the overall ability of the knee joint
- *Grade II*: Moderate injury, partially torn. The knee can "give away" periodically
- *Grade III*: Severe injury, completely torn and the knee feels very unstable.

Q. What are the clinical symptoms?

- Audible pop or crack, sensation of something going out then going back
- Extremely painful especially in the 1st few minutes—activity is discontinued
- Large tense effusion occurs in most cases due to hemarthrosis
- Restricted movement especially loss of extension
- Widespread tenderness
- Lateral joint line tenderness—subluxation
- Medial joint line may be tender due to associated MCL and medial meniscus injury.

Q. What are the special tests?

Lachman's test:

- Patient supine
- Hold the knee in between full extension and 15 degrees of flexion
- The femur is stabilized with other hand
- Firm pressure is applied to the posterior aspect of the proximal tibia to translate it anteriorly.

Pivot shift test:

- Patient supine with knee in extension
- The leg is hold up at the ankle
- The knee is flexed and internally rotated while placing the other hand behind the fibula
- A strong valgus force is placed on the knee by the upper hand
- At approximately 30 degrees of flexion, the displaced tibia will suddenly reduce, indicates a positive pivot shift test.

Anterior drawer test:

- Patient supine
- Hip flexed to 45 degrees, knee flexed to 90 degrees
- Hamstring relaxed
- Sits on the patient's foot
- Keep hands behind the proximal tibia and thumbs on the tibial plateau
- Anterior force is applied to the proximal tibia while Hamstring tendons are palpated with index fingers
- Increased tibial displacement compared with the opposite side, indicates an anterior cruciate ligament tear.

Q. What are the other associated injuries?

- Menisci (50%)
- Articular cartilage (30%)
- Collateral ligaments (30%)

(In football players and skiers, consists of injuries to the ACL, the MCL and the medial meniscus)

Q. What is O'Donoghue's triad?

- Anterior cruciate ligament injury
- Medial collateral ligament injury
- Medial meniscus injury.

Q. Why women are more susceptible to injury?

- Smaller size of ACL
- Smaller intercondylar notch
- Larger Q-angle (doubtful)
- Differences in physical condition and muscular strength (weaker Hamstring)
- Estrogens level.

Q. What are the common modes of injury?
- Sudden stop and twisting force
- Extreme hyperextension.

Q. What are the attachments of ACL?
- Femoral—on posterior part of medial surface of lateral femoral epicondyle
- Tibial—on the tibial plateau, medial to the insertion of the anterior horn of the lateral meniscus in a depressed area anterolateral to the anterior tibial spine
- Direction—from tibia to femur runs posteriorly, superiorly and laterally.

Q. What are the other investigations?
- X-ray knee: Segond sign
- USG knee: Not much of help.

Q. What are the indications of surgery and arthroscopic repair?
- Traditional ACL repair was done as soon as possible. As per recent evidence, delaying the surgery decreases postoperative risk of arthrofibrosis
- 3 weeks might be an appropriate delay.

Q. What is the protocol of conservative management?

Depends upon:
- Age of patient
- Degree of instability
- Associated injuries
- Participation in pivoting sports
- Occupation (police, defense)
- Cost of treatment /time off work.

Preoperative rehabilitation:

Goals:
- Diminish inflammation, swelling, and pain
- Restore normal ROM (especially knee extension)
- Restore voluntary muscle activation
- Provide patient education to prepare patient for surgery.

Brace:
- To prevent hyperextension.

Weight-bearing:
- As tolerated with or without crutches.

Exercises:
- Ankle pumps
- Passive knee extension to 0 degrees
- Passive knee flexion to tolerance
- SLR: Three-way, flexion, abduction, adduction
- CKC exercises: 30-degree mini-squats, lungs, step-ups.

Muscle stimulation:
- Quadriceps during voluntary quadriceps exercises (4–6 h/day).

Cryotherapy/Elevation:
- Ice for 20 minutes of every hour, elevate leg with knee in full extension (knee must be above heart).

Postoperative rehabilitation:

Goals:
- Protect graft fixation
- Minimize effects of immobilization
- Control inflammation
- Achieve full extension, 90 degrees of knee flexion
- Educate patient about rehabilitation progress.

Brace:
- Locked in extension for ambulation and sleeping (droplock brace).

Weight-bearing:
- Weight-bearing as tolerated with two crutches
- Discontinue crutches as tolerated after 7 days (with demonstrated good quadriceps control).

Postoperative phase 1 (Week 0–2):

Exercise:
- Heel slides/wall slides
- Quadriceps sets, Hamstring sets
- Patellar mobilization
- Non-weight-bearing gastrocsoleus, Hamstring stretches
- Sitting assisted flexion hangs
- Prone leg hangs for extension
- Straight leg raises (SLR) all planes with brace until quadriceps strength is sufficient to prevent extension lag.

Functional training:

A. Aerobic conditioning:
   - Upper extremity ergometry
   - Well-leg bicycling.

B. Proprioception:
   - Active/Passive joint positioning
   - Balancing activities
   - Stable platform, eyes open
   - Stable platform, eyes closed
   - Seated ball throwing and catching.

Postoperative phase 2 (Week 2–4):

Criteria for progression to phase 2:
- Good quad set, SLR without extension lag
- Approximately 90 degrees knee flexion
- Full extension
- No signs of inflammation.

Goals:
- Restore normal gait
- Restore full ROM
- Protect graft fixation
- Improve strength, endurance, and proprioception to prepare for functional activities.

A. Weight-bearing:
   - Patellar tendon graft—ambulation with brace locked in extension
   - Hamstring graft and allograft—may discontinue brace.

B. Therapeutic exercises:
   - Mini-squats 0–30 degrees
   - Stationary bike (begin with high seat, low tension)
   - Closed-chain extension (leg press 0–30 degrees)
   - Toe raises
   - Continue others.

C. Functional training:
   - Aerobic conditioning
     - Advance to two-leg bicycling
     - Continue upper extremity ergometry.
   - Plyometrics/Eccentric muscle training
     - Stair walking
     - Up/down, forward/backward.
   - Aquatherapy
     - Pool walking
     - Pool jogging (deep-water running).

Proprioception:
- Balancing activities
- Unstable platform [kinesthetic ability trainer 9KAT) or biomechanical ankle platform system (BAPS) board] with eyes open/closed
- Mini-tramp standing
- Standing ball throwing and catching.

Postoperative phase 3 (Week 6 to Month 4):

Criteria for progression to phase 3:
- Normal gait
- Full ROM
- Sufficient strength and proprioception to initiate functional activities
- Stable graft on Lachman and KT1000 testing.

Goals:
- Improve confidence in the knee
- Avoid overstressing graft fixation
- Protect the patellofemoral joint
- Progress strength, power, and proprioception to prepare for functional activities.

A. Therapeutic exercises:
   - Continue flexibility exercises as appropriate for patient
   - Advance closed-kinetic chain strengthening (one-leg squats, leg press 0–60 degrees)
   - Elliptical stepper, stair stepper.

B. Functional training:
   - Aerobic conditioning
     - Continue bicycling/upper extremity ergometry
     - Pool running/swimming
     - Stair stepper/elliptical stepper.
   - **Plyometrics:**
     - Stair jogging
     - Box jumps
     - 6- to 12-inch heights.
   - **Running:**
     - Straight ahead jogging, progressing to running
     - Figure-of-eight pattern
     - Large circles, walking or slow jogging.
   - **Proprioception:**
     - Mini-tramp bouncing
     - Pogoball balancing
     - Lateral slide board
     - Ball throwing and catching on unstable surface.

Postoperative phase 4 (Month 4):

Criteria for progression to Phase 4
- Full, painless ROM
- No evidence of patellofemoral joint irritation
- Sufficient strength and proprioception to progress functional activities
- Physician clearance to initiate advanced closed-kinetic chain exercises and functional progression
- Stable graft on Lachman and KT1000 testing.

Goal:
- Return to unrestricted activities.

A. Therapeutic exercises:
   - Continue and progress flexibility and strengthening programs.

B. Functional training:
   - Agility
     - Start at slow speed advance slowly.
     - Shuttle run.
   - Running
     - Small circles, running.
   - Plyometrics
     - Box jumps
     - 1–2 ft height.

Postoperative phase 5 (Return to sports):

Criteria for progression to phase 5—
- No patellofemoral joint or soft-tissue complaints
- Return to sports
- Physician clearance to resume full activity.

Goals:
- Safe return to athletics
- Maintenance of strength, endurance, and proprioception
- Patient education concerning any possible limitations.

A. Brace:
   - Functional brace may be recommended by physician for use during sports for the first 1-2 yr after surgery for psychological confidence.

B. Therapeutic exercises:
- Gradual return to sports participation
- Maintenance program for strength and endurance
- Agility and sport-specific drills progressed.

Posterior Cruciate Ligament Injury

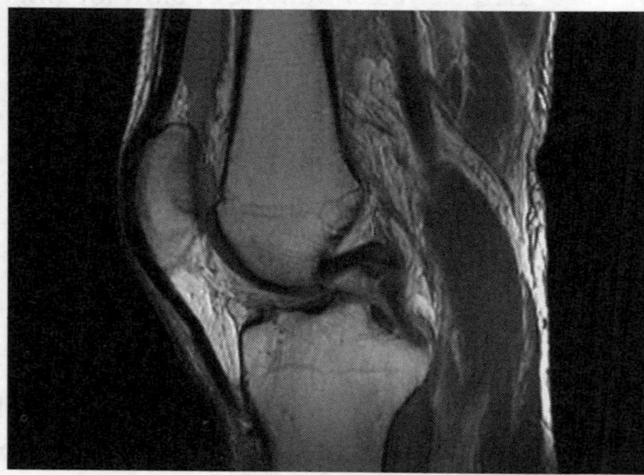

Figure 5.34: MRI of knee of T2 sequence in sagital plane showing high-intensity signal in place of posterior cruciate ligament which is difficult to identify

Figure 5.34 is a MRI of knee of T2 sequence in sagital plane showing high-intensity signal in place of posterior cruciate ligament which is difficult to identify. So, I think this is a MRI of posterior cruciate ligament (PCL) injury.

Q. What are the salient features of PCL injury?
- Usually less common
- Mode of injury:
  - Direct posterior blow to the anterior aspect of the proximal tibia
  - Hyperflexion of the knee with an anterior-directed force on the femur
  - Hyperextension of the knee.
- Clinical features:
  - Patient complains of poorly defined pain in posterior part of knee
  - Swelling is minimal.
- Investigations:
  - X-ray to rule out any bony avulsion from site of tibial insertion which is an indication of surgical repair
  - MRI of knee.
- Grading (Table 5. 5)

Table 5.5: Grading

Grade	*Posterior translation*
Grade 1	0–5 mm
Grade 2	5–10 mm
Grade 3	>10 mm

Q. What are the management protocol for PCL injury?
- Generally conservative
- Grade III injuries: Immobilization in extension for two weeks
- Surgical reconstruction: Indicated when other associated injuries, such as LCL, lateral meniscus or significant lateral instability are present
- Unlike a torn ACL and more like a torn MCL, the PCL may regain continuity with time.

Phases of rehabilitation regimen:

A. Phase 1—0–3 weeks:
   - Day 1-7:
     - ROM 0–60 degrees
     - Weight-bearing with two crutches
     - Electrical muscle stimulation to quadriceps
     - Quadriceps and SLR sets
     - Hip adduction and abduction
     - Mini-squats (0–45 degrees).
   - Weeks 2–3:
     - ROM 0–60 degrees
     - Weight-bearing without crutches
     - Progress exercises using weights
     - Pool program
     - Leg press (0–60 degrees).

B. Phase 2—4–6 weeks:
   - Week 4:
     - ROM exercise up to tolerance
     - Discontinue brace
     - Stairmaster, rowing
     - Progress exercises with weights
     - Mini-squat (0–60 degrees)
     - Step-ups
     - Hip abduction and adduction
     - Toe-calf raises.
   - Week 5-6:
     - Continue all exercises
     - Fit functional brace
     - Pool running.

C. Phase 3—7–12 weeks:
   - Begin running program
   - Continue all strengthening exercises
   - Gradual return to sports activities.

Q. What are the special test to be done in suspected PCL injury?

- **Posterior drawer test:**
  - Patient position is supine with the test hip flexed to 45 degrees, knee flexed to 90 degrees, and foot in neutral position
  - Sits on the patient's foot with both hands behind the patient's proximal tibia and thumbs on the tibial plateau
  - Posterior force is applied to the proximal tibia
  - Increased posterior tibial displacement as compared with the uninvolved side indicate to a partial or complete tear of the posterior cruciate ligament.
- **Reverse Lachmans test:**
  - Prone position with knee in 30 degree flexon
  - Stabilization of the distal femur by placing hand over distal thigh
  - Hamstring should be relaxed
  - Apply an upward pressure
  - Pain or increase translation indicates PCL strain or rupture.
- **Posterior sag test:**
  - Patient position: Supine with the hip flexed to 45 degrees and the knee flexed to 90 degrees
  - Tibia sags back on the femur if there is posterior cruciate ligament injury present.
- **Reverse pivot shift test:**
  - Patient position: Supine with knee flexed to 80–90 degree
  - Valgus and external rotation force is applied to the knee
  - If tibia is subluxated posterolaterally, then it is positive test
  - Should be compared with contralateral side
  - Normally seen in 35% cases.
- **Quadriceps active test:**
  - Done after posterior sag sign positive
  - Knee flexed in 90 degree with neutral rotation position
  - Patient contracts the quadriceps
  - Apply counter pressure over the ankle
  - If there is PCL tear then anteriorly pulled tibial tubercle will be reduced back.

Medial Meniscus Injury

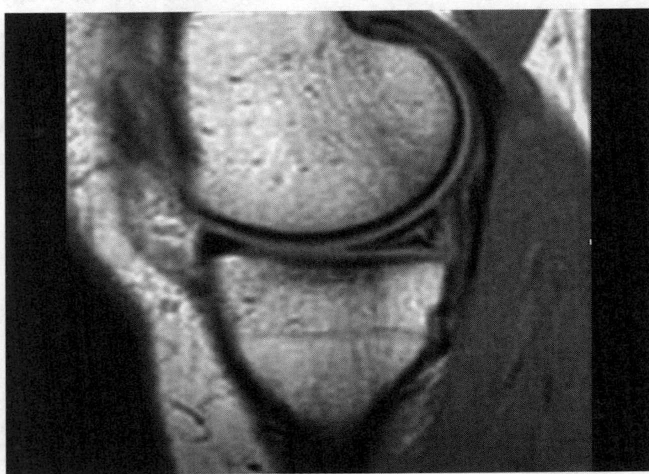

Figure 5.35: MRI of knee showing full-thickness horizontal tear of posterior horn of medial meniscus

Figure 5.35 is a MRI of knee showing full-thickness horizontal tear of posterior horn of medial meniscus. So, I think this is a MRI of meniscal injury.

Q. What are the attachments of medial meniscus?

Attached to tibia via meniscotibial ligament.

- *Anterior end*: To intercondyloid fossa, anterior to ACL
- *Posterior end*: To posterior condyloid fossa between lateral meniscus and PCL.

Q. What is the mode of injury?

- Twisting injury, foot anchored to ground and knee bent
- Commonly in contact sports by other player's body.

Q. What are the clinical symptoms and signs?

- Tearing sensation at the time of injury
- Pain
- Locking
- Swelling
- Gives away
- Restricted ROM
- Special test:
  - McMurray test:
    - Knee flexed

- Joint stabilized by one hand
- Other hand rotates leg medially and laterally while extending
- Pain and click in internal rotation indicates lateral meniscus injury while pain and click in external rotation indicates medial meniscus injury.

– Thessaly test:
  - Patient standing in one leg
  - Knee 20 degree flexion
  - Body rotate one side to another
  - Rotational stress on joint cause pain if tear present
  - 95% diagnostic accuracy.
– Apleys test:
  - Patient prone
  - 90 degree flexion of knee
  - Compression and rotational force applies on knee
  - Pain if meniscus is torn.

Q. What are the types of menisci injury?

1. Longitudinal.
2. Degenerative.
3. Flap.
4. Radial.
5. Bucket handle.
6. Horizontal cleavage.

Q. What are the investigations to be done in suspected menisci injury?

- MRI: Investigation of choice
- Arthroscopy: Both diagnostic and therapeutic advantage
- X-ray: To rule out other pathology.

Q. When you will do conservative management?

- Symptom develop over 24–48 hours after injury
- Minimal swelling
- Full ROM, with pain only at the end of ROM
- Able to bear weight
- Pain in Mc Murray test in inner range of flexion.

Q. What are the indications of surgery or arthroscopic repair?

- If the joint cannot be unlocked
- Little improvement of clinical features after 3 wks of conservative treatment
- Presence of associated ACL tear
- Positive McMurray test (palpable clunk)
- Severely twisted injury, athlete unable to continue his sports.

Q. What are the complications?

- Persistent knee pain
- Knee instability
- Restricted ROM
- Osteoarthritis of knee.

Q. What are the postoperative rehabilitation programs?

- Acute phase rehabilitation (0–2 weeks)
- Internal phase rehabilitation (2–4 weeks)
- Advance activity phase rehabilitation (4–8 weeks).

Q. Salient features of lateral meniscus.

- More mobile and less prone to injury than medial meniscus
- Associated with other injury.

Ankle

Lateral Ligament of Ankle Injury

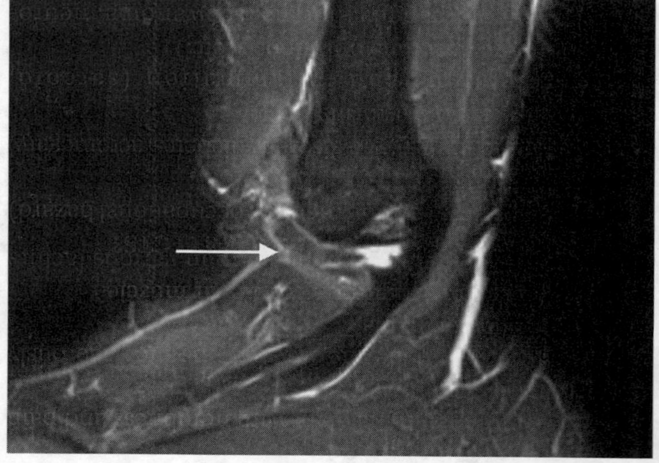

Figure 5.36: T2-weighted MRI of ankle joint showing high-signal intensity in anterior talofibular ligament

Figure 5.36 is a T2-weighted MRI of ankle joint showing high-signal intensity in anterior talofibular ligament. So, I think this is a MRI of anterior talofibular ligament injury.

Q. What are the components of lateral ligament?

- Anterior talofibular
- Anterior tibiofibular
- Bifurcate
- Calcaneofibular
- Posterior talofibular
- Posterior tibiofibular ligament.

Q. What is the most common ligament to be injured? why?

- Anterior talofibular ligament
- Cause:
  - Taut in plantar flexion
  - Can tolerate less strain.

Q. What is the attachment of the ligament?

- Lateral talar neck and tip of the fibula.

Q. What are the mechanism of injury?

- Inversion
- Plantar flexion.

Q. What are the grades?

- *Grade I*: No ligament laxity, only sprain
- *Grade II*: Some degree of laxity with partial tear
- *Grade III*: Gross laxity with full tear.

Q. What are the investigations needed?

- X-ray: to rule out associated fracture
- USG of ankle
- MRI: Investigation of choice.

Q. What are the clinical features?

- Pain
- Audible crack or snap
- Swelling with tenderness
- Difficulty or inability to weight bearing
- Painful ROM, often restricted
- Test:
  - *Anterior drawer test:*
    - Ankle in slight plantar flexion
    - Grasp lower end of leg and ankle from posterior side
    - Upward pressure
    - Anterior slippage noted compared to normal side
    - Present—positive test.
  - *Lateral talar tilt*:
    - Ankle grasped with both hand one above and one below
    - Lateral movement of talus are assessed
    - Pain indicate positive test.

Q. How you will manage it?

- Immobilization, depend upon severity up to 48 hours
- Ankle brace or binder for mobility
- Protective taping or bracing up to 6–12 months
- Ice compression
- Analgesia for pain
- Exercise:
  - ROM exercise
  - Muscle strengthening exercise
  - Propioceptive training
  - Functional exercise
- Surgery: Anatomical reconstruction, tenodosis. Full rehabilitation after surgery.

Q. What are indication of functional exercise?

- No pain
- Full ROM
- Adequate muscle strengthand propiocetion.

Q. What are the indications of surgery?

After 6 weeks of conservative injury in grade III injury:

- Recurrent instability
- Persistent pain.

Spine

Prolapsed Intervertebral Disc

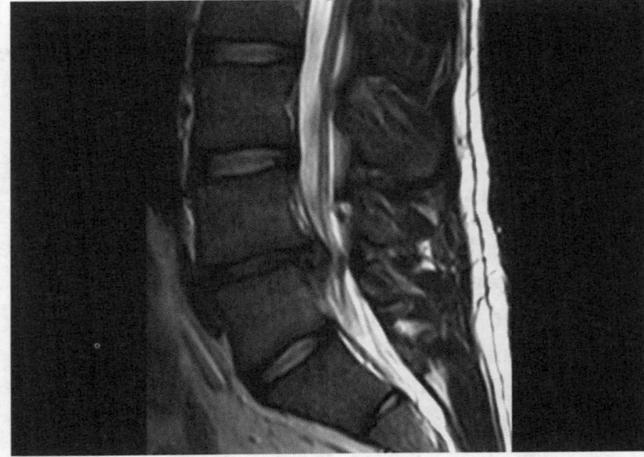

Figure 5.37: MRI of lumbosacral spine showing continuation of intervertebral disc beyond vertebral body

Figure 5.37 is a MRI of lumbosacral spine showing continuation of intervertebral disc beyond vertebral body with base distance more than edge distance and decreased height of disc space with blackening of disc suggestive of less water. So, I think this patient is having disc extrusion.

Q. What do you mean by prolapsed intervertebral disc (PIVD)?

Disc material extends beyond intervertebral disc.

Q. What are different types of PIVD?

A. **Disc bulge:** Displaced disc material is >50% of its circumference.

B. **Herniation:** Displaced disc material is <50% of its circumference.

C. **Disc protrusion:** Distance of the edges of herniated intervertebral disc material is less than the distance of the edges at its base with intact annular fiber.

D. **Disc extrusion:** Distance of the edges of the herniated intervertebral disc material is greater than the distance of the edges at its base with torn annular fiber.

E. **Sequestration**: The extruded intervertebral disc material has no continuity with the disc of origin with complete tear of annular fiber.

F. **Vertical disc herniation (Schmorl's node):** Vertical protrusion of nucleolus pulposus in adjacent vertebral body through vertebral endplate.

Q. What are the clinical features?

- Asymptomatic (may be)
- Axial back pain, radicular symptoms
- Symptoms aggravated by different movement of spine depending upon herniation-like pain by posterolateral herniation aggravated by forward bending, central herniation pain aggravated by extension
- Paresthesia or numbness in leg, muscle weakness
- Sciatic scoliosis
- Restricted spinal movement
- Bladder/Bowel symptoms may occur
- Cauda equina or conus medularis syndrome.

Q. What are the red flag and yellow flag signs?

- **Red flag signs:**
  - Age—<18 years or >55 y
  - Violent trauma
  - Nocturnal pain
  - Immunodeficiency state
  - Severe pain with restricted motion or deformity
  - Pain with compressive myelopathy
  - Inflammatory LBP.
- **Yellow flags:**
  - Female gender
  - Low income
  - High BMI
  - Previous surgery
  - Neurological deficit
  - Positive SLR
  - High-intensity leg pain
  - Pain with movement
  - Difficulties in sitting
  - High functional limitation at 4 week
  - High disability
  - Lack of appropriate signs and symptoms
  - Catastrophic thinking
  - Avoidance
  - Depression/Anxiety
  - Somatization.

Q. What are the different types of SLR?

Straight Leg Raising Test (SLRT):

- Active: The patient is asked to raise his/her leg, reproduction of radicular pain indicate positive test
- Passive: The patient lies on his back (supine). The examiner raises the leg with the knee extended straight. Normally, if the patient experiences radicular pain (sciatic nerve distribution) between 30–70 degree, the test is positive
- Crossed SLRT: If there is contralateral radicular leg pain when the uninvolved leg is raised the test is positive. It is most specific.
- Milgram test: Patient is asked to raise both legs at the same time 2–6 inches above bed and hold it for 30 second. Test is positive if there is leg pain or cannot hold it or unable to raise the legs
- Reverse SLR test: Patient is prone. Elevate the leg up to 30–60 degree. Pain radiating to anterior thigh indicate positive test. Sensitivity is high in high lumbar PIVD
- Femoral stress test—Patient is prone. Knee is flexed to 90 degree. Hip is then passively extended. Reproduction of anterior thigh pain indicate positive test.

Q. What are the clinical implications of SLRs?

- **SLR** test is positive means there is pathology in nerve root or distal to nerve root like sciatic nerve or tibial nerve
- **Crossed SLR test** is positive when nerve root is involved like by PIVD or any SOL
- **Passive SLR** test more specifically indicate nerve root pathology like disc herniation
- **Sensitivity of reverse SLR** is high in high lumbar PIVD.

Q. How you will manage the case?

- Relative rest
- Maintenance of posture
- Pharmacological—for LBP → NSAIDS, opioids, muscle relaxant, oral/ local.

For radiation: Tricyclic antidepressant-like amitryptiline, nortryptiline, anticonvulsants-like gabapentine, pregabaline, etc; SSRI-like duloxetine.

- Nonpharmacological:
  PT:
  - Exercise:
    - Strengthening exercise—paraspinal, abdominal, core muscle

  - Spinal stabilisation
  - Neural release exercise
  - Mckenzie centralization technique
  - Conditioning exercise.
- OT: Relaxation, work modification
- Modality: Superficial (dry heat, infrared therapy) and deep heat (UST)
- TENS
- PO: For stabilization like LSO.

Q. What are the other investigations?
- X-ray
- EMG NCS.

Q. What are the indications of interventions?
See Chapter 10 page number 243.

Q. What are the indications for surgery?
See Chapter 10 page number 243.

Q. What is the prognosis of PIVD?
- Resolution: 60% cases:
  - Generally within the first few months of their onset
  - Clinical improvement usually corroborative with MRI
  - Large extruded disc > small disc protrusions and disc bulges.
- Nonresolution: 20–30%.

6 Chapter

PMR Tracings

NERVE CONDUCTION STUDY

Carpal Tunnel Syndrome

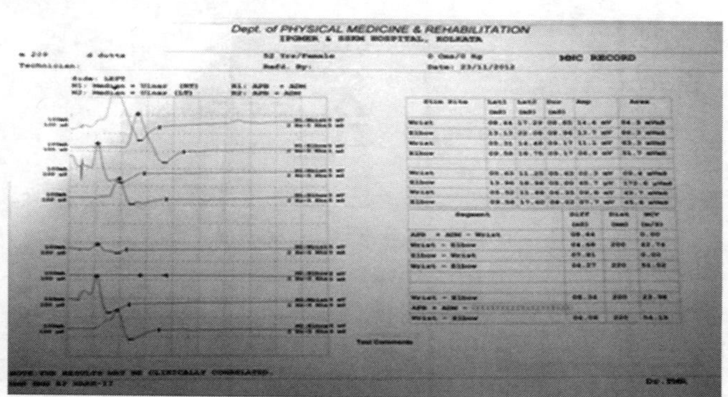

Figure 6.1: NCS tracing of CTS

This is the EMG NCS study of both upper limbs showing decreased median motor and sensory latency in left carpal tunnel. So, I think this patient is suffering from left carpal tunnel syndrome.

Q. What is carpel tunnel syndrome (CTS)?

- CTS is a compressive neuropathy affecting median nerve in carpal tunnel at wrist.

Q. What are the electrodiagnostic criteria of CTS?

- Abnormal median studies—prolonged distal motor (>4.2) and sensory latencies (>3.5 ms)
  - CMAP and SNAP amplitude decreased (in case of demyelination with axonal loss
  - Motor conduction velocity <49 ms
  - Prolonged minimum F wave latencies
  - CSI (combined sensory index) >0.9
- Normal ulnar study—
  - Ulnar sensory, motor and F wave latencies normal.

Q. How will you confirm the diagnosis of CTS in unilateral upper limb amputee patient?

By nerve conduction study (NCS) comparing the median nerve with other sound nerves (like ulnar nerve) in same hand. Small differences in between median and ulnar nerve latency are significant (0.4–0.5 ms)

Q. What are the other investigations to confirm the diagnosis of CTS?

USG of wrist (carpal tunnel).

Q. What are the advantages of USG over NCS in diagnosing CTS?

- USG is **not an alternative** to NCS but may be **complementary** to each other
- It has certain advantages like :
  - Lower cost, shorter time and non-invasive
  - Confirmation of nerve compression
  - More value in **secondary cases**, shows any lesion causing compression of nerve.

Q. Is there any fixed criteria for surgery in NCS?

Absent SNAP and CMAP showing prolonged latency with decreased amplitude.

Q. What are the other entrapment sites of median nerve?

- At ligament of Struther's
- At or immediately below elbow by pronator teres muscle
- Anterior interosseous nerve entrapment by flexor digitorum sublimis and flexor digitorum profundus muscle.

Q. What are the clinical features of CTS?

- More common in female
- Numbness and paraesthesia in the radial three and half fingers

- Awakening in the night with numbness and pain in the fingers
- **Flick sign**: Relieving of symptoms after vigorously shaking of hands
- Weakness and atrophy of thenar muscle.

Q. What are the common etiologies of CTS?

- Idiopathic (repetitive stress, occupational hazard)
- Wrist injury
- Endocrine (thyroid disorder, diabetes, acromegaly)
- Rheumatoid arthritis
- Infections and inflammation (sarcoid, tuberculosis, histoplasmosis, etc.)
- Tumors (ganglia, lipoma, schwanoma, neurofibroma, hemangioma)
- Others (pregnancy, amyloidosis, spasticity at wrist causing persistent wrist flexion, congenital, etc.).

Q. What are the classical sign of CTS?

- **Flick sign**: Relief of symptoms after vigorous shaking of hand
- **Tinel sign**: Reproduction of symptoms after percussion of median nerve at wrist
- **Phalen sign**: Reproduction of symptoms occurs after forced flexion at the wrist to 90° for 1 minute
- **Reverse phalen sign**: Reproduction of symptoms occurs after forced extension at the wrist to 90° for 1 min.
- **Tourniquet test**: Inflated BP cuff for 1 min causing reproduction of symptoms
- **Carpal compression test**: Thumb compression over the tunnel for 30 seconds reproduce symptoms.

Q. What is the minimum pressure required to provoke CTS?

Clinically evident CTS presented with average carpal pressure of >30 mm of Hg cause neuropraxia.

Q. How to manage CTS?

CTS can be managed by:

- Night time splinting
- NSAIDs, pregabalin and methylcobalamin
- Steroid—oral or locally injectable
- Tendon or nerve gliding exercise
- Occupational modification
- Surgery.

Q. What are the indications of surgery in CTS?

- Muscle atrophy
- Severe pain
- Refractory cases of nonsurgical measures (after 10 months).

Q. How are the prognostic factors of surgery?

Prognosis of surgery depend upon various factors like:

- Good prognosis—accurate diagnosis result in good prognosis
- Poor prognosis—
  - Poor surgical skill
  - Motor deficit
  - Impaired sensation
  - Secondary CTS (associated with some systemic disease like DM).

Q. What is pronator teres syndrome?

Entrapment of median nerve between two heads of pronator teres or bridging fascial band of the flexor digitorum superficialis muscle.

Q. What are the clinical features?

- Pain in proximal forearm
- Increased pain by forceful pronation or finger flexon
- Weakness can occur in muscle supplied by median nerve except pronator teres.

Q. What are the entrapment sites of ulnar nerve?

- **At arm**: Arcade of struthers.
- **At forearm**:
  - Tardy ulnar nerve palsy—after many years of distal humerus fracture
  - Cubital tunnel syndrome—compression of nerve by flexor carpi ulnaris aponeurosis or arcuate ligament.
- **At hand**: At guyon's canal.

Facial Nerve NCS

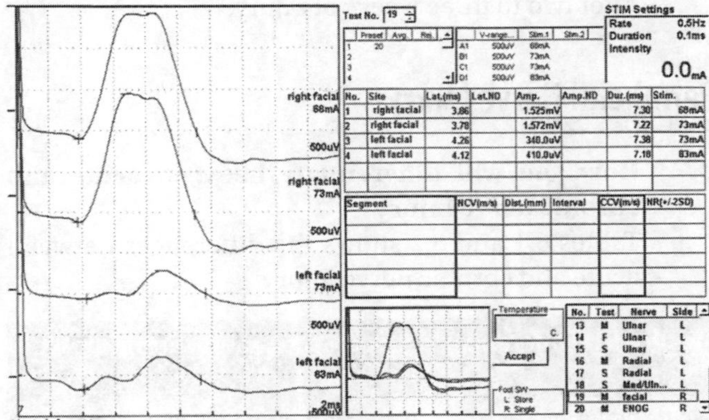

Figure 6.2: Facial nerve NCS

It is electrophysiological tracing of facial nerve showing diminished amplitude and conduction velocity of left facial nerve. So, it is probably NCS of left bell's palsy.

Q. What are the clinical features of Bell's palsy?

Clinical presentation depends on location:

- **Central lesion**: Causes contralateral weakness of lower facial muscle with relative sparing of orbicularis oculi and frontalis muscle, facial movement during crying , laughing persist.

- **Peripheral lesion**: Causes weakness of both upper and lower facial muscles resulting in:
  - Inability to wrinkle, close the eye, or smile
  - Dysfunction of tearing and saliva production
  - Hyperacusis
  - Absent taste sensation over anterior two-third of tongue depending on branch involved
  - Pain behind ear.

Q. How is it managed?

Evidence suggest that most cases of Bell's palsy are viral (herpes virus) induced cranial neuritis. It is managed by—

- Antiviral medications like acyclovir (Dose -800 mg 5 times a day for 7 days)
- Steroid: Prednisolone (Dose—started with 30 mg ODPC then gradually tapered down and stop)
- Massage
- Exercise—facial muscle exercise
- Stimulation—Galvanic stimulation.

Q. How is the prognosis?

In most cases prognosis is excellent with full recovery over several weeks to months.

Q. What are the effects of early stimulation?

- Hampered in spontaneous recovery
- Muscle spasm/tetany
- Muscle stiffness/contracture
- Crocodile tear.

Q. When should be electrical stimulation started?

After two to three weeks of injury.

Peripheral Nerve Injury

Q. How you will differentiate between acute and chronic nerve injury?

Tables 6.1 and 6.2 shows the differences between acute and chronic nerve injury.

Table 6.1: Differences between acute and chronic nerve injury

Acute nerve injury	*Chronic nerve injury*
• Seen in lesions that are more than several days but less than several weeks old • Enough time for wallerian degeneration to occur • Not enough time for denervations potential to develop • Seen after nerve trauma or infarct	• Seen months to years after occurrence of lesion • Lesion no longer active • Reinnervation is complete • Denervating potentials have disappeared • Successful reinnervation have occurred

Table 6.2: Acute vs Chronic nerve injury

	Acute nerve injury	*Chronic nerve injury*
	NCS	NCS
Motor— • Amplitude • Conduction velocity • Distal latency.	Decreased Normal/decreased Normal/decreased	Normal/decreased Normal/decreased Normal/increased
Sensory— • Amplitude • Conduction velocity • Distal latency	Decreased Normal/decreased Normal/increased	Decreased Normal/decreased Normal/increased

Q. What should be the clinical manifestation of these patients?

- Clinical features of acute nerve injury: Loss of sensation, loss of voluntary movement.

For other relevant questions see Page 98 in Chapter 3.

Myopathy

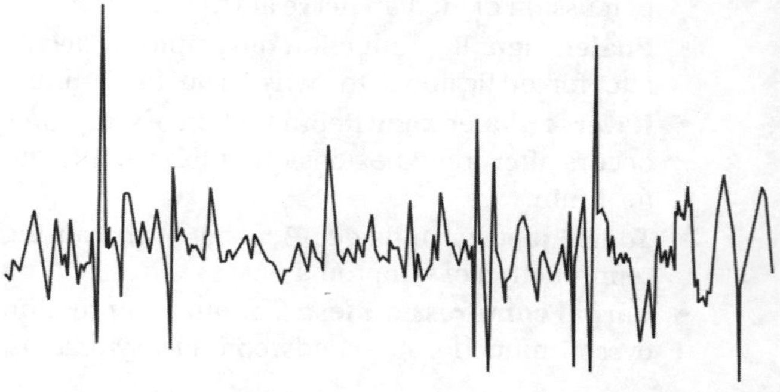

Figure 6.3: EMG study of myopathy

This is an EMG study of a muscle showing recruitment pattern of polyphasic, short-duration, low-amplitude MUAPs (motor unit action potentials). So, I think this patient is suffering from myopathy.

Q. What are the electrophysiological differentiating points between myopathy and neuropathy?

The differences in as follows (Table 6.3).

Table 6.3: Comparison between myopathy and neuropathy

	Myopathy	*Neuropathy*
NCS: SNAP CMAP	Normal Abnormal	Abnormal Abnormal
EMG: Resting activity	Abnormal depends on type	Normal/Abnormal
MUAP	Normal	Reduced
Interference pattern	Consists of short duration small amplitude MUAPs	Incomplete and consist of high amplitude MUAPs

Q. What are the clinical features of myopathy and neuropathy?

- Clinical features of myopathy:
  - Progressive muscle weakness, most commonly proximal.
  - Muscle fatigue
  - Gait abnormalities and difficulties in daily activities
  - Atrophy/hypertrophy of muscle
  - Abnormal muscle stretch response
  - Myotonia, arthrogryposis, etc.
- Clinical features of neuropathy:
  - Pain, numbness or paraesthesia or abnormal sensation
  - Impaired balance and gait difficulty
  - Muscle weakness, muscle atrophy
  - Autonomic symptoms like dysphagia, abdominal pain, fecal incontinence, diarrhea, constipation (GI system); sinus tachycardia, orthostatic hypotension, sinus arrhythmia, syncope (CVS); urinary problem and heat intolerance, gustatory sweating, etc.

Q. What are the NCS criteria of acute and chronic myopathy?

The NCS criteria of acute and chronic myopathy includes (Table 6.4):

Table 6.4: Comparison between acute and chronic myopathy

		Acute myopathy	*Chronic myopathy*
NCS	MOTOR → Amplitude	Normal/decreased	Normal/decreased
	SENSORY → Amplitude	Normal	Normal
EMG	Spontaneous activity	Norma/fibrillation potentials/ positive wave/ myotonia	Normal/fibrillation potentials/ positive waves/ CRDs (complex repetitive discharges)
	Activation	Normal	Normal
	Recruitment	Normal/early	Normal/early/ slightly decreased
	MUAP morphology	Short duration Low amplitude Polyphasic	Short duration Low amplitude Polyphasic and/or Long duration High amplitude Polyphasic

Q. What are the etiologies, management of myopathy?

Etiology of myopathy:

- Endocrine disorders: Hypothyroidism, hyperthyroidism, Cushing disease, Addison disease
- Autoimmune disorders: Myasthenia gravis, thyroiditis, scleroderma
- Infections: HIV, Lyme disease, trichinosis
- Metabolic: Glycogen and lipid storage disease
- Vitamin D deficiency, Vitamin E and A toxicity
- Medications: Corticosteroid.

Management of myopathy:

- **Rehabilitation is crucial in prolonging and maintaining locomotion**
- **Strenthening exercise in rapidly progressive myopathy: Submaximal strengthening** is recommended (eccentric and lengthening contraction cause mechanical stress)
- **Strenthening in slowly progressive myopathy**: Supervised moderate resistance home exercise is recommended
- **Aerobic exercise**: Home based aerobic walking program.

Alternative exercise: Aquatic based therapy, endurance training

- **Contracture prevention**:
  - Stretching:
    - Early stretching program slows progression of contracture
    - ROM program most useful in ambulatory patient with mild tightness
    - Passive stretching : 3 sitting/day, 10 to 15 times repetition/sitting
    - 2–3 hours standing (wheelchair dependent).
  - Bracing:
    - Night time resting splint or AFO to prevent tendoachilis contracture
    - KAFO with solid ankle at 90°, drop lock knee joints and ischial weight bearing upper thigh component: Help to maintain upright posture with reduced lumbar lordosis
    - Static wrist-hand orthosis to prevent hand contracture.
  - Transfer and mobility aids:
    - Standing frame, standing wheelchair, swivel walker occasionally used
    - Walkers where arm strength less affected
    - Wheelchair: Power needed for independence
    - Transfer board
    - Indoor lift, van with lift, roll in shower.
  - Surgery:
    - Tendon release
    - Ankle deformity corrected by TA lengthening/tendon transfer
    - Hamstring and iliotibial band release by low Yount fasciotomy, high Ober fasciotomy—allows better gait compensation
    - Scapular fixation surgery/scapulopexy
    - Scoliosis correcting surgery.

- **Management based on systemic involvement:**
  - Respiratory:
    - Breathing exercises
    - In-exsufflator for airway clearance
    - Influenza and pneumococcal vaccine
    - Assisted ventilation.
  - Cardiological:
    - Pacemaker for conduction defect and arrhythmia
    - Digoxin for cardiomyopathy.
  - Ocular:
    - Artificial tear drop
    - Tarsorrhaphy.
  - Nutrition:
    - Weight maintenance
    - Protein and caloric supplements
    - Percutaneus feeding tube for rapid provision of calorie and fluid.
  - Osteopenia/osteoporosis:
    - Encourage weight bearing and physical activity
    - Calcium supplements 80 mg/kg/d
    - Phosphate 40 mg/kg/d
    - Vitamin - D: 400 IU/day above RDA (required daily allowances).
  - Psychosocial issues:
    - Formal education, special education for accommodation and modification
    - Counseling is a very important factor.

Myotonica Dystrophica

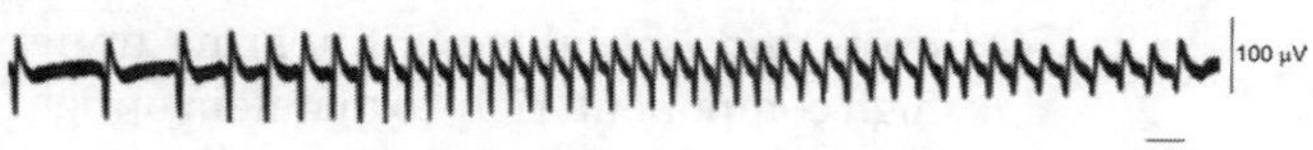

Figure 6.4: EMG study of myotonica dystrophica

This is an EMG study of a muscle showing waxing and waning of both frequency and amplitude. So, I think this is EMG of myotonica dystrophica.

Q. What is myotonia, paramyotonia and dystonia?

- **Myotonia**: It is a state of delayed relaxation or prolonged contraction of muscle
- **Paramyotonia**: It is paradoxical increased myotonia with exercise and exposure to cold
- **Dystonia:** It is slow sustained muscle contractions that frequently cause repetitive movement or abnormal posture.

Q. What are the diseases which can present with myotonia?

- Myotonia congenita
- Paramyotonia congenita
- Schwartz Jampel syndrome.

Q. What are the salient features of myotonica dystrophica?

- Myotonia including percussion myotonia.
- Frontal balding
- Lugubrious facies (long thin face with temporal and masseter wasting, ptosis)
- Posterior subscapular cataract
- Predominantly distal muscle weakness
- Cardiac conduction defects
- Restrictive lung disease
- Difficulty in swallowing and constipation
- Insulin insensitivity, higher incidence of diabetes
- Primary gonadal dysfunction with infertility
- Thyroid dysfunction
- Wide range of IQ variation.

Q. What are the investigations needed for it?

- For diagnosis:
  - Blood for CPK
  - EMG NCS of all four limbs
  - Genetic screening.
- Others:
  - ECG, echocardiography
  - Workup for thyroid and DM
  - Video fluoroscopy during swallowing
  - Ophthalmological test
  - IQ testing.

Q. Is there any pharmacological management for myotonica dystrophy?

If myotonia become severe enough a number of drugs can be used which are proved to be effective in relieving symptoms—Mexiletine, quinine, procainamide, tegretol and phenytoin, etc.

Q. What is the genetic linkage of myotonia dystrophy?

- DM1—19q13.3
- DM2—3q21.

Q. What are the nonpharmacological management of myotonica dystrophy?

- Avoidance of stimulator of myotonic attack
- Moderate resistance strengthen program
- Aerobic exercise
- Breathing exercise
- Spinal bracing for scoliosis and other orthosis for muscle weakness like AFO for foot drop.

Repetitive Nerve Stimulation Curve

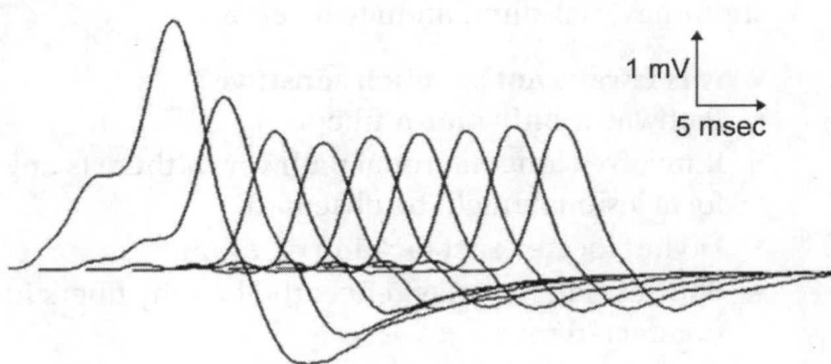

Figure 6.5: RNS curve

It is a repetitive stimulation curve (RNS) showing decrement pattern on repetitive stimulation of muscle. So, I think this is a RNS curve of neuromuscular junction disorder probably MG.

Q. What is myasthenia gravis (MG)?

- It is an autoimmune neuromuscular disorder resulting in decreased quantal response due to an autoimmune response against postsynaptic acetylcholine (Ach) receptors.

Q. What are the diagnostic criteria of MG?

- There are now widely accepted diagnostic criteria for MG. The most important element of diagnosis are history and clinical findings which is supported by laboratory testing.

A. Characteristic signs and symptoms:
One or more of the following—
- Ptosis, diplopia, dysphagia, dysarthria
- Exacerbation of weakness during exercise and repetitive use with at least partially restored strength after period of rest
- Dramatic improvement in strength following anticholinergic drugs (edrophonium).

***And one or more of the following*:**

B. EMG NCS: Repetitive stimulation at a rate of 2 per second shows at least 10% decrement. In EMG shows unstable MUAP.
C. Antibody to acetylcholine receptor.

Q. What are the types of MG?

- Generalized MG
- Ocular MG
- Congenital MG
- Transient neonatal.

Q. What are the other neuromuscular diseases?

- Eaton-Lambart syndrome
- Botulism.

Q. What are the clinical features of MG?

- Proximal fatigue and weakness increasing after exercise, heat and at the end of day
- Weakness improved with rest
- Facial or bulbar symptoms:
  - Ptosis
  - Diplopia
  - Dysphagia
  - Dysarthria.

Q. What are the investigations needed for diagnosis of MG?

- Tensilon test
- Blood: Anti-Ach receptor antibody
- Muscle biopsy
- EMG NCS: Repetitive nerve stimulation.

Q. What are the drugs used for treatment of MG?

- Cholinesterase inhibitor: **Pyridostigmine**—60 mg orally three times per day then maintenance by 60–1500 mg divided 3–6 times per day; increased dose as needed with at least 48 hours interval.

  Neostigmine—15 mg to 375 mg orally daily.
- Corticosteroids: Prednisone—0.05–2 mg/kg/day divided 1 to 4 times/day
- Immunosuppressant: Azathioprine, mycophenolate mofetil, cyclosporine.

Q. How can MG be managed nonpharmacologically?

- As muscle fatigue is a most common problem people with MG should exercise in morning.
  - Submaximal strengthening exercise
  - ROM exercise
  - Stretching to maintain flexibility
  - Breathing exercise
  - Swimming
  - Endurance training.

Q. What are the drugs that should be avoided in MG?

- Beta blockers
- Calcium channel blockers: Verapamil
- Statins
- Other cardiac drugs like procainamide, quinidine, quinine
- Anticonvulsants: Phenytoin, gabapentine, carbamazepine
- Antipsychotics: Phenothiazines, lithium
- Antibiotics: Aminoglycosides, tetracyclines, sulfonamides, penicillins, amino acid antibiotics, nitrofurantoi, fluoroquinolones, colistin
- Chloroquine
- Ophthalmologic medications: Timolol.

Q. Where you will find continuous increment pattern in RNS?

When the increment pattern becomes progressively greater and continuous, the patient is more likely having **Lambert–Eaten syndrome**.

Q. What are the differences between the two?

The differences is as follows (Table 6.5):

Table 6.5: Difference between MG and LEMS

	MG	*LEMS*
Ocular	Usually first	Unlikely
Muscle weakness	Proximal to distal	Distal to proximal
Only arm weakness	Present	Unusual

F Wave

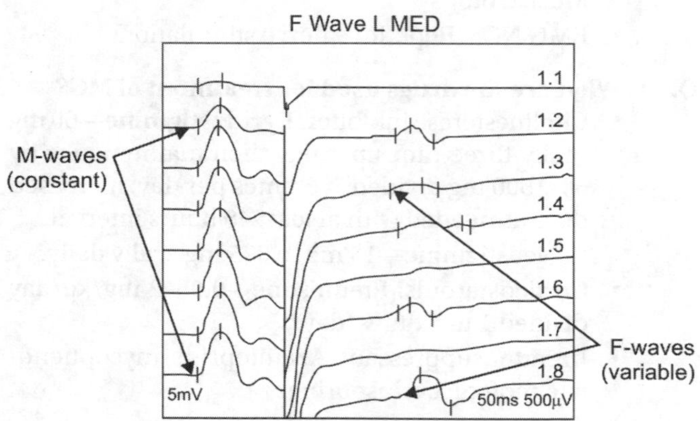

Figure 6.6: F wave

This is a NCS of study of left median nerve showing F wave after supramaximal stimulation.

Q. What is F wave?

It is a long latency muscle action potential seen after supramaximal stimulation to a nerve.

Q. Why is F wave not so much sensitive?

- Pathway is **only motor** fibers
- It involves long neuronal pathway. If there is any focal lesion it might be obscured
- Do not locate exact location of lesion
- Shortest latency may reflect the healthy fibers in unaffected root
- **Variable** latency and amplitude: Multiple stimulation required to find the shortest latency.

Q. What is F wave ratio?

Alternative F wave technique which do not require distance measurement. It develops as an error which can occur while measuring distance for F wave conduction velocity.

Q. What is the implication of this graph?

- It is a sensitive measurement parameter for polyneuropathy and radiculopathy
- In case of GB syndrome it helps in diagnosis where distal motor latency and conduction velocity is normal
- Reduced persistence of F wave is attributed to Anterior Horn cell loss.

Q. How you differ between radiculopathy, plexopathy and neuropathy?

The difference between the three are given in Table 6.6.

Table 6.6: Comparison between radiculopathy, plexopathy and neuropathy

	Radiculopathy	*Plexopathy*	*Neuropathy*
Pathology	Within the neural foramina or spinal canal involving proximally to nerve root	Plexus itself, distal nerve roots and proximal nerve trunks	Peripheral nerves
NCS	**Axonal lesion:** Decreased distal latency and CV, CMAP may be decreased. Demyelinating lesion—Normal distal latency, CV, CMAP and abnormal F wave. F wave: • Abnormal if C8-T1 roots are involved • Normal if C5, C6 or C7 root involved • Abnormal in L5–S1 radiculopathy (tibial and peroneal F wave). H reflex: • In S1 radiculopathy it is abnormal when recorded from soleus	Sensory NCS play a central role in plexopathy. **SNAP**—abnormal Motor studies are less helpful. Primarily used to exclude entrapment neuropathy. In axonal brachial plexus lesion affecting lower trunk and medial cord, median and ulnar CMAP may have reduced amplitude with mild slowing of distal latency and CV. Median and ulnar F responses prolonged	**Demyelinating lesion—** Prolonged distal latency, slowed conduction velocity, conduction block, increased temporal dispersion Axonal injury—Reduced CMAP amp, reduced SNAP amplitude, normal distal latency and CV
EMG	• 1 Week—Decreased recruitment of MUAP in clinically weak muscle. • 2 Week— Fibrillation potential and positive wave develops in muscles proximal to lesion • 3-4 Week—Similar changes in proximal group muscles • 5-6 Week—Most distally innervated group of muscles	Assessment of most proximal muscle is of importance as to differentiate a plexus from root lesion as the nerve supply directly comes from root	**Demyelinating lesion**—No fibrillation potentials or positive sharp waves, myokinatic discharge, decreased recruitment **Axonal injury**—Fibrillation potentials and positive sharp waves, decreased recruitement, LDLA polyphasic potentials
	Reinnervation occurs with development of large amplitude, long duration polyphasic MUAP develop. Fibrillation potential diminish, large reinnervated MUAP with decreased recruitment		

Q. What are the common etiologies of radiculopathies?

- Structural lesion:
  - PIVD
  - Bony impingement from spondylosis
  - Mass lesions like epidural abscess, metastatic tumor, vascular lesion.
- Infiltration by tumor, granulomatous lesion like sarcoid
- Infection like lyme disease, herpes zoster
- DME: Rarely early GB syndrome as cases of pure radiculopathy or polyradiculopathy.

Q. What are the baseline investigations?

- X-ray of spine
- EMG-NCS of all four limbs
- MRI of spine.

H Reflex

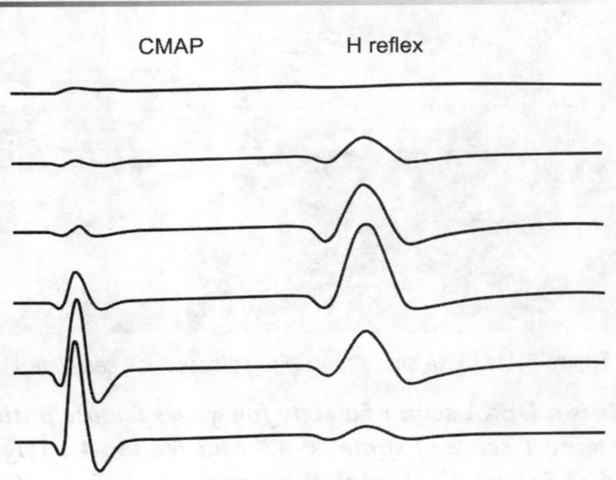

Figure 6.7: H reflex

It is an NCS of gastrosoleus muscle showing presence of H reflex with gradual decreased H latency and decreased amplitude.

Q. What is the clinical implication?

- It is a sensitive measure to assess radiculopathy
- The H reflex primarily assesses afferent and efferent S1 fibers.
- H reflexes help to distinguish S1 from L5 radiculopathy.

Q. What are the other investigations to confirm this?

- MRI scan of lumbosacral spine.

Q. Compare between H reflex and F wave?

Comparison between H reflex and F wave is given in Table 6.7.

Table 6.7: Comparison between H reflex and F wave

	H reflex	*F wave*
Originally described	By Hoffman	Obtained in foot muscles
Synapses	Monosynaptic or oligosynaptic	Polysynaptic
Pathway	• Sensory orthodromic • Motor antidromic	• Motor antidromic • Motor orthodromic
Stimulus required	Submaximal	Supramaximal
Elicited in	Soleus and Flexor Carpi Radialis	Most neurons
Stimulation site	Posterior tibial nerve in popliteal fossa	Any peripheral nerve

STRENGTH DURATION CURVE

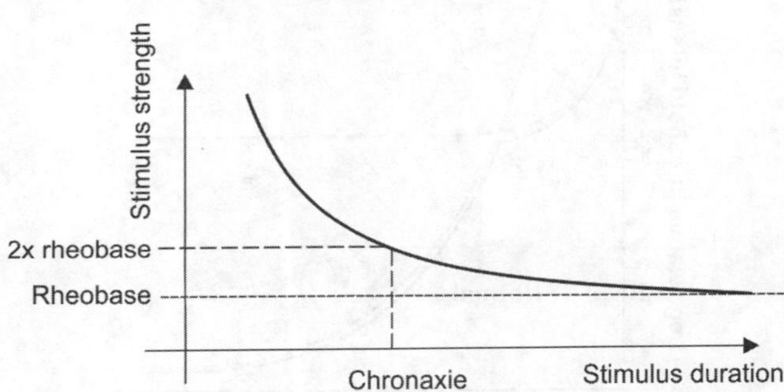

Figure 6.8: Strength duration curve for stimulers of an exictable tissue

This is a strength duration (SD) curve showing increased stimulus strength requires for shorter duration and longer duration current requires less stimulus strength to produce same response. So, I think this is an SD curve of normally innervated muscle.

Q. What is SD curve?

- It is a strength duration graph representing the relationship between intensity and duration of a current to determine if a muscle is innervated or not.

Q. What is rheobase and chronaxie?

- **Rheobase**: Minimal current strength below which no response from a muscle can be elicited
- **Chronaxie**: Minimal duration of direct current pulse that is required to contract the muscle at twice the rheobase strength.

Q. How you will interpret the curve?

- When all the nerves supplying muscle are intact the SD curve has shape given in Figure 6.8.
- In case of denervated muscle the curve shows below characteristic shape (Fig. 6.9)

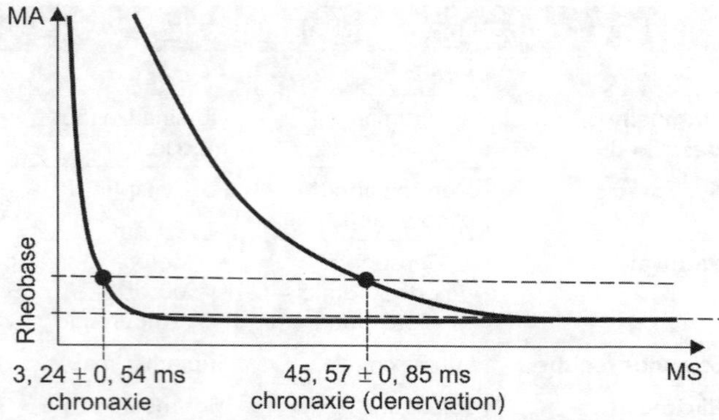

Figure 6.9: Strength duration curve of a denervated muscle

- In partial denervated muscle the curve is like below (Fig. 6.10)

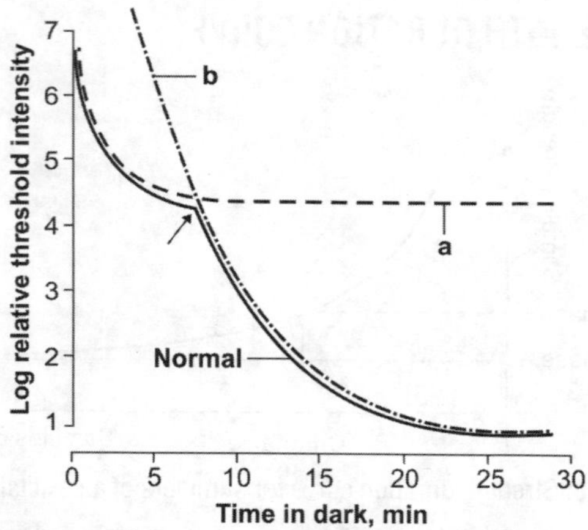

Figure 6.10: Strength duration curve of a partially innervated muscle

- So, from above curve we can see the interdependence between stimulus strength and time required to activate the muscle. In normally, innervated muscle same strength of stimulus is required to produce a response of all the responses of longer duration and shorter duration requires an increase in strength of stimulus
- In denervated muscle the strength of stimulus must be increased each time the duration decreased and for short duration no impulse is obtained
- In partially denervated muscle longer duration impulses are required for denervated muscle fiber and shorter duration required for innervated muscle fibers.

Q. What are the advantages of SD curve?

- Simple
- Reliable
- Shows a proportion of denervation.

Q. What are the disadvantages of SD curve?

- Site of denervation cannot be localized
- Cannot show the full picture of a large muscle, only a proportion can be stimulated.

Q. When can the SD curve be done?

SD curve can be done after 10 to 14 days of injury has occurred.

DEXA SCAN

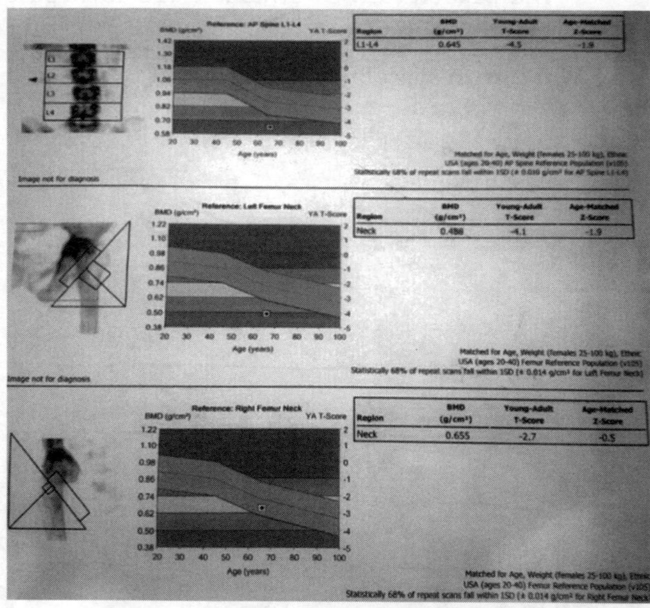

Figure 6.11: DEXA scan report *(For color version see plate 1)*

This is a DEXA scan of a sixty five years female patient showing T score of spine is -4.5 and femur -4.1 (right) and -2.7 (left). So, I think this patient is suffering from osteoporosis.

Q. What is T score?

T score is bone density of a person compared with what is expected in a healthy young adult of same sex at his or her age.

Q. What is Z score?

Z score is the number of standard deviations above or below what's normally expected for a person of his age, sex, weight and ethnic and racial origin.

Q. Which one is more valuable?

T score is more valuable because Z score can be normal as it is compared with same age and sex person but T score is measured compared with a normal young healthy person.

Q. How do you differentiate osteopenia from osteoporosis?

Table 6.8: Differentiation between osteoporosis and osteopenia

Osteopenia	*Osteoporosis*
BMD is between 1 and 2.5 SDs below that of a young normal adult. T score between -1.0 to -2.5	BMD is 2.5 SDs below that of a young normal adult. T score -2.5 or below

Q. What are the risk factors for osteoporosis?
- Advanced age
- Female sex
- Inadequate physical activity
- Low body weight
- Current smoker
- Estrogen deficiency
- Corticosteroid use
- Testosterone deficiency
- Vitamin D deficiency
- Low calcium intake
- Alcoholism
- Positive family history
- Previous fracture
- Anticonvulsive medication
- Excessive thyroxin replacement
- Recurrent fall
- Dementia.

Q. What are the common presentations of osteoporosis?
- Osteoporosis is typically a silent disease.
  - Vertebral, hip, distal forearm fractures are most common
  - Pain.

Q. What are the X-ray features of osteoporosis?
- Increased lucency of vertebral bodies with horizontal trabeculae loss
- Increased prominence of cortical end plate
- Vertically oriented trabeculae
- Cortex thickness reduction
- Anterior wedging of vertebral bodies.

Q. What is the role of MRI in osteoporosis?
- It not only shows trabecular architectures of bone but it also has the capacity to study other bony physiology not measurable by other technique. It can measure marrow fat content, perfusion and molecular diffusion
- It also detects first sign of inflammation associated with vertebral micro fracture
- Also helpful in neurologic involvement with compression fracture
- Also helpful to identify avascular necrosis, disc herniations and facet pathology post fracture.

Q. What are the drugs used in treatment of osteoporosis?
- Calcium
- Vitamin D2 or D3
- Bisphosphonate:
  - Alendronate—70 mg once in a week
  - Risedronate—35 mg once weekly
  - Ibandronate—150 mg once monthly
  - Zoledronic acid—5 mg once yearly.
- Teriparatide—20 microgram S/C daily for 3 to 6 months
- Calcitonin nasal spray
- Estrogen with or without progesterone
- Estrogen agonist/ antagonist-raloxifen—breast CA
- RANKL Inhibitor-Denosumab.

Q. Name of some new drugs.
- Teriparatide
- RANKL inhibitor.

Q. What are the nonpharmacological management of osteoporosis?
- Postural care: Improve posture, proper bed positioning and mobility technique, fall reduction technique and safe ADLs
- PT for muscle strengthening and flexibility
- PO- Spinal brace like CASH brace.

Q. What is the role of Ca^{2+}, PO^{4-}, ALP estimation?

To differentiate osteoporosis with other diseases (See Table 6.9 below):

Table 6.9: Role of Ca^{2+}, PO^{4-}, ALP estimation in different disease

	Ca^{2+}	*PO^{4-}*	*ALP*	*PTH*
Osteoporosis	Normal	Normal	Normal	
Primary hyper-parathyroidism	Increased	Decreased	Increased	
Secondary hyperparathy-roidism	Decreased/ normal	Increased	Increased	
Hypoparathy-roidism	Decreased	Increased	Normal	Decreased
Pseudohypopar-athyroidism	Decreased	Increased	normal	Increasing
Pseudopseudo-hypoparathy-roidism	Normal	Normal	Normal	

Contd...

Contd...

	Ca^{2+}	*PO^{4-}*	*ALP*	*PTH*
Vitamin D deficiency	Decreased	Decreased	Increasing	
Myeloma	Increased	Normal	Normal	
Pagets disease	Normal	Normal	Markedly Increased	
	Ca^{2+}	*PO^{4-}*	*ALP*	*PTH*
Metastasis	Increased	Normal/ Increased	Increased	
Sarcoidosis	Increased	Normal	Normal	
Vitamin D intoxication	Increased	Increased	Normal	

PULMONARY FUNCTION TEXT

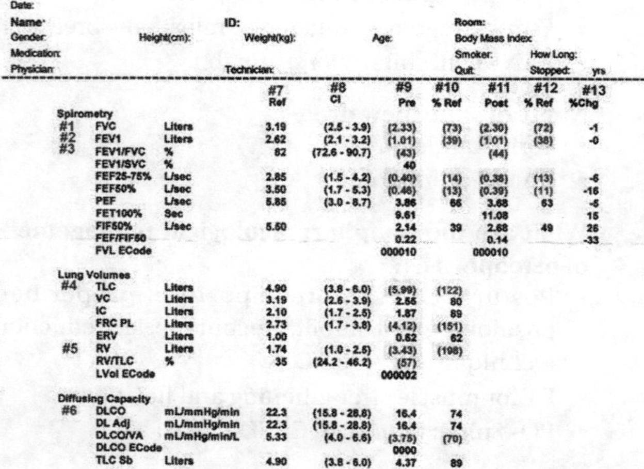

Pulmonary Function Lab

Date:
Name: ID: Room:
Gender: Height(cm): Weight(kg): Age: Body Mass Index:
Medication: Smoker: How Long:
Physician: Technician: Quit: Stopped: yrs

			#7 Ref	#8 CI	#9 Pre	#10 % Ref	#11 Post	#12 % Ref	#13 %Chg
Spirometry									
#1	FVC	Liters	3.19	(2.5 - 3.9)	(2.33)	(73)	(2.30)	(72)	-1
#2	FEV1	Liters	2.62	(2.1 - 3.2)	(1.01)	(39)	(1.01)	(38)	-0
#3	FEV1/FVC	%	82	(72.6 - 90.7)	(43)		(44)		
	FEV1/SVC	%			40				
	FEF25-75%	L/sec	2.85	(1.5 - 4.2)	(0.40)	(14)	(0.38)	(13)	-6
	FEF50%	L/sec	3.50	(1.7 - 5.3)	(0.46)	(13)	(0.39)	(11)	-16
	PEF	L/sec	5.85	(3.0 - 8.7)	3.86	66	3.68	63	-5
	FET100%	Sec			9.61		11.08		15
	FIF50%	L/sec	5.50		2.14	39	2.68	49	25
	FEF/FIF50				0.22		0.14		-33
	FVL ECode				000010		000010		
Lung Volumes									
#4	TLC	Liters	4.90	(3.8 - 6.0)	(5.99)	(122)			
	VC	Liters	3.19	(2.6 - 3.9)	2.55	80			
	IC	Liters	2.10	(1.7 - 2.5)	1.87	89			
	FRC PL	Liters	2.73	(1.7 - 3.8)	(4.12)	(151)			
	ERV	Liters	1.00		0.62	62			
#5	RV	Liters	1.74	(1.0 - 2.5)	(3.43)	(198)			
	RV/TLC	%	35	(24.2 - 46.2)	(57)				
	LVol ECode				000002				
Diffusing Capacity									
#6	DLCO	mL/mmHg/min	22.3	(15.8 - 28.8)	16.4	74			
	DL Adj	mL/mmHg/min	22.3	(15.8 - 28.8)	16.4	74			
	DLCO/VA	mL/mHg/min/L	5.33	(4.0 - 6.6)	(3.75)	(70)			
	DLCO ECode				0000				
	TLC Sb	Liters	4.90	(3.8 - 6.0)	4.37	89			

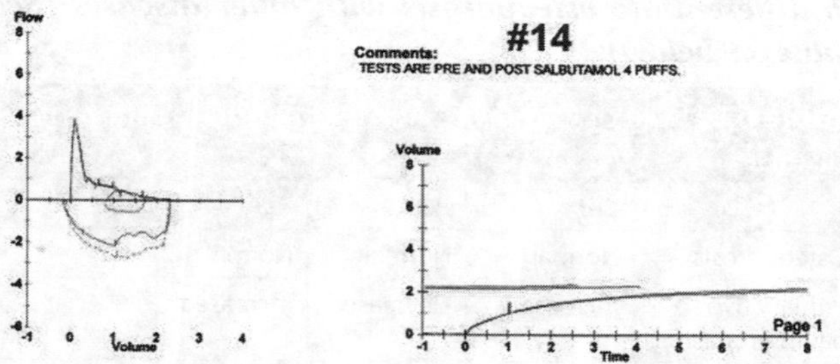

Figure 6.12: Pulmonary function text

It is a graph of PFT showing decreased FEV1 and FVC as well FEV1/FVC without any significant change of pre and post salbutamol puffs and also 'dog leg' pattern graph. So, I think this is curve of chronic obstructive lung disease.

Q. What is obstructive and restrictive lung disease?

Obstructive lung disease: Irreversible airflow limitation to lungs.

Restrictive lung disease: Impaired lung ventilation as a result of:

- Loss of normal elastic recoil of the lungs and the chest wall
- Associated with respiratory muscle dysfunction
- Stiffness of the chest wall or the lung tissue itself.

Q. What are the diseases caused obstructive lung disease?

- Emphysema
- Chronic bronchitis with chronic airflow obstruction
- Small airway disease.

Q. How to differentiate between chronic obstructive pulmonary disease (COPD) and bronchial asthma (BA)?

See Table 6.10 below.

Table 6.10: Differentiation between COPD and BA

	FEV1	*FVC*	*FEV1/ FVC*	*TLC*	*RV*	*KCO*
COPD	↓↓	↓	<70%	↑	↑	↓
BA	↓	↓↓	>80%	↓	↓	↓

Increased KCO seen in—

- Polycythemia rubra vera (PRV)
- Pleural hemorrhage
- Left to right shunt
- Asthma.

Decreased KCO seen in—

- Interstitial lung disease
- Primary pulmonary hypertension
- Pulmonary edema
- Anemia
- COPD.

Q. What is emphysema?

COPD caused by destruction of gas exchanging air spaces of lung (bronchioles, alveolar ducts, alveoli).

Q. What are the types of emphysema?

- Centriacinar
- Panacinar
- Paraseptal.

Q. What are the differentiating features of chronic bronchitis and emphysema?

Distinguishing features of chronic bronchitis and emphysema are given in Table 6.11.

Table 6.11: Comparison between emphysema and chronic bronchitis

	Emphysema	*Chronic bronchitis*
Onset	Usually 6th decade	Onset is usually 5th decade
Severity	Severe dyspnea	Moderate dyspnea
Cynosis	Pink puffers	Blue bloaters
Sputum	Scanty mucoid cough, occurs after dyspnea	Copious and purulent cough, occurs before dyspnea
Respiratory distress	Terminally attacks of respiratory distress	Repeated attacks of respiratory distress
Chest X-ray	Hyperinflation +/-bulous changes of lung with small heart	Increased bronchovascular markings with large heart
Complications: • Infections • Pulmonary hypertension • Cor pulmonale	• Less common • Mild • Occurs in terminal stage	• Very common • Moderate to severe • Common occurrence of cor pulmonale

Q. What is GOLD criteria?

Global Initiative of Lung Disease criteria used for grading of severity of COPD.

The grading of severity of COPD is given in Table 6.12.

Table 6.12: GOLD criteria of COPD

Grade	*Severity*	*Spirometry*
I	Mild	FEV1/FVC <0.7 and FEV1 ≥80% predicted
II	Moderate	FEV1/FVC <0.7 and FEV1 –50% to 80% predicted
III	Severe	FEV1/FVC <0.7 and FEV1 –30% to 50% predicted
IV	Very severe	FEV1/FVC <0.7 and FEV1 <30% predicted

Q. What are the complications of COPD?

- Lung infections
- Bronchiectasis
- Pulmonary hypertension
- Heart failure (cor pulmonale)
- Osteoporosis.

Q. What are the other investigations required?

- Chest X-ray
- ABG
- Echocardiography
- CT thorax.

Q. What is the role and benefit of oxygenation in COPD?

- Decrease pulmonary hypertension
- Decrease polycythemia
- Prevent hypoxemia
- Increase effort during exercise
- Prolong life
- Improve quality of life.

Q. What are the drugs used in treatment of COPD?

Bronchodilators—

- Short acting:
  - ***Anticholenergic***—Ipratropium bromide, oxytropium is the mainstay of treatment.
  - ***Beta-2 agonist***—Albuterol, Levalbuterol, Metaprotrenol, Pirbutrenol.
- Long acting:
  - ***Anticholenergic***—Iotropium, Glycopyrronium
  - ***Beta-2 agonist***—Salmeterol, Formoterol, Indacaterol.
  - **Corticosteroids**—Budesonide, fluticasone, baclomethasone, mometasone, ciclesonide, triamcinolone
  - **Phosphodiesterase-4 inhibitor**—Theophyline, etophylline, doxophylline, acebrophylline, roflumilast.
  - **Antibiotic.**

Q. What are the steps in nonpharmacological management?

A. Primry and secondary prevention

- Smoking cessation
- Immunization
- Prevention of exacerbation
- Pulmonary toilet: Maintaining hygiene, cough technique, chest PT
- Maintain proper nutrition
- Family training.

B. Dyspnea relief

- Exercise—
  - Strengthening exercise
  - Conditioning
  - Respiratory muscle training
  - Upper limb strengthening exercise
  - ADL training.
- Lifestyle modification—
  - Breathing training
  - Relaxation technique
  - Confidence build-up.

C. Disease management

- Coping and acceptance
- Quality of life improvement
- Encouragement
- Compliance.

Q. What are the different types of breathing?

- Normal
- **Dyspnea**—Difficult and laboured breathing
- **Tachypnea**—Increased rate of breathing
- **Bradypnea**—Decreased rate of breathing
- **Hyperventilation**—Rapid, deep breathing
- **Apnea**—Suspension of breathing by voluntary and mechanical compression or neurological disease process
- **Apneusis**—Cessation of breathing in inspiratory phase
- **Cheyne-stokes breathing**—Periodic breathing characterized by alternate tachypnea and apnea
- **Kussamaul's respiration**—Gasping and very deep labored breathing
- **Biot respiration**—Unpredictable irregular breathing alternates with period of apnea
- **Obstructive breathing**—Trapping of air in airway, seen in COPD
- **Sighing respiration**—Breathing with frequent sighs.

Q. What are different types of breathing exercises?

For respiratory retraining:

- **Diaphragmatic breathing**—Breathing by optimal use of diaphragm and decreased use of accessory muscles
- **Segmental breathing**—Expansion of localized area of lung while keeping the other areas quite
- **Pursed lip breathing**—Controlled expiration while keeping the lip lightly pursed
- **Air shifting technique**—After taking a deep inspiration, it is held with the glottis closed for 5 seconds, during which time the air shifts to lesser-ventilated areas of the lung, then expiration is done via pursed lips.

For mobilization of secretion:

- **Positive expiratory pressure breathing**—Expiration against resistance to airflow, patient expires through a specially designed mask or mouthpiece.
- **Flutter breathing**—It is combination of PEP and oscillation applied at the mouth. The patient expires through a small pipe and a small stainless steel ball rests on the expiratory end of the pipe which is pushed upward during expiration, producing PEP, and falls downward again, interrupting flow

Respiratory resistance training

- **Inspiratory resistive training**—Done by using pressure or flow based devices to provide resistance to airflow. It improves the strength and endurance of the inspiratory muscles and decreases the occurrence of inspiratory muscle fatigue.
- **Incentive respiratory spirometry**--Ventilatory training that emphasizes sustained maximum inspirations. The purpose is to increase the volume of air inspired by inhaling as deeply as possible through a small, handheld spirometer. It is used primarily to prevent alveolar collapse and atelectasis in postoperative patients.

Glossopharyngeal breathing:

Used in ventilator dependent patient whose diaphragm is not/partially functioning due to high spinal cord injury or other neuromuscular disease. It involves taking of several gulps of air in mouth then mouth is closed. After that tongue pushes the air back and it traps in pharynx then air is forced into the lungs when glottis is opened.

Increases depth of inspiration and improves vital capacity.

Q. Tell some different types of inspiratory technique.

- **Inspiratory resistance training—**Inspiration using pressure or flow based device to provide resistance to airflow.
- **Incentive respiratory spirometry—**Training of sustained maximum inspiration usually using a spirometry. It can also be done without spirometry.
- **Glossopharyngeal breathing—**Technique of increasing capacity in case severe weakness of muscle of inspiration.

Q. What are the indications of LTOT (long-term oxygen therapy)?

- Cor pulmonale
- Hypoxia in COPD (SPO2 <88%, PaO2<55 mg of Hg)
- Terminally ill patient.

*Patient must be stable and appropriate treatment by antibiotic, bronchodilators and PT has already been done.

Smoking cessation is a prerequisite.

Q. What are the role of occupational therapy in pulmonary rehabilitation?

- Upper extremity mobility, strength, endurance
- Self-care activities and training in ADLs
- Energy conservation and work simplification
- Workplace and home modification assessment
- Relaxation technique.

ELECTROCARDIOGRAM

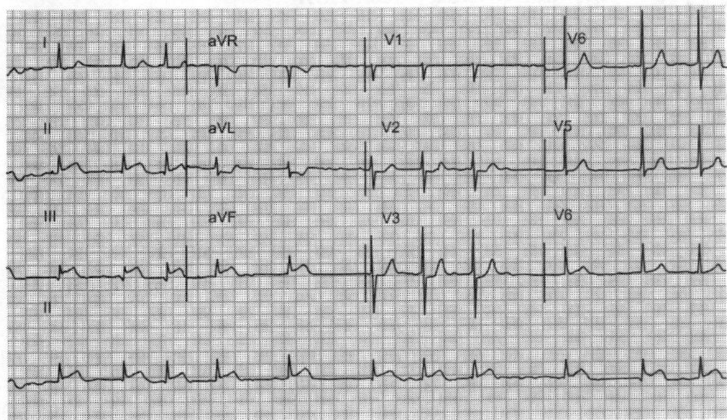

Figure 6.13: ECG tracing of acute inferior wall infarction

It is an electrocardiogram (ECG) of a 65-year-old male patient showing ST elevation in II, III and aVF and Q wave in II, III. So, I think this is an ECG indicate acute inferior wall infarction.

Q. What are the presentations of this patient?

Patient of MI can present with—
- Chest pain/discomfort not relieved by rest, position change or even medication like nitrate. Sometimes pain may radiate to shoulder or neck or jaw.
- Nausea and vomiting
- Sweating, palpitation. LOC
- Signs—initially high BP and tachycardia, or with heart failure like low BP, lung crackles, elevated jugular pressure
- May be completely asymptomatic.

Q. What are the other investigations to be done to confirm it?

Blood for cardiac enzyme like:
- Troponine T-stay elevated for 2 weeks.
- CPK: Begins to rise 3–12 hours after acute MI, which may peak in 24 hours
- Serum LDH—Start to rise after 12–24 hours, that may peak at 72 hours and back to normal at 10–14 days.

Q. How do you assess the patient initially apart from ECG?
- Checking of vital signs and O_2 saturation
- History and physical examination
- Blood investigations for cardiac enzyme markers, electrolytes and coagulation profile.

Q. What are the drugs used in treatment of this condition?
- Morphine
- Oxygen
- Nitroglycerin
- Aspirin
- Statin
- Low molecular weight heparin
- Beta blocker/ACE inhibitor/CCB accordingly.

Q. What are the risk factors?

Nonmodifiable:
- Age
- Sex
- Family history.

Modifiable:
- Smoking
- Hypertension
- Diabetes
- Dyslipidemia, obesity
- Sedentary lifestyle.

Q. How will you rehabilitate the patient with MI?

Acute Phase (Phase I):
- Goals:
  - Prevent physiologic deconditioning
  - Achieve safe mobility
  - Determine disposition

Cardiac rehabilitation (CR) is initiated as soon as the patient is medically stable following a cardiac event.
- Passive range of motion exercises
- Early mobilization to 2–3 METs prevents loss of cardiovascular reflexes associated with prolonged bed rest
- Chest physical therapy, including breathing exercises, incentive spirometer and manual techniques to promote secretion clearance
- Nasal cannula oxygen is prescribed to keep oxygen saturations over 90%
- Telemetry monitored seated activities, standing, and ambulation at 3–4 METs
- **Training in ADL to 4–6 METs is initiated,** focusing on **energy conservation** and pacing
- **Education is initiated regarding nutrition, risk factor modification,** potential medical complications, and the ongoing CR process
- Patients transition home or to in patient CR.

Inpatient Rehabilitation Phase (Phase IB):
- According to the recovery the admission to either an acute or a subacute rehabilitation facility prior to discharge home is considered phase IB rehabilitation
- Commonly seen as patients with cardiac disease often are of advanced age or with comorbidities that make mobilization more difficult
- The guidelines for exercise are often the same as they are for the strict phase I patients, but the period of recovery is longer

- Exercise intensity is **generally limited to a target heart rate** which is known to be safe
- The target HR is determined during a low level ETT (exercise tolerance test)
  - The level of exercise is usually done at a level of approximately 70% MHR or an MET level of 5.
  - Age >40 ≈ MHR of 130 bpm or 5METs
  - Age <40 ≈MHR 140 bpm or 7 METs
  - A Borg rating of perceived exertion scale of 7 (modified scale) or 15 (old scale) can also be used to determine the maximum tolerated exercise.

Training Phase (Phase II):

- It is started after a symptom limited full level ETT or completion of a revascularization procedure and return to full activities
- The MHR from the cardiac exercise test can be used to determine the maximum exertion during aerobic training
- Patients in the low risk group, 85% MHR is safe
- Patients with higher risk, a target 65–75% MHR is safe and target rates as low as 60% can still yield a training benefit.

Q. What will be rehabilitative management goal for early uncomplicated MI.

- For those able to return to work:
  - Return to productive employment as soon as possible
  - Improve and maintain a good cardiovascular fitness.
- For those not able to return to work:
  - Maintain a life as active as possible
  - Establish new areas of interest to improve quality of life.
- Patient education and reduction of coronary risk factors.

Q. What is the Wenger protocol for early mobilization?

DAY 1–2 →

- Step 1—Passive range of motion, ankle pumps, introduction of the program, self-feeding
- Step 2—As above, also dangle at side of bed
- Step 3—Active assisted ROM, sitting upright in a chair, light recreation and use of bedside commode
- Step 4—Increased sitting time, light activities with minimal resistance, patient education
- Step 5—Light activities with moderate resistance, unlimited sitting, seated ADL activities.

DAY 2–3 →

- Step 6—Increased resistance, walking to bathroom, standing ADL, up to 1 hour long group meetings
- Step 7—Walking up to 100 ft, standing, warm-up exercises
- Step 8—Increased walking, walk down stairs (not up), continued education
- Step 9—Increased exercise program, review energy conservation and pacing techniques.

DAY 3 →

- Step 10—Increase exercises with light weights and ambulation, begin education on home exercise program
- Step 11—Increased duration of activities
- Step 12—Walk down two flights of stairs, continue to increase resistance in exercises
- Step 13—Continue activities, education and home exercise program teaching.

DAY 4–5 →

- Step 14—Walk up and down two flights of stairs, complete instruction in home exercise program and in energy conservation and pacing techniques.

Q. What are the indications of CABG?

Coronary artery (2011 ACCF/AHA/SCAI guidline):

- **In left main CAD revascularization—**
  - In class I:
    - Significant (>/= 50%) reduction in lumen diameter of left main coronary artery.
- **In non-left main CAD revascularization—**
  - In class I:
    - Significant stenosis (>/=70% diameter) in 3 major coronary artery or proximal LAD plus 1 other major coronary artey
    - Survival of sudden cardiac death caused by significant stenosis in a major coronary artery.
  - In class IIa:
    - Significant stenosis in 2 major coronary arteries with severe or extensive MI
    - Mild-moderate left ventricular systolic dysfunction (EF 35-50%)and significant multivessel CAD or left LAD stenosis with viable myocardium at the site of revascularization
    - Complex 3 vessel CAD.
  - In class IIb: SIHD with EF <35%:

Revascularization to improve symptoms—

- In class I:
  - 1 OR more significant (>/=70%) coronary artery stenosis with unacceptable angina despite SDMT.
- In class IIa:
  - 1 OR more significant (>/=70%) coronary artery stenosis with unacceptable angina and contraindication to SDMT

- 1 OR more significant (>/=70%) coronary artery stenosis with ischemia and unacceptable angina despite SDMT
- Complex 3 vessel CAD.
- In class IIb: With previous CABG, 1 OR more significant (>/=70%) coronary artery stenosis not amenable to PCI and with unacceptable angina and contraindication to SDMT.

Q. How you will treat the further angina during cardiac rehabilitation?

- Exclude unstable angina/another MI/arrhythmias—if positive - referral to respective cardiologist
- Otherwise topping up the doses of anti angina like increased dose of nitrate as needed
- May be add on CCB/beta-blocker/nicorandil, etc. with liaison with cardiologist.

Q. What are the protocols of TMT?

The most frequently used stepped treadmill protocols are the:

1. Bruce
2. Modified Bruce
3. Naughton protocols
4. Weber protocol
5. Asymptomatic cardiac ischemia pilot (ACIP)
6. Modified ACIP.

Q. What are the contraindications of TMT?

Absolute Contraindications:

- Acute myocardial infarction (within 2 days)
- High-risk unstable angina
- Uncontrolled cardiac arrhythmia with hemodynamic compromise
- Active endocarditis
- Symptomatic severe aortic stenosis
- Decompensated heart failure
- Acute pulmonary embolism or pulmonary infarction
- Acute myocarditis or pericarditis
- Physical disability precluding safe and adequate testing.

Relative Contraindications:

- Known left main coronary artery stenosis
- Moderate aortic stenosis with uncertain relationship to symptoms
- Tachyarrhythmia with uncontrolled ventricular rates
- Acquired complete heart block
- Hypertrophic cardiomyopathy with a severe resting gradient
- Mental impairment with limited ability to cooperate.

URODYNAMIC STUDY

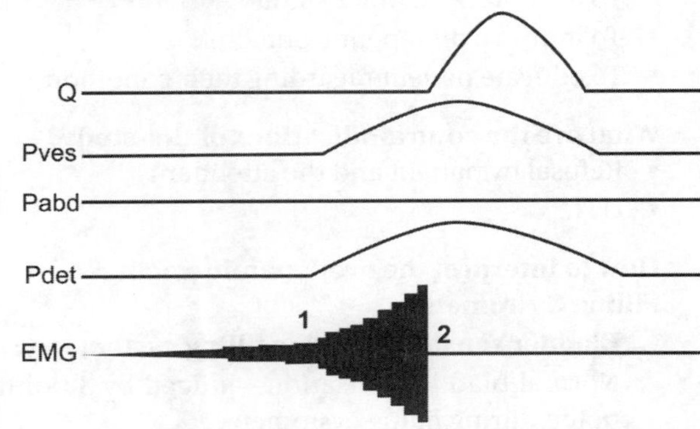

Figure 6.14: UDS tracing of sphincter dyssynergia

This is a urodynamic Study (UDS) tracing showing sphincter dyssynergia with detrusor contraction as evidenced by progressive increase in external urethral sphincter contraction activity that peaks at maximal detrusor contraction followed by sudden relaxation of the external urethral sphincter when the detrusor pressure declines allowing urination.

Q. What are the parameters?

- Cystometry
- Leak point pressure measurement
- Video urodynamics
- Ambulatory urodynamics
- Urethral pressure measurement.

Q. What are the components of UDS study?

- Simple cystometry
- Subtraction cystometry
- Video cystometrography
- Ambulatory urodynamics
- Filling cystometry—Sensation of bladder, compliance of bladder, capacity of bladder, stability of bladder leak
- Voiding cystometry—Detrusor pressure at maximum flow rate, bladder contractility index.

Q. Where should you place the probe?

- For abdominal pressure—rectum/vagina/stoma
- For vesical pressure—bladder
- For filling—bladder.

Q. What are the prerequisite?

- Consent of patient or legal guardian in case of minor
- Urine should be sterile.

Q. Why urine should be sterile?

- One of the most common cause of lower urinary tract symptoms is urinary tract infection. So, in presence of UTI, misinterpretation of UDS can occurs.

Q. What are the indications for this study?

- To diagnose underlying cause of lower urinary dysfunction

- To classify lower urinary tract dysfunction
- To formulate treatment strategy
- To improve therapeutic outcome
- To educate patient regarding their condition.

Q. What are the contraindications of this study?

- Refusal by patient and the attendant
- UTI.

Q. How to interpret the urodynamic tracing?

Filling Cystometry:

A. Bladder sensation during filling cystometry:

Normal bladder sensation—judged by 3 points noted during filling cystometry.

- *First sensation of bladder filling*—Feeling of the patient while he/she first becomes aware of bladder filling.
- *First desire to void*—Feeling that lead the patient to pass the urine in next convenient moment.
- *Strong desire to void*—Patient desire to void without fear of leakage
- *Increased bladder sensation*—An early first sensation of bladder filling and or an early desire to void occurred at low bladder volume and which persist.
- *Reduced bladder sensation*—Diminished sensation throughout bladder filling
- *Absent bladder sensation*—Has no bladder sensation
- *Nonspecific bladder sensation*—Make the individual aware of bladder filling (abdominal fullness or vegetative symptoms)
- *Bladder pain*—Self explatory term and an abnormal finding.
- *Urgency*—Sudden compelling desire to void.
- *The vesical/urethral sensory threshold*—Least current which consistently produces a sensation perceived by the patient during stimulation at the site under investigation.

B. Detrusor function during filling cystometry:

- *Normal detrusor function*—Bladder filling with little or no change in pressure
- *Detrusor overactivity*—Involuntary detrusor contractions during the filling phase, spontaneous or provoked
- Detrusor overactivity can be—
  1. *Phasic waveform detrusor overactivity*—Involuntary detrusor contraction leading to voiding but patient can suppress the leak.
  2. *Terminal*—Involuntary detrusor contraction occurring at cystometric capacity, which cannot be suppressed resulting in incontinence/voiding.
  3. *DO incontinence*—Incontinence due to an involuntary contraction.
  4. *Idiopathic*—No defined cause of DO.
  5. *Neurogenic*—Underlying neurological cause present.

C. Bladder compliance during filling cystometry:

Describes relationships between change in bladder volume and change in detrusor pressure.

- Compliance=change in volume/change in detrusor pressure.
- Points:
  1. At the start of filling—Pdet is 0, volume is 0.
  2. At cystometric capacity or immediately before any detrusor contraction that caused significant leakage.

D. Bladder capacity during filling cystometry:

- *Cystometric capacity*—Bladder volume at the end of filling cystometrogram when permission to void given
- *Maximum cystometric capacity*—Volume at which patient feels he/she can no longer delay micturition patient with normal sensation
- *Maximum anesthetic bladder capacity*—Volume to which bladder can be filled under deep anesthesia and should be classified according to anesthesia used.

E. Urethral function during filling cystometry:

- *Normal urethral closure mechanism*—Maintains a positive urethral closure during bladder filling even in the presence of increased abdominal pressure
- *Incompetent urethral closure mechanism*—Which allows leakage of urine
- *Urethral relaxation incontinence*—Leakage due to urethral relaxation
- *Urodynamic stress incontinence*—Involuntary leakage of urine during increased abdominal pressure.

F. Assessment of urethral pressure measurement:

- *Urethral pressure*—Fluid pressure needed to just open the urethra
- *Urethral pressure profile*—Graph indicating the intraluminal pressure along the length of urethra
- *Urethral closure pressure*—(urethral pressure -intravesical pressure)
- **Maximum urethral pressure** —The maximum pressure of the measured profile
- **Maximum urethral closure pressure (MUCP)** —Maximum difference between the urethral pressure and the intravesical pressure
- **Functional profile length**—Length of the urethra along which the urethral pressure exceeds intravesical pressure in women.

Pressure flow study

A. Measurement of urine flow.

- *Flow rate*—Volume of fluid expelled via the urethra per unit time. It is expressed in mL/s.

- *Voided volume*—Total volume expelled via the urethra
- *Maximum flow rate*—Maximum measured value of the flow rate after correction for artefacts
- *Voiding time*—Total duration of micturition
- *Flow time*—Time over which measurable flow actually occurs
- *Average flow rate*—Voided volume divided by flow time
- *Time to maximum flow*—The elapsed time from onset of flow to maximum flow.

B. Pressure measurement during pressure flow study:

Following are applicable for each pressure curves:

- *Premicturition pressure*—Pressure recorded immediately before the initial isovolumetric contraction
- *Opening pressure*—Pressure recorded at the onset of urine flow
- *Opening time*—Elapsed time from initial rise in detrusor pressure to onset of flow
- *Maximum pressure*—Maximum value of the measured pressure
- *Pressure at maximum flow*—Lowest pressure recorded at maximum measured flow rate
- *Closing pressure*—Pressure measured at the end of measured flow
- *Minimum voiding pressure*—Minimum pressure during measurable flow but is not necessarily equal to either the opening or closing pressures
- *Flow delay*—Time delay between a change in bladder pressure and the corresponding change in measured flow rate.

C. Detrusor function during voiding:

- ***Normal detrusor function***—Normal voiding is achieved by a voluntarily continuous detrusor contraction that leads to complete bladder emptying within a normal time span, and in the absence of bladder outlet obstruction.
- ***Abnormal detrusor activity***—
  - *Detrusor underactivity*—Contraction of reduced strength and/or duration, resulting in prolonged bladder emptying and/or a failure to achieve complete bladder emptying within a normal time span
  - *Acontractile detrusor*—Does not demonstrate contractile activity during urodynamic studies.
- ***Post void residual (PVR)***—Volume of urine left in the bladder at the end of micturition.

D. Urethral function during voiding:

- **Normal urethra function**—Urethra that opens and is continuously relaxed to allow the bladder to be emptied at a normal intravesical pressure
- ***Abnormal urethra function***—
  - *Bladder outlet obstruction*—Generic term for obstruction during voiding and is characterized by increased detrusor pressure and reduced urine flow rate. It is usually diagnosed by studying the synchronous values of flow rate and detrusor pressure
  - *Dysfunctional voiding*—Characterized by an intermittent and/or fluctuating flow rate due to involuntary intermittent contractions of the peri-urethral striated muscle during voiding in neurologically normal individuals
  - *Detrusor sphincter dyssynergia*—A detrusor contraction concurrent with an involuntary contraction of the urethral and/or peri-urethral striated muscle. Occasionally, expulsion of urine may be prevented altogether.
  - *Non-relaxing urethral sphincter obstruction*—Characterized by a non relaxing, obstructing urethra resulting in reduced urine flow. Usually occurs in individuals with a sacral or infrasacral neurological lesion.

Q. What are the normal values of parameters?

- **Uroflowmetry:**

  Men under 40 years = Q_{max} >25mL/sec

  Men over 60 years = Q_{max} >15mL/sec

  Females = Q_{max}>30–35mL/sec
- **Pressure or flow studies:**

  A. Storage—

  Maximum cystometric capacity (MCC) =350–600 mL

  Volume at first sensation = approx 50% of the MCC

  Volume at normal desire = approx 75% of MCC

  Volume at strong desire = approx 90% of the MCC

  Normal compliance= >30 mL/cm H_2O

  B. Voiding—

  Maximum detrusor pressure = 25–60 cm H_2O

  Pdetr@Q_{max} in men = 40–60 cm H_2O

  Pdet@Q_{max} in females = 20–40 cm H_2O

  Post void residual volume = <25 mL

Q. What are the target pressures?

See above.

Q. How you will describe the different curve pattern?

1. Normal (Fig. 6.15):

This is a normal UDS tracing showing gradually increased detrusor pressure leading to adequate

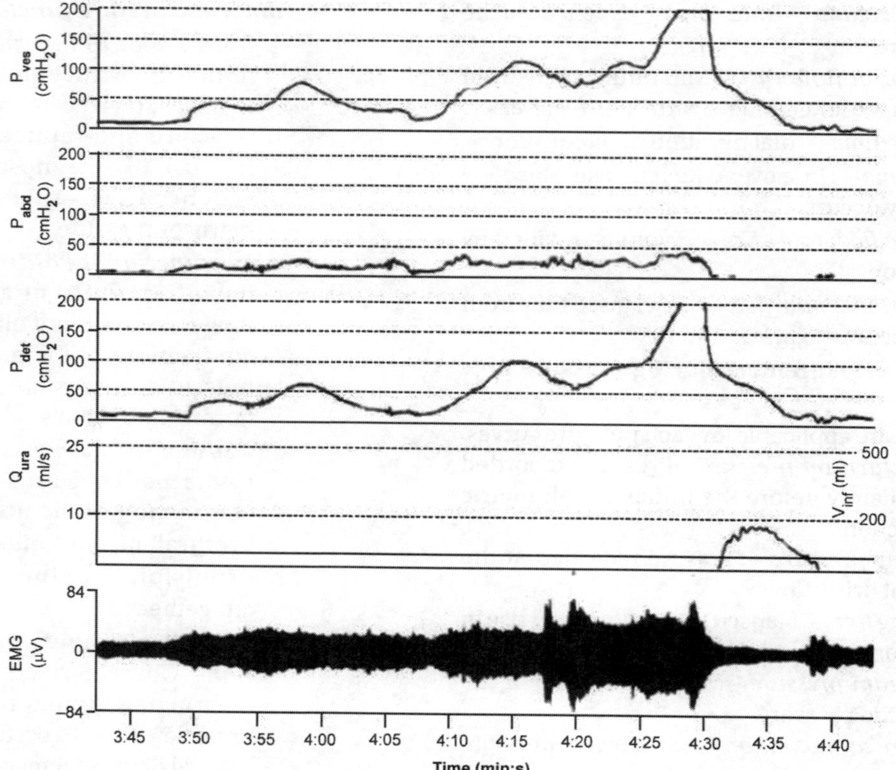

Figure 6.15: Normal UDS tracings

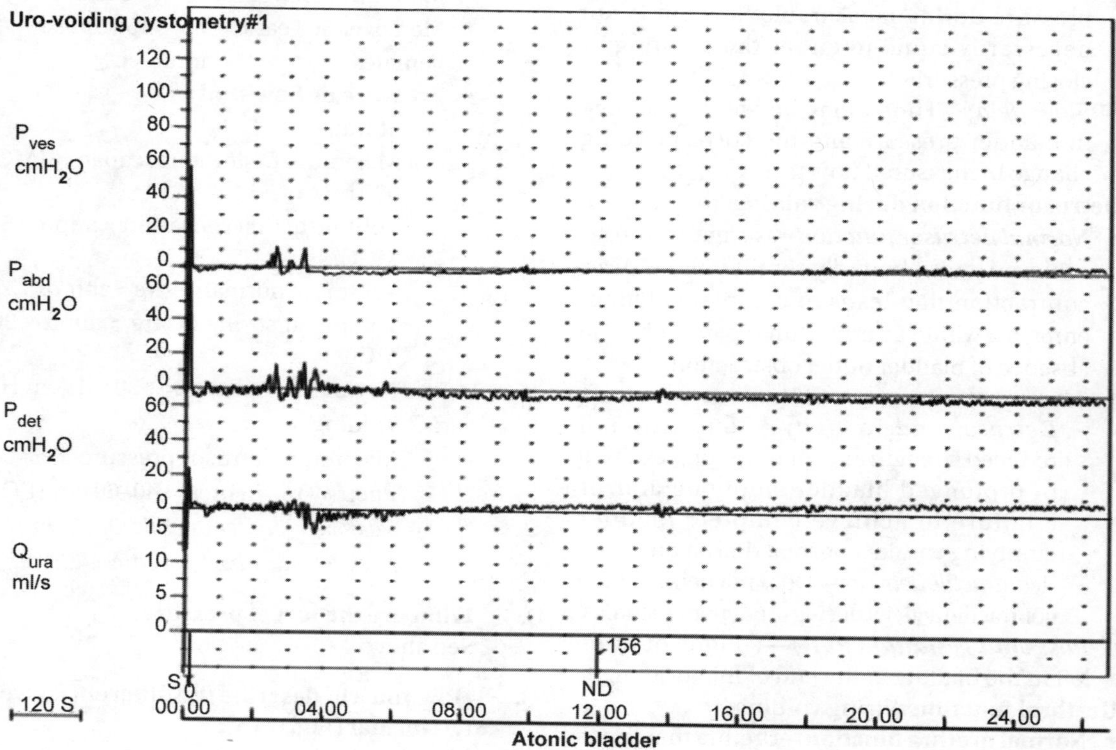

Figure 6.16: UDS tracings of atonic bladder

gradually increased intravesical pressure with relaxation of urethral sphincter which lead to voiding of urine with normal flow pattern.

2. **Atonic Bladder (Fig. 6.16)*:***

This is a UDS tracing of atonic bladder in which no contraction of detrusor leading to inability to rise adequate intravesical pressure resulting in no voiding of urine.

3. **Detrusor Hyperactivity (Fig. 6.17)*:***

This is a UDS tracing of detrusor hyperactivity showing characteristic repeated waveform of detrusor contraction during filling phase of bladder.

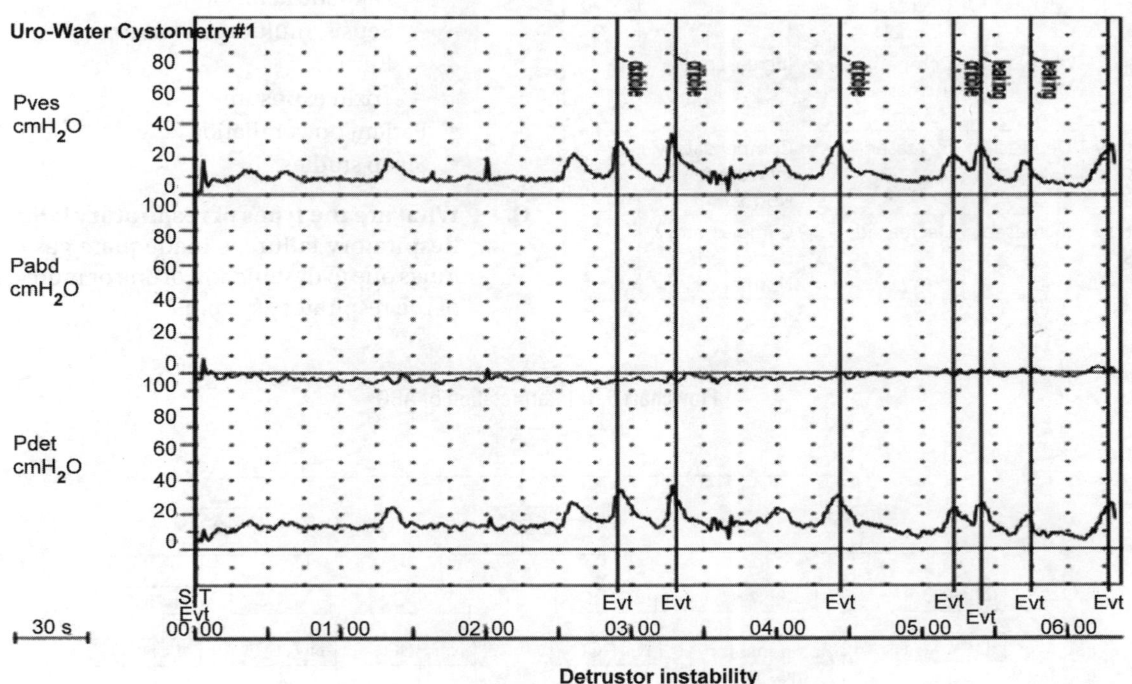

Figure 6.17: UDS tracings of detrusor Instability

ABG

Table 6.13: Sample ABG report

	Blood gas	
pCO_2	38.6 mmHg	[35.0 – 45.0]
pO_2	92.7 mmHg	[80.0 – 100.0]
pH	7.213	[7.350 – 7.450]
Hct	53.0 % (+)	[35.0 – 50.0]
SO_2	96.3%	[75.0 – 99.0]
$cHCo_3$	15.2 mmol/L	
	Electrolytes	
Na^+	134.7 mmol/L (-)	[135.0 – 148.0]
K^+	4.69 mmol/L (+)	[3.50 – 4.50]
Ca^+	0.436 mmol/L (- -)	[1.120 – 1.320]
Cl^-	102.3 mmol/L	[98.0 – 107.0]

Contd...

Contd...

	Hb derivatives	
tHb	15.8 g/dL	[11.5 – 17.4]
O_2Hb	94.7 % (-)	[95.0 – 99.0]
COHb	1.0 % #	[0.5 – 2.5]
HHb	3.6%	[1.0 – 5.0]
MetHb	0.7%	[0.4 – 1.5]
Bili	out of rang (-)	[3.0 – 49.7]
	Metabolites	
Glu	159 mg/dL (++)	[60 – 110]
Lac	14 mg/dL	[4 – 20]
Urea	not calibrated	[15 – 38]

This (Table 6.13) is an ABG report showing pH <7.35 with decreased HCO_3 and normal PCO_2 and normal PO_2. So, this patient is having noncompensatory metabolic acidosis.

Q. How will you interpret?

In summary (Table 6.14and Flowchart 6.1):

Table 6.14: Interpretation of ABG

	pH	*pCO_2*	*HCO^-_3*	*pO_2*
Normal	7.35–7.45	35–45 mm Hg	22-26meq/l	80–100%
Metabolic acidosis	Decreased	Compensatory Decreased/ Normal	Decreased	
Metabolic alkalosis	Increased	Compensatory increased/ normal	Increased	
Respiratory acidosis	Decreased	Increased	Compensatory increased/ Normal	
Respiratory alkalosis	Increased	Decreased	Compensatory decreased/ Normal	

Q. What are the normal values?

See above.

Q. When you will do it?

- Respiratory failure
- Any illness leading to metabolic derangement—
  - Cardiac, hepatic, renal failure
  - Diabetic ketoacidosis
  - Sepsis, multiorgan failure
  - Burns
  - Toxin exposure
- Patient on ventilation
- Sleep studies.

Q. What are the types of respiratory failure?

Respiratory failure is inadequate gas exchange by lungs due to dysfunction of one or more components of the respiratory system.

Flowchart 6.1: Interpretation of ABG

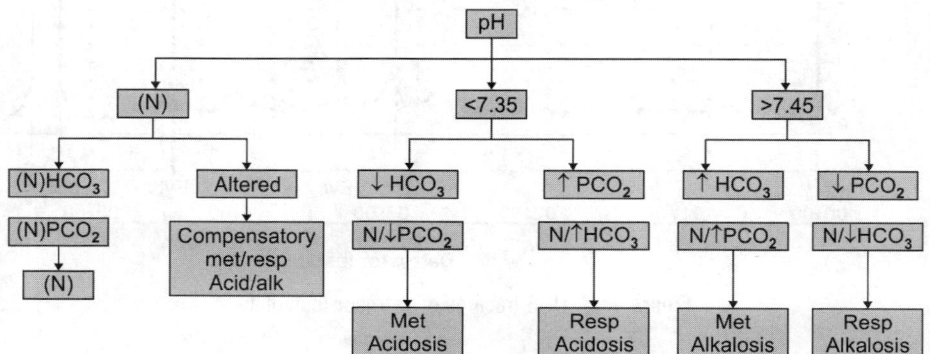

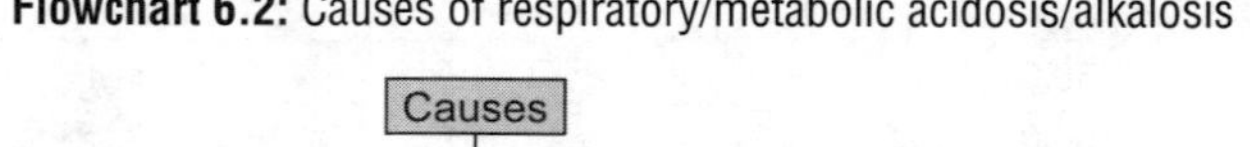

Abbreviation: Resp; Respiratory; Alk, Alkalosis; Met, Metabolic; Acid, Acidosis

Flowchart 6.2: Causes of respiratory/metabolic acidosis/alkalosis

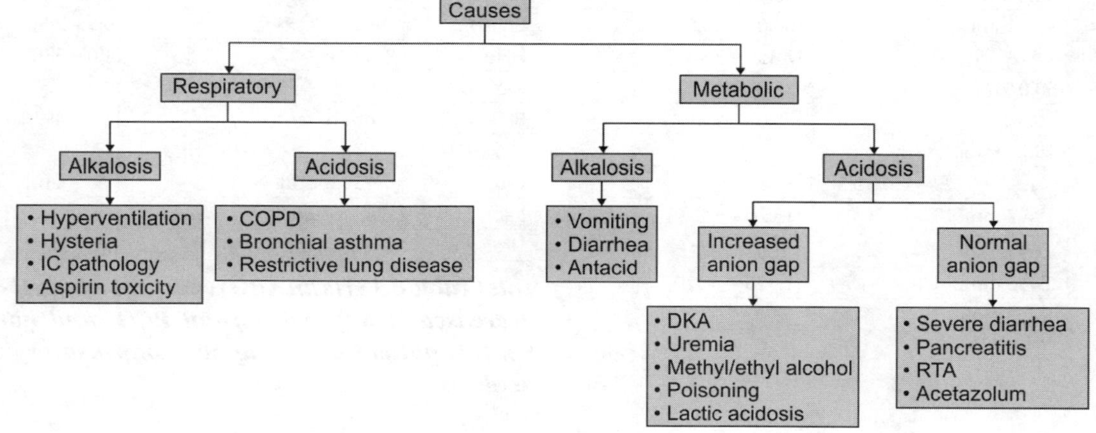

Q. What is respiratory failure?

- **Type 1 or hypoxemic respiratory failure:** Failure of oxygen exchange, normal PCO_2 decreased PO_2.
- **Type 2 or hypercapnic respiratory failure:** Failure to remove carbon dioxide, increased PCO_2, decreased PO_2.
- **Type 3 respiratory failure:** Perioperative respiratory failure caused by increased atelectasis due to low FRC in a setting abnormal abdominal wall mechanics.
- **Type 4 respiratory failure:** In patient of shock and patient is intubated and on ventilation.
- **Cause of lactic acidosis:**
  - Sepsis
  - Liver failure
  - Metformin.

7 Chapter

PMR Specimen

BRONCHIECTASIS OF LUNG

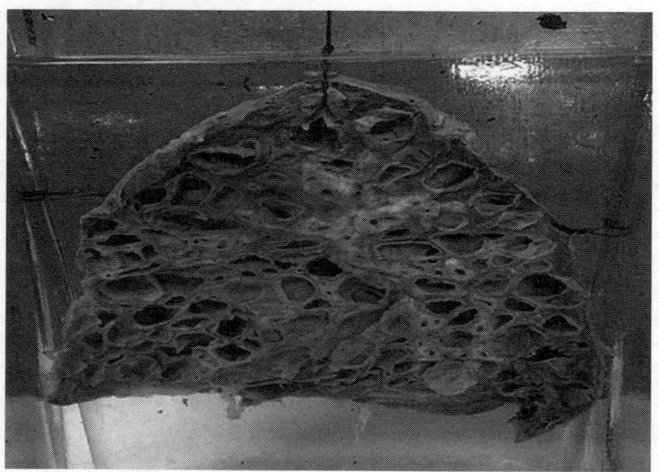

Figure 7.1: Bronchiectasis of lung *(For color version see plate 1)*

Figure 7.1 is a specimen showing markedly distended peripheral brochi with thickened bronchial wall. So, I think this is a specimen of lung bronchiectasis.

Q. What is bronchiectasis?

Bronchiectasis refers to an irreversible airway dilatation of the lung focally or diffusely.

Q. What are the etiologies?

- Endobronchial obstruction due to foreign body or mass
- Recurrent aspiration
- Infection: Bacterial (nontubercular), mycobacteria
- Immunodeficiency: HIV, lung transplantation
- Genetic causes: Cystic fibrosis, Kartagener's syndrome
- Autoimmune or rheumatic diseases: RA, Sjogren syndrome, inflammatory bowel disease
- Immunomediated disease: Allergic bronchopulmonary aspergillosis (ABPA)
- Recurrent infection
- Yellow nail syndrome
- Marfan syndrome
- Idiopathic.

Q. What are the symptoms of bronchiectasis?

- Persistent productive cough with thick tenacious sputum
- Recurrent hemoptysis
- Clubbing of digits occasionally
- Coarse crackles on lung auscultation.

Q. What are the complications of bronchiectasis?

- Recurrent infection
- Pulmonary hypertension
- Cor pulmonale
- Amyloidosis
- Respiratory failure.

Q. What are the investigations done in bronchiectasis?

- Chest X-ray: Tram track sign in longitudinal section, ring shadow in cross-sectional section
- HRCT of chest for confirmation (tram tracks, signet ring sign, tree in bud pattern).

Q. How you will manage this case?

- Patient education and counseling
- Pharmacological
  - Antibiotic in exacerbated cases

- Anti-inflammatory therapy by inhalation
- Mucolytic agents
- Nonpharmacological: ***Postural drainage***
- Breathing exercises.

Q. What is Kartagener's syndrome?

Triad consists of:

- Primary cilliary dyskinesia
- Situs inversus
- Chronic sinusitis.

Q. What is postural drainage?

- Postural drainage is the gravitational clearance of secretions from specific bronchial segments by using one or more of different positions.

Q. What are the prerequisites of postural drainage?

- Patient is to be placed with the dependent lung segment as vertical as possible
- A position is medically unsafe or causes increased patient discomfort, position must be modified to suit the clinical situation

Q. What are the different positions?

Apical segment of upper lobe:

- Patient in semi-Fowler's position with head of the bed raised 45°.

Anterior segment of both upper lobes:

- Patient supine with the bed flat.

Posterior segment of right upper lobe:

- Patient one-quarter turn from prone with the right side up, supported by pillows with head of the bed flat.

Posterior segment of left upper lobe:

- Patient one quarter turn from prone with left side up, supported by pillows with head of the bed elevated 30°.

Medial and lateral segment of right middle lobe:

- Patient one quarter turn from supine with right side up and foot of the bed elevated 12–14 inches.

Superior and inferior segments of left lingula:

- Patient one quarter turn from supine with left side up and foot of the bed elevated 12–14 inches.

Superior segments of both lower lobes:

- Prone on a flat bed with a pillow under abdominal area.

Anterior basal segment of both lower lobes:

- Patient supine with foot of the bed elevated 18–20 inches.

Posterior basal segments of both lower lobes:

- Patient prone with foot of the bed elevated 18–20 inches.

Lateral basal of left lower lobe and medial basal of right lower lobe:

- Patient in right lateral position with foot of the bed elevated 18–20 inches.
- Summary of different position is given in flowchart 7.1.

Flowchart 7.1: Summary of different position

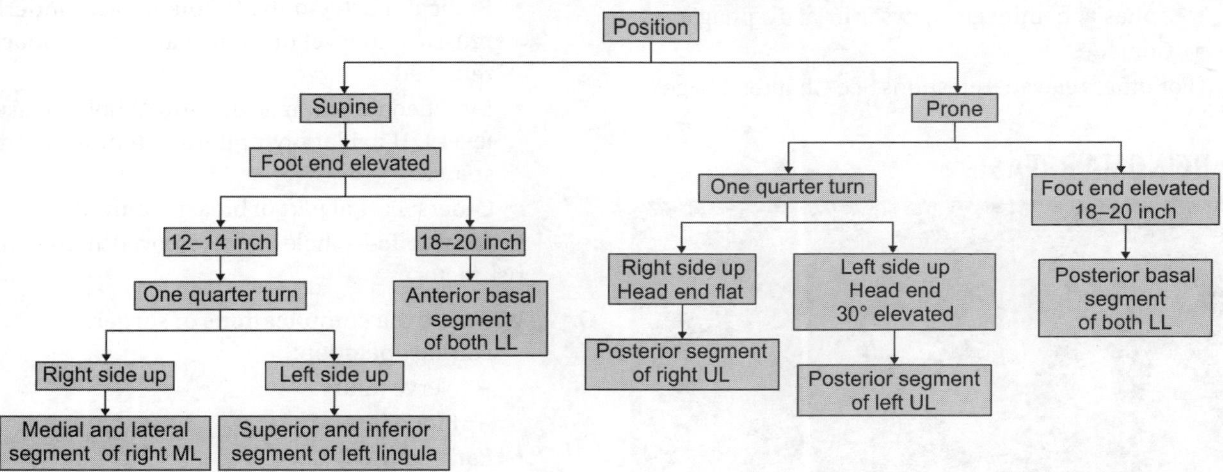

Q. What are the indications of surgery in bronchiectasis?

- ***Surgical resection*** done in case of:
  - Severely affected segments
  - Bleeding segments.
- ***Lung transplantation*** done in case of advanced cases:
  - Oxygen dependent respiratory failure
  - Hypercapnia
  - Pulmonary hypertension.

BRAIN HEMORRHAGE

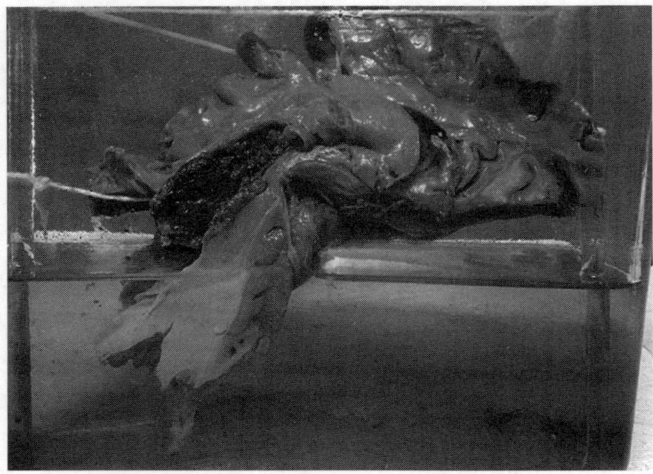

Figure 7.2: Brain hemorrhage *(For color version see plate 1)*

Figure 7.2 is a specimen of brain showing blackish hematoma in occipital and parietal lobe.

Q. What is the incidence?

15% of all strokes.

Q. What are the clinical features of this condition?

- Features of increased ICT like sudden onset of headache and/or loss of consciousness, vomiting, seizure
- Neck rigidity can occur
- Hemiplegia along with cranial nerve palsy
- Aphasia, hemineglect, dysarthria, dysphagia
- Coma.

(For other relevant questions See Chapter 2 Page 6).

CARCINOMA BREAST

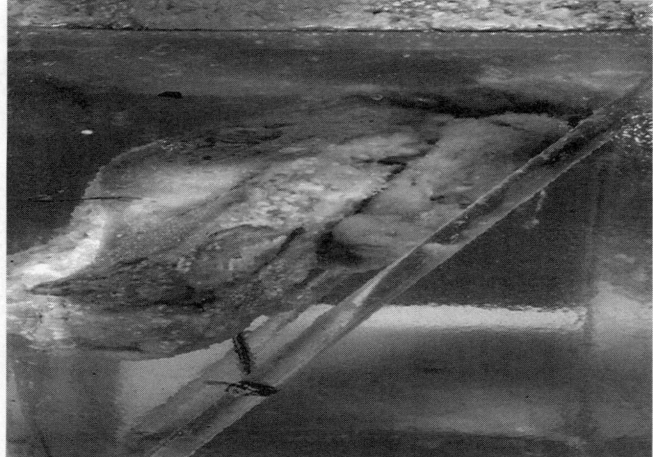

Figure 7.3: Carcinoma breast *(For color version see plate 1)*

Figure 7.3 is a specimen of breast showing an irregular SOL in the breast with skin involvement peau d'orange skin. So, I think this is a specimen of breast carcinoma (CA).

Q. Name different types of CA breast.

- Ductal carcinoma in situ
- Invasive ductal carcinoma
- Invasive lobular carcinoma
- Inflammatory breast cancer
- Paget's disease of nipple
- Phylloids tumor
- Angiosarcoma
- Adenoid cystic carcinoma
- Medullary carcinoma
- Mucinous carcinoma
- Papillary carcinoma
- Tubular carcinoma.

Q. What is the treatment of choice?

Treatment of breast CA depends upon type of breast cancer, stages of breast cancer and other associated medical illness and also personal preferences.

- Surgery
- Radiation therapy
- Adjuvant therapy by chemotherapy, hormone therapy.

Q. What are the types of mastectomy?

- Simple mastectomy: Whole breast and lymph node if present removed
- Radical mastectomy: Whole breast, underlying muscle and level I,II,III axillary lymph nodes are removed
- Modified radical mastectomy: Whole breast and level I, II axillary lymph node removed, muscle spared.

  Others: Partial part of breast removed.

Prophylactic—Whole breast removed in women with risk factor.

Q. What are the complications of surgery?

- During operation:
  - Nerve injury
  - Blood loss.
- Early complications:
  - Infection
  - Wound dehiscence
  - Discharge.
- Late complications:
  - Hypertrophy of scar
  - Contracture with deformity of shoulder and back
  - Lymphoedema.

Q. What is postmastectomy lymphoedema?

It is a disorder of lymhphatic fluid accumulation resulting in swelling of affected area after mastectomy operation due to removal or damage of lymph nodes.

Q. Write brief notes about breast reconstructive surgery.

- Breast reconstruction surgery is to restore the shape and feel of the breast after mastectomy operation
- It can be done by either flap reconstruction or using an implant.

Flap reconstruction:

- Reconstruction done with patient's own tissues
- Good option for women with bulky muscle
- Longer duration and more challenging operation
- Matching surgery of opposite breast may require
- Easier to match the opposite breast compared to implant.

Implant reconstruction:

- Implant is placed under pectoralis muscle
- Do not last lifetime
- It requires less time
- Good option for lean and thin women
- Rupture, deflation, capsular contracture may occur
- Often opposite healthy breast needs surgery to match
- In case of radiation it should be avoided.

Q. What are the types of flap reconstruction?

- TRAM flap
- DIEP flap
- SIEA flap
- Latissimus dorsi flap, etc.

Q. What are the different types of breast prosthesis?

1. Saline
2. Silicone gel
3. Combination of two.

CARRIE'S SPINE

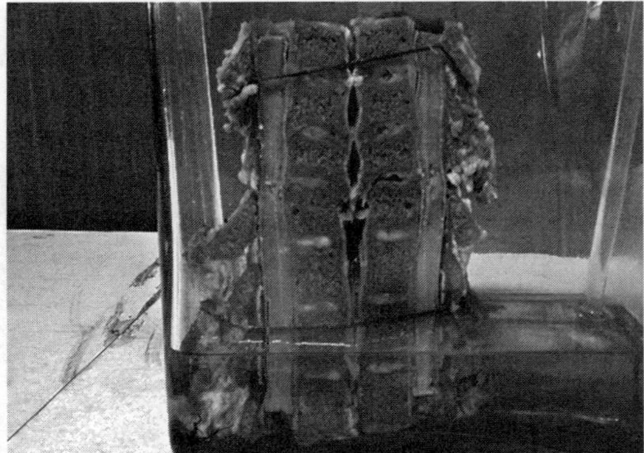

Figure 7.4: Carrie's spine *(For color version see plate 2)*

Figure 7.4 is a specimen of spine showing destruction of multiple vertebral bodies along with involvement of intravertebral disk but pedicle is normal. So, I think this is a specimen of Carrie's spine.

Q. What do you mean by Carrie's spine?

- Tubercular spondylitis, destruction of vertebral body and intervertebral disk by *Mycobacterium tuberculosis.*

Q. What are the routes of transmission?

The bacteria can spread via:

- Hematogenous route from lungs or lymph nodes
- Paravertebral plexus of veins, i.e. Batson's plexus from abdominal visceral plexus.

Q. What may be the clinical features of this case?

The clinical features of Carrie's spine vary in different patient.

- Back pain
- Weight loss, fever, fatigue, malaise
- Stiffness of back
- Cold abscess
- Deformity : Knuckle (deformity due to wedging of **one vertebrae**), gibbus (one form of kyphosis caused by **more than one vertebral** wedging), kyphus
- Paraplegia.

Q. How do you diagnose the case?

Carrie's spine is diagnosed by history, clinical examination and investigations.

Investigations done are—

- Routine blood investigations to see elevated ESR and CRP
- Mantoux test
- X-ray of spine, chest
- CT scan
- MRI of spine is investigation of choice.

Q. What are the X-ray and MRI features?

X-ray features of Carrie's spine:

- Focal areas of erosion and osseous destruction of anterior vertebral bodies
- Destruction of intervertebral disk
- Vertebral body collapse
- Skip lesions of vertebral body collapse
- Vertebra plana deformity in case single vertebra involvement
- Paraspinal abscess as fusiform soft tissue swelling around spine.

MRI features of Carrie's spine:

- *T1 weighted images*: Decreased signal for affected vertebral bodies, disk height loss, paraspinal soft tissue masses

- *T2 weighted images*: Usually nonspecific increased signal in bony and soft tissues
- *Contrast enhanced MRI*: Presence of thick rim of enhancement around paraspinal and intraosseous abscesses.

Q. What type of ankylosis occurs in this case?

In case of Carrie's spine bony ankylosis occurs.

Q. What is the role of ATD in Carrie's spine?

Biological control of causative agents by ATD lead to relief of pain, stoppage of further destruction of vertebrae and consequently further complications like neurological deficit and deformity and improves quality of life.

Q. What are the regimens?

- For new cases:
  - *Intensive phase*—8 weeks isoniazid, rifampicin, pyrazinamide and ethambutol in daily fixed dose combinations in four weight bands
  - *Continuation phase*—isoniazid, rifampicin, ethambutol for 16 weeks and can be extended by 28–40 weeks based on clinical decision by treating physician.
- For defaulter or recurrence cases:
  - *Intensive phase*—Injection streptomycin, INH, rifampicin, pyrazinamide and ethambutol. Injection streptomycin for 8 weeks and rest for another 4 weeks
  - *Continuation phase*—Rifampicin, INH, ethambutol for 20 weeks and can be extended by 3–6 months depending on clinical decision by treating physician.

Q. Tell me about dose and side effects of first line ATD.

Dose of ATD:

Drugs name	*Daily dose (mg/kg body wt)*
Isoniazid	5 mg/kg (4–6 mg/kg)
Rifampicin	10 mg/kg (8–12 mg/kg)
Pyrazinamide	25 mg/kg (20–30 mg/kg)
Streptomycin	15 mg/kg (12–18 mg/k)
Ethambutol	15 mg/kg (15–20 mg/kg)

Adverse effects:

- Isoniazid—Peripheral neuritis, hepatitis, rashes, fever, acne, arthralgia
- Rifampicin—Hepatitis, respiratory syndrome (breathlessness with shock and collapse), purpura, hemolysis, renal failure, flushing, pruritis, rashes, flu-like syndromes, nausea, vomiting, abdominal cramps
- Pyrazinamide—Hepatitis, hyperuricemia, arthralgia, flushing, rashes, fever, poor glycemic control
- Ethambutol—Optic neuritis, hyperuricemia, neurological changes, rashes, fever.
- Streptomycin—Ototoxicity, nephrotoxicity.

Q. What are the causes of paraplegia in Carrie's spine?

Causes of paraplegia in Carrie's spine are mainly due to compression. The causes are:

- Cold abscess
- Bony deformity
- Granulation tissue
- Tuberculous focus
- Posterior spinal disease
- Infective thrombosis spinal vein.

Late onset paraplegia can occur due to recurrent disease, fibrous septae following healing.

Q. What are the implications of Mantoux test and role in diagnosis?

- The Mantoux test measures degree of hypersensitivity to tuberculin protein. There is no relationship between size of indurations and current active disease and its correlation with the future development of TB
- Associated health factor determine the size of induration
- There is no correlation between the size of post-vaccination Mantoux reaction and protection against TB
- Role in diagnosis
- Induration larger than 15 mm likely to be due to active disease in a person with not known risk factor of TB
- Formation of vesicles, bullae, necrosis indicate high likelihood of infection with TB.

Q. How you will do it?

One unit of purified protein derivative (1.5 mL) is injected subcutaneously by proper technique forming a 6–10 mm wheal.

Reading is done after 72 hours.

Q. Where you will find false negative result?

- Cutaneous anergy
- Recent TB

- Very old TB infection
- Less than 6 months old baby
- Recent live vaccination
- Viral illness
- Overwhelming TB infection
- Incorrect interpretation and administration.

Q. Where you will find false positive result?
- Previous BCG vaccination
- Infection with nontuberculous mycobacteria
- Incorrect method of administration
- Misinterpretation of result
- Incorrect antigen used.

Q. How will you stabilize the spine?
- Externally by proper orthotic support
- Internally by surgical fixation.

Q. What are the exercise regimens in Carrie's spine?
Exercise regimens of Carrie's spine are same as SCI by any cause.
(For further information See Chapter 2, Page 17.)

Q. What is the role of immobilization in Carrie's spine?
- Pain relief
- Aids in healing of vertebral lesion
- Support of spine till the vertebrae became stable.

OSTEOMYELITIS

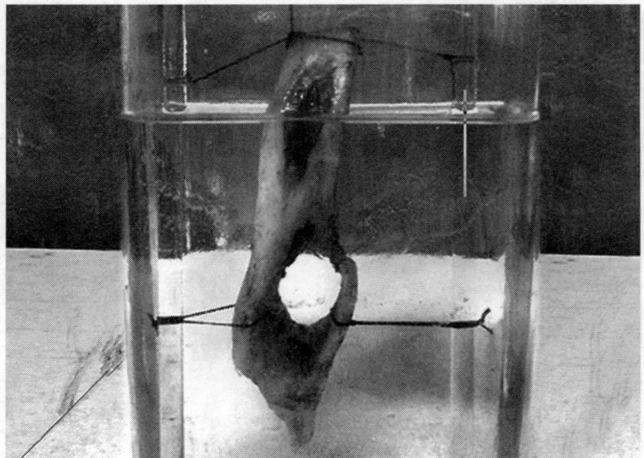

Figure 7.5: Osteomyelitis *(For color version see plate 2)*

Figure 7.5 is a specimen of long bone showing destruction of part of bone with presence of sinus tract and dead bone (sequestrum). So, I think this is a specimen of chronic osteomyelitis.

Q. What are the common presentations of acute and chronic osteomyelitis?
Acute osteomyelitis:
- Acute onset pain and swelling of bone
- Systemic features of infection like fever.

Chronic osteomyelitis:
- Minimal pain
- Chronic discharging sinuses
- In acute exacerbations systemic features like fever may occur.

Q. What are the common pathogens of osteomyelitis?
- *Staphylococcus aureus* is the most common *organism*
- *Streptococcus*
- *Pneumococcus.*

Q. What investigations should be done to diagnose the case?
- Blood: Routine blood investigations to see leukocytosis, elevated ESR and CRP
- Pus culture and sensitivity
- X-rays
- Bone scan.

Q. What is sequestrum?
- It is a piece of dead bone.

Q. What is involucrum?
- It is the dense sclerotic bone over a sequestrum.

Q. How you will manage the case medically?
- Rest by splint or traction
- Broad spectrum antibiotic and in case of pus discharge preferably after culture sensitivity.

Q. What are the indications of surgery in osteomyelitis?
- In case of acute osteomyelitis if there is no response after 48 hours of treatment surgical intervention is required
- In case of chronic osteomyelitis surgery is the treatment of choice.

Q. How you will rehabilitate the patient after surgery?

Goal of rehabilitations after surgery is—

- Prevent pathological fracture
- Augmentation of healing
- Prevention of deformity like contracture, joint stiffness
- Regimen:
  - Rest –relative rest and non-weight bearing of affected limb progressing to gradual weight bearing
  - Strengthening exercise to prevent wasting and atrophy as well as of upper limb
  - ROM and stretching exercise to prevent contracture and deformity.
  - Endurance training
  - Balance and gait training
  - Maintain proper nutrition.

Q. What are the complications of osteomyelitis?

- Acute osteomyelitis:
  - Chronic osteomyelitis
  - Pathological fractures
  - Limb length discrepancy and deformity
  - Acute pyogenic arthritis.
- Chronic osteomyelitis:
  - Acute exacerbation of infection
  - Pathological fracture
  - Limb length discrepancy
  - Contracture or deformity of joint
  - Sinus tract malignancy
  - Amyloidosis.

8 Chapter

PT Instruments

HEAT THERAPY

Superficial Heat Therapy

Infrared Therapy

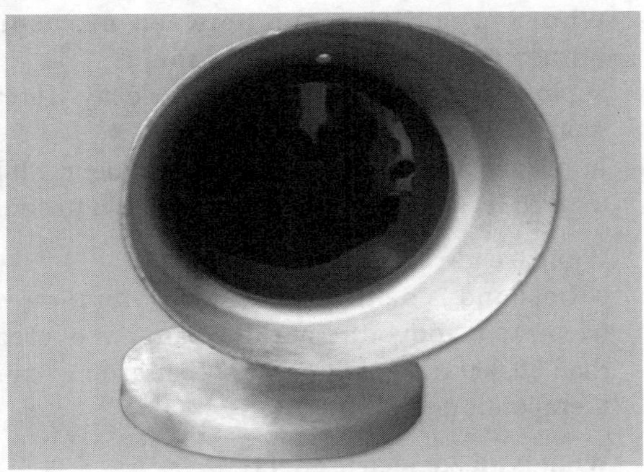

Figure 8.1: Infrared therapy

Figure 8.1 is a reddish lamp that uses infrared ray, a part of electromagnetic spectrum that gives rise to heat when absorbed by other tissues. So I think this is infrared lamp.

Q. What are the types of infrared (IR)?

- IR A from 760 to 1,400 nm (short wave IR)
- IR B from 1,400 to 3,000 nm (medium wave IR)
- IR C from 3,000 to 10,000 nm (long wave IR

Q. What is the wavelength of infrared?

See above.

Q. What are the type of IR generators?

- Non-luminous type IR generators (750 nm to 15,000 nm)
- Luminous type IR generators (350 nm to 4,000 nm).

Q. What is the application procedure?

- Position the lamp so that the rays strike the affected area at right angle
- Distance maintained is to be between 50–70 cm (Hand shake distance).

Q. What are the indications?

- Relief of pain (in mild doses), due to sedative effect on superficial sensory nerve endings
- Relieving muscle spasms
- Small joint pains
- To increase blood circulation
- Fibromyalgia syndrome.

Q. What are the contraindications?

- Pacemaker/Defibrillator
- Open injuries
- Impaired arterial blood supply
- Impaired skin sensation
- Pregnancy
- Fever
- Hemophiliacs.

Q. What are the complications?

1. Superficial heat burns
2. Electrical shock
3. Gangrene
4. Headache
5. Faintness: *To prevent this, the patient should rise slowly from the recumbent position after a session of extensive treatment.*

Paraffin Bath

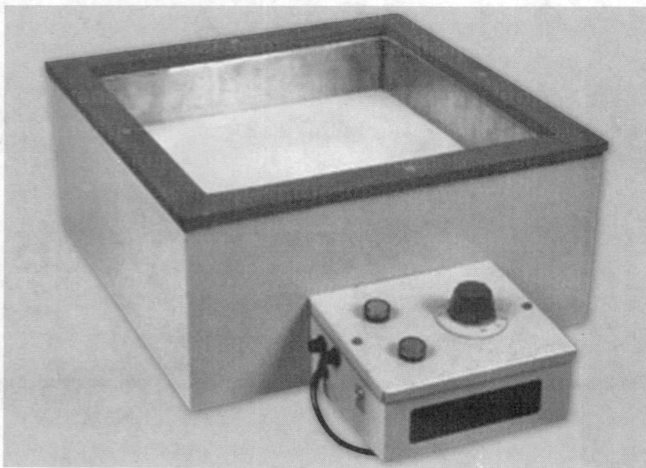

Figure 8.2: Paraffin bath

Q. How does a paraffin bath work?
A paraffin bath is a superficial heating agent that uses conduction as primary form of heat transfer.

Q. What are the ingredients?
Ingredients—paraffin: mineral oil = 6:1 or 7:1.

Q. How much heat can be obtained?
Temperature: 52.2–54.4 °C (126–130 °F)

Q. What are the methods of application?
- Dipping (most common): 12 dips then wrapping in plastic
- Immersion: 6–8 dips, then immersion for 30 minutes
- Brushing: Brushing coats of paraffin, in inaccessible areas and children.

Q. How is the safety?
- Temperature of thermometer: 48 °C
- A thin film of unmelted paraffin on tank wall indicates safe temperature.

Q. What are the indications ?
- Hand contracture secondary to burns, injury
- Edema.

Q. What are the contraindications?
- General heat precautions
- Open wounds
- Infected areas.

Deep Heat

Ultrasonic Therapy

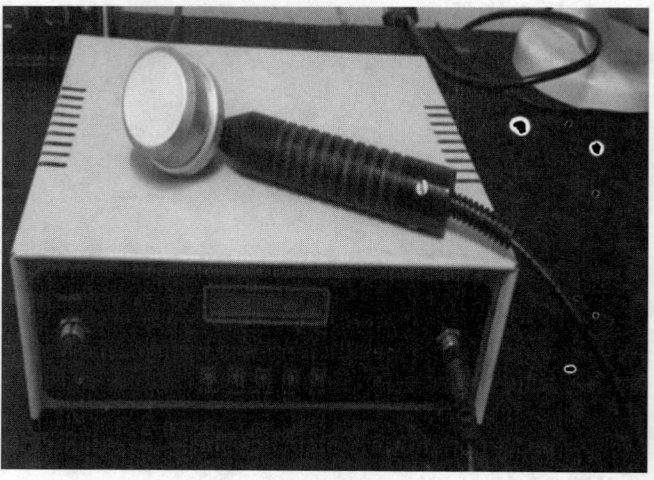

Figure 8.3: Ultrasonic therapy

Figure 8.3 is a machine attached with a round shaped metallic applicator. So I think this is an ultrasonic therapy machine.

Q. What is the difference between ultrasonic, infrasonic, supersonic and subsonic?
Supersonic and subsonic refers to velocity. If greater than speed of sound, it is supersonic.
Infrasonic and ultrasonic refer to frequency. If less than 20 Hz it is subsonic and >20,000 is ultrasonic.

Q. What are ultrasound waves?
Ultrasound is defined as acoustic vibration with frequency above the audible range, i.e. greater than 20,000 Hz. Medical uses of ultrasound can be therapeutic and diagnostic.

Q. What is piezoelectric effect?
Some substance when subjected to mechanical stress produce electric current. The reverse occurs when an electric field is applied to the crystal producing vibrations at specific frequency, this is called reverse piezoelectric effect.

Q. What are the effects of ultrasound on tissue?
- **Thermal effect** (US waves absorbed by the tissue are converted into heat). It depends on -
  - Nature of tissue (high for protein)

- Degree of vascularization
- Frequency of US (Frequency is directly proportional to absorption)
- Should be able to increase local blood flow and reduce pain and joint stiffness.

• **Non-thermal effect**
- Cavitation
- Acoustic streaming (stimulates cell activity, membrane permeability)
- Mechanical effect/micromassage
- Biological effect in all three stages of tissue repair, i.e. inflammatory, proliferative and remodeling stages.

Q. What is the application procedure?

Regular surface

- Circular
- Longitudinal
- Stationary.

Irregular surface

- Under water both transducer and surface with a gap of 1 cm in between.

Q. What are the indications?

- Recent injuries and inflammation
- Release of scar tissue
- Chronic indurated edema
- Chronic wound healing
- Trigger points.

Q. What are the contraindications?

- General heat precautions
- Near brain, eyes, reproductive organs
- Gravid or menstruating uterus
- Near pacemaker
- Near laminectomy sites
- Malignancy
- Skeletal immaturity—growing metaphyses
- Acute infection
- Bleeding disorders
- Over hollow viscera
- Peripheral vascular disease
- Arthroplasties
- Methyl methacrylate or high-density polyethylene
- Directly on plexus or nerve.

Q. What are the complications?

- Burns
- Unstable cavitations
- Vascular complication
- Tumor spread
- Spread of infection
- Fetal damage in pregnancy
- Microfracture in osteoporotic bone.

Q. What is coupling media?

To minimize the impedence difference, a suitable coupling medium has to be utilized. If even a small air gap exists between the transducer and the skin, the proportion of US that will be reflected approaches 99.998% which means that there will be no effective transmission.

The coupling media used in this context include water, various oils, creams and gels. Ideally, the coupling medium should be fluid so as to fill all available spaces, relatively viscous so that it stays in place, have an impedance appropriate to the media it connects, and should allow transmission of US with minimal absorption, attenuation or disturbance.

Q. Give some examples of coupling media.

1. Aqasonic gel - 72.6 %
2. Glycerol - 67 %
3. Distilled water - 59 %
4. Liquid paraffin - 19 %

Q. What is impedence?

It is the resistance to the passage of sound waves

Q. What are the best absorbing tissues?

The best absorbing tissues in terms of clinical practice are those with high collagen content—**ligament, tendon, fascia, joint capsule and scar tissue.**

Q. What are the precautions to be taken?

1. Always use the lowest intensity which produces a therapeutic response.
2. Ensure that the applicator is moved throughout the treatment.
3. Ensure that the patient is aware of the nature of the treatment and its expected outcome.

Q. What is phonophoresis?

Phonophoresis involves use of ultrasound to facilitate transdermal migration of topically administered medications.

Q. What are the drugs used in phonophoresis?

- Corticosteroid
- Antiinflammatory agents.

Q. Describe the use of UST on pressure ulcer?

It is generally applied over the regions adjacent to pressure ulcer which helps in reducing induration and edema.

Short Wave Diathermy

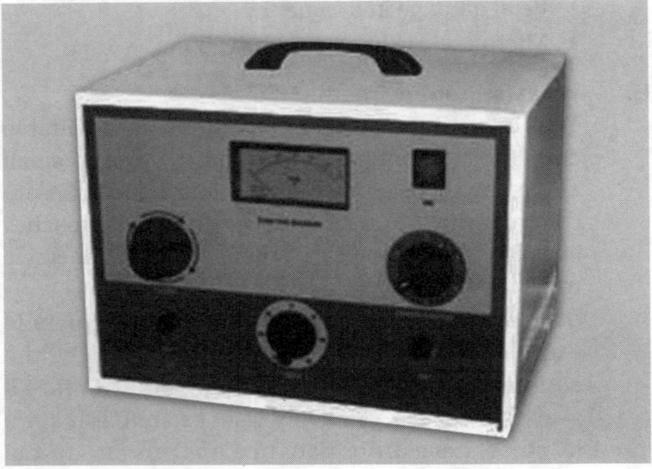

Figure 8.4: Short wave diathermy machine

Figure 8.4 is a machine which provides deep heating attached with pads for application of heat. So this is a short wave diathermy machine.

Q. What is diathermy?

In diathermy, a high-frequency electric current is delivered via shortwave, microwave and ultrasound to generate deep heat in body tissues.

Q. What is the wavelength and frequency?

Frequencies	*Wavelength*
• 13.56 MHz	22 m
• 27.12 MHz	11 m (Most common)
• 40.68 MHz	7.5 m

Q. What are the effects of diathermy?

- Effect on inflammation:
  - *Acute condition*—In acute condition, SWD is applied with caution to the treatment area in which there is already vasodilatation and exudation of the fluid increase in these processes may aggrevate the symptoms.
  - *Subacute condition*—In subacute condition stronger doses may be applied with considerable benefits.
  - *Chronic condition*—In chronic condition a thermal dose with longer duration must be used to be effective.

  Uses:
  - Lumbosacral strain
  - Degenerative disc disease
  - Tendinitis
  - Capsulitis
  - Pelvic inflammatory diseases.
- Relief of pain

  The mechanism of pain relief can be explained by the following ways:
  - *Sedative effect* due to mild degree of heating removal of noxious chemical which are the waste products of metabolism due to the increase blood flow
  - *Counter irritation* effect due to the strong superficial heating which blocks the pain transmission at the pain gate
  - Relief of pain also occur due to *resolution of inflammation* by SWD.
- Effects on traumatic condition

  Increased exudation of fluid, increased metabolism and increased blood flow help in the removal of waste products and increased availability of nutritive material which enhance healing process. In acute traumatic condition, caution should be taken.

  For joint stiffness which occurs through trauma, SWD is applied in stronger dose to cause a thermal effect in the tissue which enhances the extensibility of the collagen fibers.

  Uses:
  - Recent ankle injury
  - Meniscus injury in the knee
  - Post traumatic stiffness of the knee joint, etc.
- Induction of muscle relaxation:

  The increase of tissue temperature up to 42°C is being found to cause a decrease of the firing rate of type II muscle spindles efferent and γ - efferent and increase firing rate of type Ib fibers from the Golgi tendon organs. These changes in nerve fibers decrease the firing rate of α-motor neurons and thus reduce the muscle spasm.

  Uses:
  - Spasm of the post vertebral muscles
  - Low back pain.

Q. What is the application procedure?

- Inductive/inducto-thermic
- Capacitive

Q. What are the indications?

- Localized musculoskeletal pain
- Inflammation
- Pain/spasm
- Sprains/strains
- Tendonitis
- Tenosynovitis
- Bursitis
- Capsulitis.

Q. What are the contraindications?

1. Patient with implanted (total hip replacement, etc).
2. Pacemaker.
3. Impaired thermal sensation.
4. Pregnancy.
5. Any kind of hemorrhagic/Ischemic tissues.
6. Malignant tumors/Recent radiotherapy.
7. Active epiphysis of children.
8. Fever.

Q. What are the complications?

1. Burn.
2. Concentration of electric field.
3. Impaired blood flow.
4. Precipitation of gangrene.
5. Electric shock.
6. Damage to nearby electrical equipments.

Q. What is the depth of penetration?

3 cm.

Q. How can burn be prevented?

1. Judicious use by experienced therapist
2. Use of towel over the surface.

Ultraviolet Rays

Q. What is UVR?

Ultraviolet radiation (UVR) covers a small part of electromagnetic spectrum lying between the violet end of the visible light and X-ray region.

Q. What are general responses to UVR exposure?

1. Sunburn (**UVB**)/Erythema (Reddening of the skin).
2. Tanning of the skin/Pigmentation.
3. Decrease in sensitivity of the skin (Increased epidermal thickness).
4. Premature aging of the skin (**UVA**).
5. Skin cancer (**UVB**).
6. Exposure to the eye causes photokeratitis (**UVB**).
7. Photosynthesis of vitamin D.

Q. What are types of UVR?

1. UVA (Long UV): 400–315 nm (penetrates to dermis, responsible for development of slow natural tan).
2. UVB (medium UV, erythemal UV): 315–280 nm. (Produces new pigment formation, sunburn, vitamin D synthesis responsible for inducing skin cancer)
3. UVC (short UV, germicidal UV): 280 - 100 nm.

Q. What are the types of UVR generator?

1. High pressure mercury vapor lamp—Air cooled.
2. High pressure mercury vapor lamp—Water cooled (Kromayer lamp).
3. Fluorescent lamps.

Q. What are the physiological effects of UVR?

- Local effects—effects which produced locally in the area:
  - Erythema
  - Pigmentation/Tanning
  - Thickening of epidermis
  - Desquamation/Peeling of dead cells from skin surface
  - Antibiotic effect
- General effects—Results from a widespread irradiation:
  - Vitamin D production
  - The esophylactic effect (increase in the resistance of the body to infection)
  - General tonic effect (improvement of appetite and sleep, decrease in irritability)

Q. What is the wavelength of UV rays?

See above.

Q. What is the application procedure?

- Handheld device
- Theraktin tunnel.

Q. What are the indications?

1. Psoriasis (PUVA therapy).
2. Acne vulgaris.
3. Eczema (here also PUVA therapy may be helpful).
4. Ulcers, pressure sores, surgical incisions.
5. Vitiligo (Both UVA and UVB stimulate melanocyte activity).
6. Non-infected wounds (Venous/Arterial ulcers).
7. Deep seated pain.

Q. What are the contraindications?

1. Pulmonary tuberculosis.
2. Severe cardiac disturbances.
3. Systemic lupus erythematosis.
4. Uncontrolled diabetes.
5. Certain dermatological conditions.
6. Photosensitivity.
7. Photosensitizing medication.
8. Acute febrile illness.
9. Recent skin grafts.

Q. What are the complications?

- Premature aging
- Nonmelanoma skin cancer
- Cataracts.

CRYOTHERAPY

Q. Enlist salient points on cryotherapy?

Types:

- Cold pack
- Ice massage
- Water immersion
- Cryo compress unit
- Vapocoolant spray
- Whirlpool bath

Precaution:

- Cold intolerance
- Cryotherapy induced neuropraxia
- Arterial insufficiency
- Impaired sensation
- Cryopathies
- Paroxysmal cold hemoglobinuia
- Raynaud's phenomenon
- Cold allergy
- Impaired sensation.

TRANSCUTANEOUS ELECTRICAL NERVE STIMULATION MACHINE

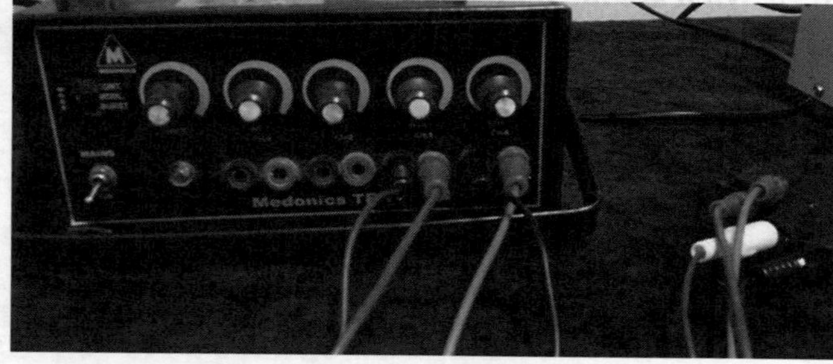

Figure 8.5: Transcutaneous electrical nerve stimulation machine

Figure 8.5 is an electrical instrument with small pads for application. I think this is TENS (Transcutaneous electrical nerve stimulation machine).

Q. What is the mechanism of action?

- Gating of pain (gate control theory)
- Endogenous opiods
- Physiological block
- Placebo.

Q. What are the types of TENS?

Conventional

- **High-frequency, low-intensity** stimulation—most effective type of stimulation
- **Duration** of treatment: 30 minutes to hours
- **Amplitude** is adjusted to produce minimal sensory discomfort
- Pain relief begins in **10–15** minutes and stops shortly after removing stimulation
- Useful for **neuropathic pain.**

Acupuncture

- **Low-frequency, high-intensity** stimulation
- Duration: 30–60 minutes
- Amplitude high enough to produce muscle contraction
- Onset of pain relief can be delayed several hours
- Pain relief persists hours after removing stimulation
- Useful for **acute musculoskeletal conditions.**

Hyperstimulation

- High-frequency, high-intensity stimulation
- Duration: Rarely tolerated more than 15–30 minutes
- It is considered that this mode stimulates C-fibers and causes counterirritation

Pulse (burst) mode

- High-frequency stimulation bursts at low-frequency intervals
- Duration: 30–60 minutes
- Delayed onset of pain relief.

Modulated

- Impulses vary in intensity and frequency
- Attempts to avoid neuro-habituation.

Q. What are the indications?

- Acute pain
  - Postoperative pain
  - Dysmenorrhea
  - Orofascial pain
  - Physical trauma (like fractured ribs)
- Chronic pain
  - Radiating low back pain
  - Arthritic pain (OA, RA)
  - Myofascial pain
  - Neuropathic pain (trigeminal neuralgia, phantom pain)

Q. What are the contraindications?

- Non cooperative patients
- Pregnancy

- Pacemaker or any other implanted electronic device
- Allergic response to the electrodes, gel
- Impaired skin sensation and active infections
- Neurological conditions like epilepsy and stroke (CVA)
- Malignancy.

Q. Where are the electrodes placed?

- Stimulation of appropriate nerve root(s)
- Stimulate the peripheral nerve (best if proximal to the pain area)
- Stimulate motor point (innervated by the same root level)
- Stimulate trigger point(s) or acupuncture point(s)
- Stimulate the appropriate dermatome, myotome or sclerotome
- May be crossed or uncrossed (using two channel mode)
- May be placed horizontally or vertically and coplaner or contra-planer.

Q. What are the complications?

- Skin irritation
- Muscle soreness.

INTERFERENTIAL THERAPY

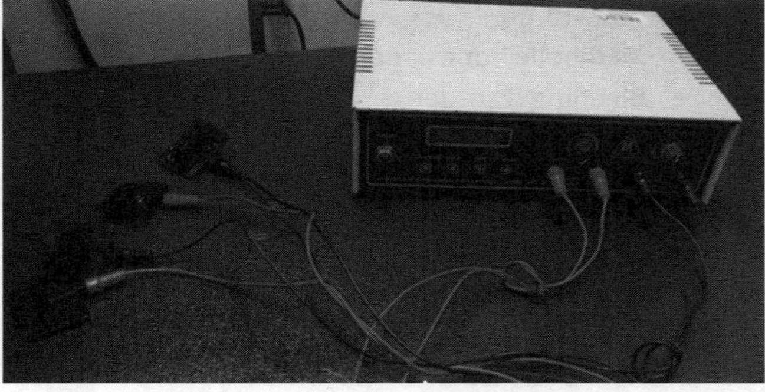

Figure 8.6: Interferential therapy machine

Figure 8.6 is a machine with 4 rubber pads for application. So I think this is interferential therapy machine.

Q. What is high frequency current?

The current having frequency above 10000 Hz is called high frequency current.

Q. What is beat frequency?

- IFT is a form of electrotherapy in which two medium frequency currents are used to produce a low frequency effect
- The difference between the frequency of the two medium frequency current gives the beat frequency.

Q. What are the effects ?

Stimulation of the peripheral nerves.

Q. What is the application procedure?

- Electrode placements should be such that the crossing point of the two currents (each of medium frequency), is over/within the target area (lesion)
- Frequencies of 80–100 Hz is used to reduce pain, whereas 1–10 Hz is used to reduce edema/swelling
- Treatment time ranges from 5–10 minutes in acute conditions and 20–30 minutes for others.

Q. What are the indications?

- Pain relief in many musculoskeletal conditions (OA knee, LBP/PIVD, fibromyalgia, shoulder disorders, fracture pain, etc.)
- Muscle (motor) stimulation
- To increase local blood flow
- Reduction of edema/effusion/swelling (as in OA knee, ankle sprain)
- Stimulation as part of the management of incontinence and pelvic floor training
- Trigger point intervention
- Debatable role in fracture healing.

Q. What are the contraindications?

- Patients unable to understand the instructions of the therapist/non-cooperative patients.
- Deep vein thrombosis/pulmonary embolism
- Pacemaker/defibrillator/other cardiac conditions
- Bacterial infections
- Malignancy
- Dermatological conditions
- Pregnancy
- Application to active epiphyseal regions in children.

Q. What are the complications?

- Skin irritation
- Burns.

EXTRACORPOREAL SHOCKWAVE THERAPY

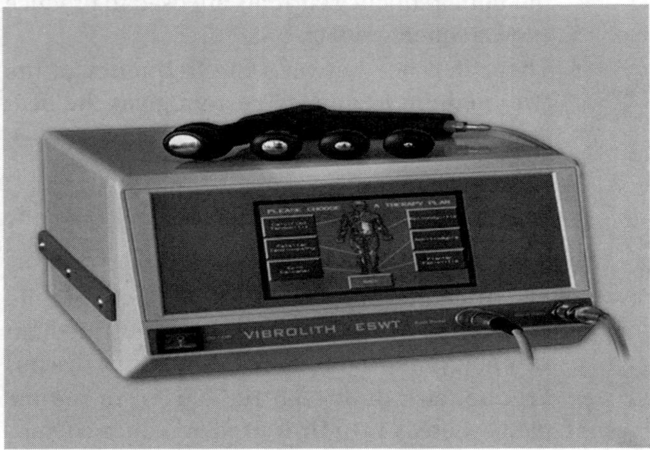

Figure 8.7: Extracorporeal shockwave therapy device

Figure 8.7 is a machine to carry out extracorporeal shockwave therapy (or ESWT), which is a new technology using shockwaves to treat chronic, painful conditions of the musculoskeletal system. A shockwave is an intense, but very short energy wave traveling faster than the speed of sound.

Q. Why is it called shockwave?

In order for a shockwave to truly be defined as a shockwave, the energy wave must literally be faster than the speed of sound, or 1,500 meters per second. This is the speed at which the "shock" of the shockwave is generated, from breaking the sound barrier.

Q. How much is the strength of the energy wave?

5–100 MPa.

Q. What are the effects of ESWT?

- Increase in cell membrane permeability and subsequent dissolution of pathological calcific deposits
- Cavitation bubbles they tend to expand to a maximum size, then collapse, much like a bubble popping help break down pathological deposits of calcification in soft tissues
- As cavitation bubbles collapse, they create smaller, secondary energy waves known as microjets also create a lot of force that also breaks down pathological deposits of calcification in the soft tissues through direct, mechanical means
- Stimulate fibroblasts
- Hyperstimulation anesthesia
- "Gate-control" mechanism.

Q. What are the indications?

- Complaints involving attachment points for tendons and ligaments in major joints like the:
  - Shoulder (such as the rotator cuff) diseases
  - Elbow (epicondylitis or tennis elbow)
  - Hip
  - Knee (tendinitis or "jumper's knee) are common sites for ESWT.
- One of the areas most frequently treated with ESWT, however, is the foot.
  - Plantar fasciitis
  - Achilles tendinitis
  - Calcific tendinitis or tendinosis
  - Connective tissue pain and degeneration
  - Muscle pain and injuries
  - Ankle joint injuries.
- Encourages bone healing, it has been used to help treat:
  - Stress fractures
  - Avascular necrosis (a dead portion of bone)
  - Slow-healing bone (delayed unions)
  - Non-healing bone (non-unions).

Q. What are the contraindications?

- Bone tumors
- Metabolic bone conditions
- Bleeding disorder
- Pregnancy
- Open growth plate
- Infection
- Where gas or air is present in the body.

ELECTROMUSCULAR STIMULATION

Q. What are the types?

- Faradic stimulation
  - Continuous faradic
  - Surged faradic
- Galvanic stimulation
  - Plain/continuous galvanic
  - Interrupted galvanic.

Faradic Current

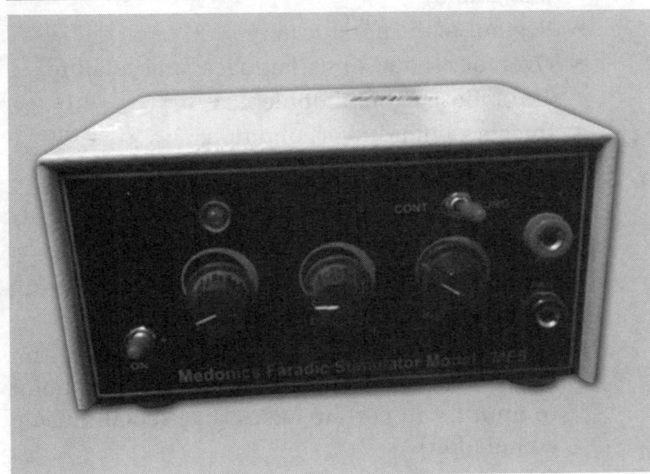

Figure 8.8: Faradic stimulator

Q. What is Faradic current?

It is a short-duration interrupted current, with a pulse duration ranging from 0.1 and 1 ms and a frequency of 30 to 100 Hz.

Q. What are the different waveforms?

- Induced asymmetrical alternating current
- Biphasic, asymmetrical, unbalanced, spiked
- Positive portion—short duration, high amplitude and spiked
- Negative portion—long duration, low amplitude and curved.

Q. What are the effects of Faradic current?

1. Sensory effects (sensory nerve stimulation): Mild prickling sensation and erythema due to vasodilatation of superficial vessels.
2. Motor effects (motor nerve stimulation): Produce tetanic contraction. The tetanic contraction causes muscle fatigue. So to avoid this, current is surged to allow muscular relaxation.
3. Effect on muscle contraction: Muscle contraction similar to the normal muscle contraction. Contraction and relaxation of muscles produce pumping action which increases blood supply to the muscles as a result of increased demand and supply of oxygen and nutrition.
4. Effect on denervated muscles: For the stimulation of denervated muscles, the impulse/duration required is more than 1 ms. In other words, the nerve supply to the muscle being treated must be intact, because the intensity of the current needed to depolarize the muscle membrane is too great to be comfortably tolerated by the patient, in the absence of the nerve. Hence, faradic stimulation is not a modality choice for denervated muscles.

Q. What are the application technique?

- Group muscle stimulation
  - Stationary stimulation
  - Both active and passive electrodes will be kept stationary.
- Motor point stimulation (with the passive electrode, i.e. the positive electrode at a stationary position at the vicinity of the motor point/at the point of origin of the muscle and the active electrode, i.e. the negative electrode will be placed at the motor point of that particular muscle or may be moved around to the motor points of different muscles having a near common origin and a common nerve supply).

Q. What are the indications of Faradic current?

1. Facilitation of muscle contraction inhibited by pain: Stimulation must be stopped when good voluntary contraction is obtained.
2. Muscle re-education: In cases of prolonged disuse or incorrect use; and in muscle transfer.
3. Training a new muscle action: After tendon transplantation, muscle may be required to perform a different action from that previously carried out.
4. Nerve damage: To stimulate muscle innervated by partially regenerated nerves
5. Improvement of venous and lymphatic drainage: In edema and gravitational ulcers, the venous and lymphatic return should be encouraged by the pumping action of the alternate muscle contraction and relaxation (Faradism under pressure, with use of a crepe bandage, with maximum pressure applied from distal to proximal)
6. Prevention and loosening of adhesions: After effusion, adhesions are liable to form, which can be prevented by keeping structures moving with respect to each other. Formed adhesions may be stretched and loosened by muscle contraction.
7. Painful knee syndromes: After trauma, there is inhibition of muscle contraction, leading to muscle atrophy. Faradism may be helpful to strengthen the atrophied muscle.
8. Training/strengthening of the intrinsic muscles of hand/foot (hand/foot bath).
9. Re-education of pelvic floor muscles.

Q. What are the contraindications of Faradic current?

1. Skin lesions.

2. Certain dermatological conditions (psoriasis, eczema).
3. Thrombosis.
4. Impaired skin sensation.
5. Cardiac pacemakers.
6. Acute infections and inflammations.
7. Any superficial metal implants.
8. Active epiphyseal region of children.

Galvanic Current

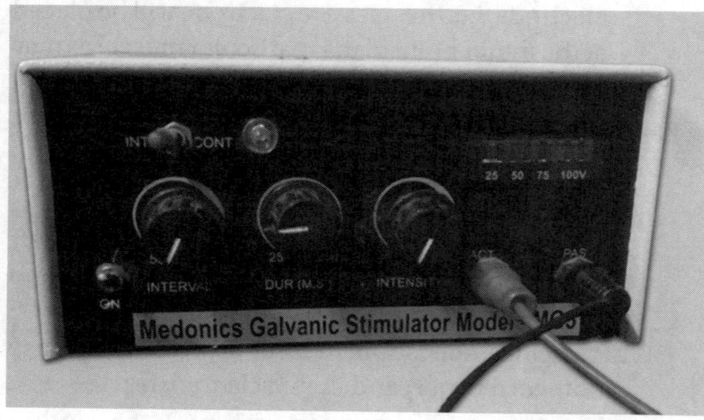

Figure 8.9: Galvanic stimulator

Q. What is galvanic current?
It is an interrupted direct (unidirectional) current also called long duration current having more than 1 ms up to 300 ms or 600 ms.

Q. What is direct current?
It is an electric current flowing in one direction only.

Q. What are the effects of galvanic current?
- Contraction of denervated muscle
- Stimulation of sensory nerves—burning sensation
- Stimulation of motor nerves.

Q. What are the indications of galvanic current?
- Iontophoresis
- 'Modified/interrupted direct or galvanic currents are used to stimulate denervated muscles
- Maintaining the properties of the muscle
- Minimizing denervation atrophy
- Improves absorption and activates pumping function of muscles
- Prevents venous and lymphatic stasis
- Maintains the extensibility of muscles.

Q. What are the contraindications of galvanic current?
- Placement of electrodes tangential/across to the heart
- Cardiac pacemakers
- Malignancy
- Regions of the phrenic nerve
- Over the carotid sinus/laryngeal musculature
- Thrombosis/thrombophlebitis
- Infected wound/skin condition.

Q. What are the precautions to be taken?
- Do not use over skin eruptions, swollen, infected/inflamed areas
- Turn the unit off when applying / removing electrodes
- Turn the intensity to zero while moving the active electrode (cathode) from one motor point to another in certain cases (like facial muscle stimulation)
- Do not use over eyelids.

LASER

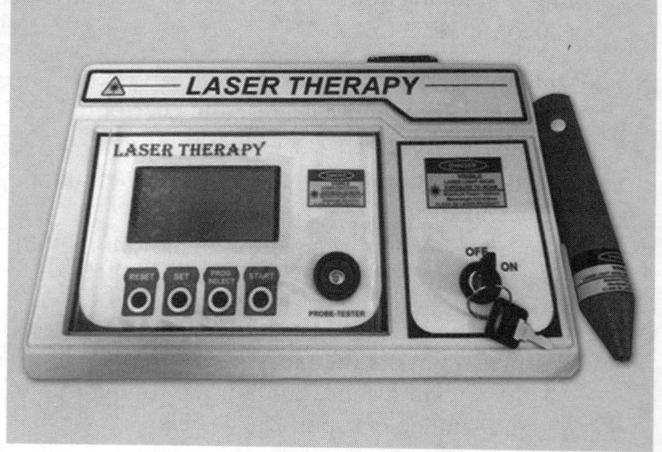

Figure 8.10: Laser therapy machine

Q. What is the full name of LASER?
Light Amplification by Stimulated Emission of Radiation.

Q. What are the types of LASER?
- Power laser: Used for the destruction of tissues or surgical purposes
- Soft laser: Used in skin diseases
- Mid laser: Used for the therapeutic purpose and is sufficient to produce biological effects in deeper tissues without damaging the skin.

Q. What is the wavelength of mid laser?
Helium: Neon laser combined with infrared laser having wavelengths of 630 nm and 904 nm, respectively.

Q. What is the depth of penetration?
30 mm from surface.

Q. What are the effects of LASER?
Cellular effects:
It activated the electron transport chain, increases ATP synthesis and reduction of the cellular pH. Laser also initiate reactions at cell membrane through its photochemical effect on the Ca channels. These biochemical effects (electron transport chain, ATP synthesis and decrease cellular pH) and cell membrane changes cause increase macrophages, fibroblasts and lymphocyte activities (wound and fracture healing)

- **Effect on nerve conduction and nerve regeneration:**
  Some studies shows that it increases the nerve conduction, some shows that it decreases the nerve conduction and some shows that it has no effect on nerve conduction. It decreases the sensory latency
- **Effects on vasodilatation:**
  It increases microcirculation which may help in wound healing by the phenomenon of vasodilatation at capillary level.

Q. What are the indications of LASER?
- Wound and fracture healing
- Arthritic conditions at distal extremities
- Enthesopathy.

Q. What are the contraindications?
- Patient with active or suspected carcinoma
- Recent radiotherapy (4–6 months)
- Areas of hemorrhage
- Direct irradiation over a pregnant uterus
- Over endocrine glands

Q. What are the conditions when supervised therapy is indicated?
- Epilepsy
- Fever
- Confused or disoriented patient.

Q. What are the regions where LASER is avoided?
- Infected tissues
- Sympathetic ganglion
- Vagus nerve
- Cardiac region in cardiac patients
- Eye (glasses to be worn by both therapist and patient).

SPINAL TRACTION

Q. What do you mean by traction?
Traction is the act of drawing or pulling and relates to forces applied to the body to stretch a given part or to separate 2 or more parts.

Q. What are the various types of traction?
1. Mechanical forms of traction use a hydraulic or motorized pulley system with weights, along with a harness or sling device to attach to the patient's body.
2. Manual traction involves the therapist using his or her hands on the patient's body, with the body weight of the therapist providing the tractive force.
3. Autotraction is controlled by the patient pulling on bars or handles at the head of the table, without direct involvement of a therapist.
4. Gravitational traction with a tilt table and underwater variations of traction are also in clinical and home use but are less frequently employed than the other forms described.

Q. What are the effects of traction in cervical and lumbar spine?
Cervical spine:
- In the cervical spine, the most reproducible result of traction is elongation
- Optimum weight for cervical traction to accomplish vertebral separation is 25 pounds
- Additionally, 2-20 mm elongation of the cervical spine has been shown to be achievable with 25 or more pounds of traction force
- Anterior intervertebral space shows the most increase in cervical flexion of 30°.

Note: Traction in the extended position generally is not recommended, because it is often painful and may increase risk of complications from vertebral basilar insufficiency or spinal instability.

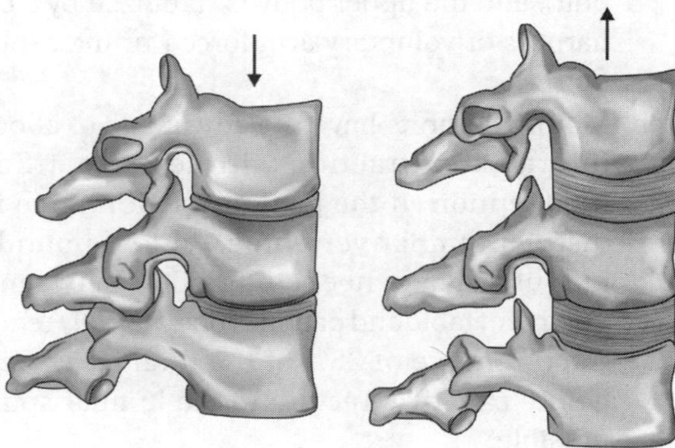

Figure 8.11: Elongation of spine

Lumbar spine:

- Once friction is overcome in the lumbar spine, the major physiologic effect of traction is elongation
- Widening of lumbar interspaces requiring between 70–300 pounds of pull up to slightly more than 3 mm at one intervertebral level.
- The length of time that the separation persists remains indeterminate, with studies documenting distraction durations of 10–30 minutes after treatment.

Note: Data on dimensional and pressure changes of lumbar disks caused by traction are not conclusive. Therefore, evidence is inconclusive, with much information favoring at least temporary reduction of the herniated component of an abnormal lumbar disk with concomitant traction.

Q. What are the different techniques of giving traction?

Cervical traction:

a. Accomplished with a free-weight-and-pulley system or an electrical, motorized device. Adequate pull is achieved by using a head or chin sling attached to a system that can provide pull in a cephalic direction

b. Motorized devices are applied easily but require the patient to be attended. Free-weight-and-pulley systems often are used in the home with 20 or more pounds of water or sand and a pulley system attached to a door.

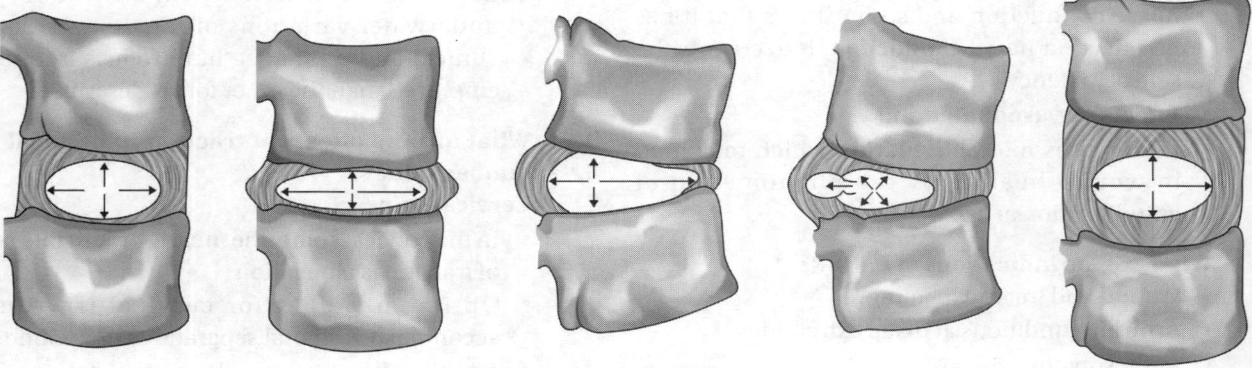

Figure 8.12: Traction in PIVD

Lumbar Traction

a. In the lumbar spine, adequate pull with weights and pulleys or motorized devices to achieve vertebral distraction usually can be obtained with the proper apparatus. Generally, a harness is attached around the pelvis (to deliver a caudal pull), and the upper body is stabilized by a chest harness or voluntary arm force (for the cephalic pull).

b. Motorized units have the advantage of allowing intermittent traction with less practitioner intervention. If the goal of traction force is to distract lumbar vertebrae, 70–150 pounds of pull usually are needed. Friction between the treatment table and patient's body usually requires traction force of 26% of the total body weight before effective traction to the lumbar spine is possible.

c. Many traction devices use a split table that eliminates the lower body segment friction.

d. Body weight theoretically should provide enough pull to distract lumbar vertebrae and eliminate mechanical devices.

e. Gravity traction is applied almost exclusively in the lumbar region. After 10 minutes of inversion traction, documented increases in intervertebral separation are noted. However, side effects also are frequently reported, including increased blood pressure, headaches, blurred vision, and contact lens discomfort.

Q. What are the indications of traction?

International studies strongly suggest that traction does not produce significant influence on long-term outcome of neck pain or low back pain.

Practitioners who rely on sound scientific advice may use traction rarely. However, no consensus has been reached among clinicians or researchers in this area.

However traction may be used for:

1. Cervical spine conditions
   A. Cervical spondylosis

   B. Cervical disk herniation
   C. Cervicogenic headaches
2. Lumbar spine conditions
   A. Lumbar spondylosis
   B. Lumbar disk herniation
   c. General low back pain (occurring due to muscle spasms / stiffness).

Q. What are the contraindication of traction?

1. Old age is a relative contraindication (due to presence of osteoporotic bones).
2. Most practitioners agree that contraindications to cervical or lumbar traction include the following:
   a. Ligamentous instability
   b. Osteomyelitis
   c. Diskitis
   d. Primary or metastatic tumor
   e. Spinal cord tumor
   f. Clinical signs of myelopathy
   g. Untreated hypertension
3. Relative contraindications:
   a. Midline herniated nucleus pulposus
   b. Ankylosing spondylitis
   c. Acute torticollis
   d. Restrictive lung disease
   e. Active peptic ulcer
   f. Pregnancy.

9 Chapter

Surgical Instruments

SPONGE HOLDING FORCEPS

Q. What is this?

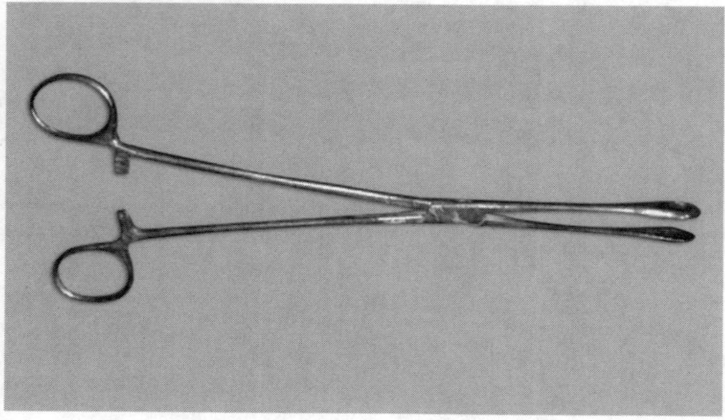

Figure 9.1: Sponge holding forceps

This (Fig. 9.1) is a long instrument (average 9.5" in length) provided with finger bows and a pair of long shaft. The shaft has a rachet, a joint and a pair of blades. The blades are oval, fenestrated and have serrations on the inner aspect.

So, it is sponge holding forceps (Rampley's curved/straight swab holding forceps).

Q. What are its uses?

1. Used for cleansing the skin after dipping the swab in antiseptic solution before all operations.
2. Used for blunt dissection in many operations. E.g. lumbar sympathectomy.
3. Used to clean the blood in a surgical field. E.g. during suture lining.

MAYO'S SCISSORS

Q. What is this?

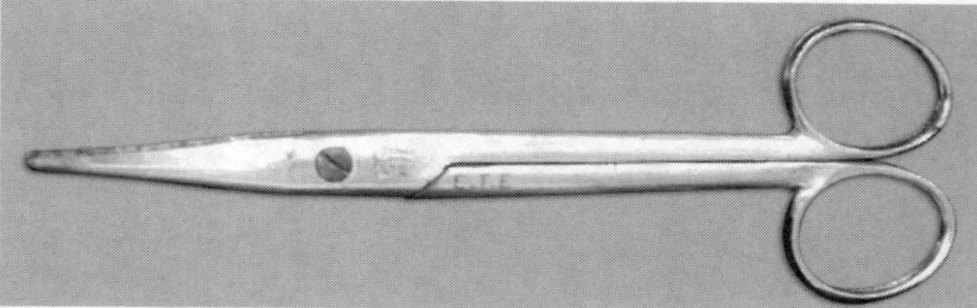

Figure 9.2: Mayo's scissors

This (Fig. 9.2) is a usually long and stout scissors. They may be blunt pointed or sharp pointed and they may be either straight or curved. So it is Mayo's scissors (straight and curved).

Q. What are its uses?

1. Used for cutting sutures.
2. Used to cut tough structures like tough fascia between muscle compartments in limbs, etc.
3. May be used to cut dressing and corrugated rubber sheet drain.

DISSECTING FORCEPS

Plain Dissecting Forceps

Q. What is this?

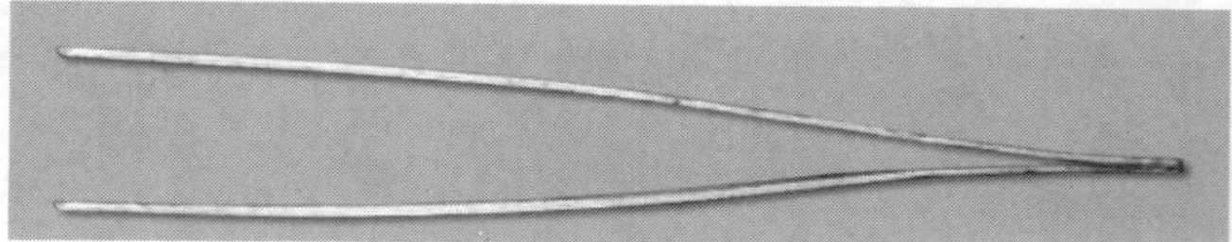

Figure 9.3: Plain dissecting forceps

This (Fig. 9.3) is made up of two limbs with grooves on the shaft to allow easy gripping and with transverse serrations at the tip to grasp the tissue and needle during suturing. There are no tooth at the tip. So, it is plain dissecting forceps.

Q. What are its uses?

1. Used during almost all operations to hold delicate structures like peritoneum, vessels, nerves, muscles, it is commonly used during dissection and suturing.
2. Fine tipped forceps are used during nerve repair and vascular anastomosis.

Toothed Dissecting Forceps

Q. What is this?

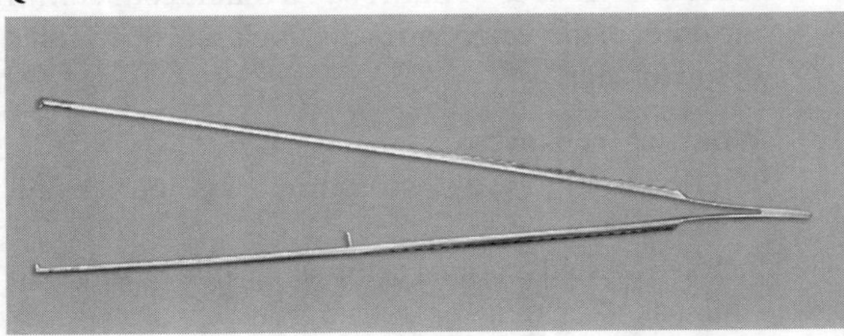

Figure 9.4: Toothed dissecting forceps

Instrument design in Figure 9.4 is same as plain dissecting forceps but with a tooth at the tip of one blade which fits into the grove at the tip of the other blade when approximated. So it is toothed dissecting forceps.

Q. What are its uses?

1. Used during almost all operations to grasp tough structures like skin, fascia, aponeurosis, tendons.
2. Used to hold cut skin margin during suturing.

SCALPEL HANDLE

Q. What is this?

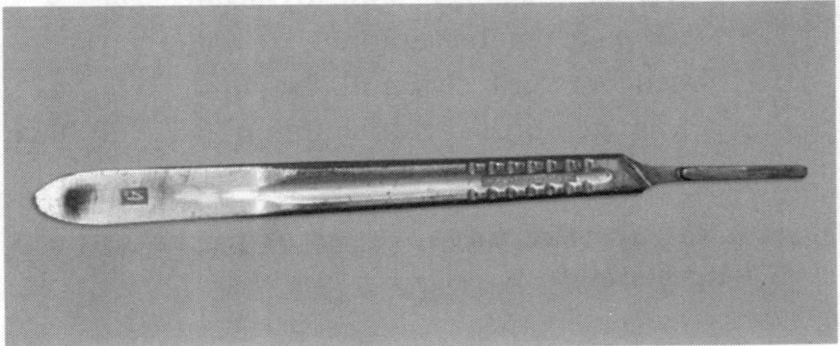

Figure 9.5: Scalpel handle

This (Fig. 9.5) is a flat stainless steel instrument with one end narrower with a slot on one side for attachment of scalpel blade. So it is scalpel handle (Bard parker's handles).

Q. What are its uses?

1. Making an incision
2. To raise skin flaps during operations.

Q. Name some CTEV surgeries?

- Tendo achilis tenotomy
- Z-plasty posteromedial release (Turco).

Q. What are the steps of TA tenotomy?

- Incision: A small incision is made at the medial aspect of the tendo achilles using a No.15 blade
- The tendon is then transected, (Caution: Posterior tibial vessels injury)
- Simple interrupted sutures are given followed by bandaging.

Q. What are the postoperative care given?

- Application of plaster cast (wound is checked prior to application of cast)
- Sutures: Removal at 2 weeks.

Q. What are the steps of posteromedial release?

- Incision: Medial incision 8–9 cm long from the base of the 1st metatarsal to the tendocalcaneus curving it just inferior to the medial malleolus without undermining skin
- Tibialis posterior, flexor digitorum longus, flexor hallucis longus, the tendo achilles tendons are mobilized and exposed
- Incision is continued in the sheaths of FDL and FHL dividing the master knot of Henry beneath the navicular
- Spring ligament is divided, detaching it from the sustentaculu mtali and the origin of abductor hallucis
- Remaining contractures are released from posterior end
- Tendo Achilles (Z plasty) is lengthened by detaching the medial half of the tendon insertion
- Subtalar capsule and calcaneofibular ligaments are divided
- Neurovascular bundle is retracted posteriorly and the tibiocalcaneal part of the deltoid ligament is divided
- Tibialis posterior if contracted, is lengthened.
- Talonavicular joint is opened and its capsule divided, then subtalar ligaments are released and

the navicular is reduced onto the head of the talus which should properly align the other tarsal bones.
- Relationship of the talus to the calcaneus and navicular is corrected
- Foot is stabilized with 'K' wires with the first wire being passed from the dorsum of the foot across the first metatarsal shaft, the medial cuneiform, the navicular and into the talus
- A second wire fixes the subtalar joint and this should maintain the foot in the corrected position.

Q. What are the postoperative care?
- A above knee POP is applied which is changed at 3 weeks and maintained to 6 weeks
- The foot is initially held in slight equinus if there is tension on the skin closure, which is corrected at the time of change of POP
- Splinting is continued for at least 4 months after surgery followed by night splints.

MOSQUITO HEMOSTATIC FORCEPS

Q. What is this?

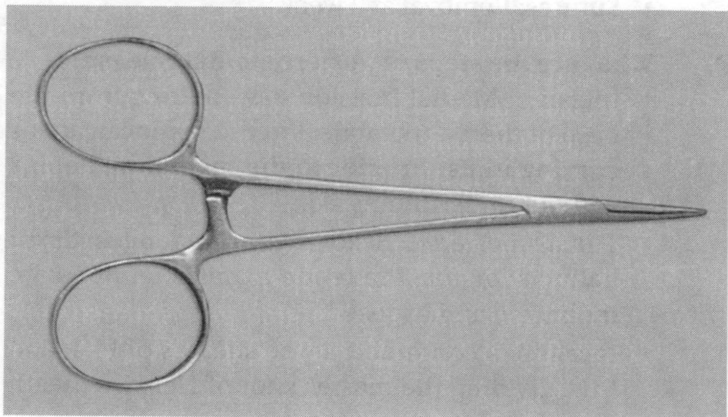

Figure 9.6: Mosquito hemostatic forceps

Instrument in Figure 9.6 is a very light, small and delicate with fine transverse serrations in the blades. The tip of the blades are conical and nontoothed. So it is mosquito hemostatic forceps.

Q. What are its uses?
Used to hold fine bleeding vessels.

ALLIS TISSUE FORCEPS

Q. What is this?

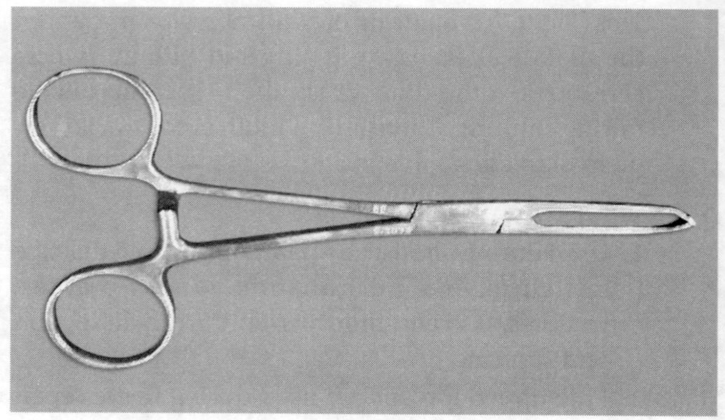

Figure 9.7: Allis tissue forceps

It (Fig. 9.7) is a light instrument with long blades and a gap between the blades to accommodate some tissue. The tips of the blades are provided with sharp teeth and grooves in between so that it coapts with the other blade when the rachet is closed. So it is allis tissue forceps.

Q. What are its uses?
1. Used to hold tough structures. E.g. retract skin margins.
2. Used to hold margins of the skin while raising skin flaps.
3. Used to hold tendons.
4. Used for *TA tendon release operations.*

Q. What are the types of TA release operation?
- Open lengthening
- Percutaneous lengthening.

Q. What are the advantages of open lengthening?
The procedure allows for correction of more severe equinus deformities due to its ability to treat the gastrocnemius and soleus muscles, precisely determination of the amount of correction gained due to the same parameters that accompany the traditional Z-type tendon can be done.

Q. What are the disadvantages of open lengthening?
- Over-lengthening leading to calcaneal gait
- Complete tendon rupture
- Need for large incision/dissection
- Prolonged postoperative immobilization have mitigated its usage.

Q. What are the advantages of percutaneous lengthening?

It is simple, efficient and requires minimal tissue dissection.

Q. What are the steps of percutaneous lengthening?

- Incision: Longitudinal stab incision midline 2 cm proximal to the tendon insertion
- The knife is rotated medially and approximately half of the tendon is transected
- This is then repeated at two separate incision locations 2–3 cm proximal to the previous, with the next directed laterally, and the final again directed medially
- Force is then applied to the lower extremity in a controlled manner to complete the tendo Achilis lengthening (TAL).

Extreme care should be taken to avoid traumatic/ iatrogenic rupture.

Q. When will you plan for Achilles tenotomy?

In case of severe contracture of tendo achillis.

- The concept of complete surgical transection of the Achilles tendon has fallen out of favor.

Q. What are the specific scenarios where TA tenotomy is helpful?

- Patients who are non-ambulatory and/or require complex near-total foot amputations often benefit from tenotomy due to its ability to balance the residual "stump".
- Patients requiring complex rear foot arthrodesis, tibio-talo-calcaneal arthrodesis, or Charcot/post-traumatic deformity correction can benefit from tenotomy to allow for intraoperative positioning of a plantar-grade foot.

BABCOCK'S TISSUE FORCEPS

Q. What is this?

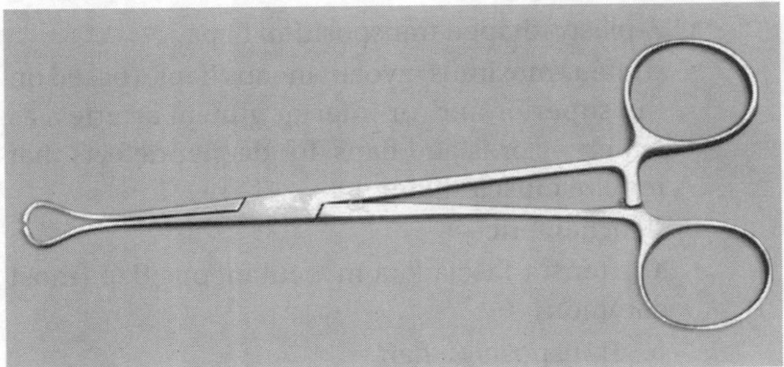

Figure 9.8: Babcock's tissue forceps

It (Fig. 9.8) is a light instrument with long blades that are curved and fenestrated. The tips of the blades are provided with a ridge on one blade and a groove in the other. This is a nontraumatic forceps. So it is Babcock's tissue forceps.

Q. What are its uses?

- Used to hold muscles and tendons during limb surgery.
- It may be used in Z-plasty lengthening of Achilles tendon.

Q. What are the steps of Z-plasty lengthening of Achilles tendon?

- *Anesthesia*: General anesthesia
- *Position:* Supine
- *Incision:* Posteromedial incision is made midway between the Achilles tendon and the posterior aspect of medial malleolus. The lower extant of the incision is at the superior border of the calcaneus and then extended proximally for 4–5 cm
- Achilles tendon is *exposed* and its sheath split longitudinally and the tendon is freed from the surrounding tissues
- A *longitudinal incision* is made in the center of the Achilles tendon from proximal to distal, and the scalpel is turned medially distally
- Half of the tendon is *divided transversely*
- The cut portion is held with forceps and the scalpel is brought to the proximal part of the longitudinal incision in the tendon
- The scalpel is turned opposite to the distal cut and the half of the tendon is cut transversely to free the Achilles tendon completely
- The plantaris tendon on the medial aspect of Achilles tendon is divided transversely
- Passive excursion of triceps surae muscle is evaluated by pulling the proximal stump of the tendon to its maximally stretched length
- The tendon is allowed to retract halfway back to its resting length and then *sutured to the distal tendon by keeping ankle at 10–15 °C of dorsiflexion*
- The repair is performed with heavy absorbable sutures
- The wound is closed and long leg cast was applied.

Q. What are the postoperative advices?

- Ambulation is allowed soon as the patient became pain free
- Long leg cast is continued for 4 weeks and then changed to short leg cast which is continued for further 2 weeks
- Brace is advised for 6 months.

HUMBY'S KNIFE

Q. What is this?

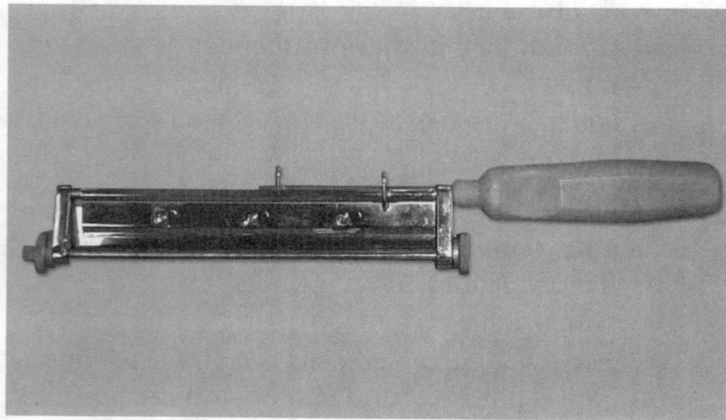

Figure 9.9: Humby's knife

Q. What are its uses?

Used in split thickness skin grafting for pressure sores.

Q. What are the steps of split thickness skin grafting?

- Preparation of the recepient area:
  - A clean, fresh and tidy wound: No problem if hemostasis is secured
  - Untidy wounds and granulating areas must be prepared
  - Adherent slough must be excised and the exuberant granulation must be scraped off
  - Bleeding can be controlled with moist warm packs.

  Contraindication: Presence of beta haemolytic streptococci or a heavy growth of any organism.
- Cutting and preparing the graft:
  - The donor site should be shaved
  - Grafts can be harvested with a hand-held knife (Humby's knife) but more dermatome device is more consistent
  - The blade of the knife and the donor site are smeared with lubricant such as liquid paraffin
  - The limb should be held firmly by the assistant, whose hands provide counterpressure from behind to present the surgeon a flat surface from which to cut the graft
  - The surgeon creates tension on the donor site just in front of the skin grafting knife with a wooden board
- The handheld skin grafting knife is pressed firmly against the skin and with a steady to and fro sawing motion the knife and wooden board move forward.
- The thickness of the graft must be assessed by the pattern of bleeding on the donor site (bleeding points will be closely packed and confluent)
- The donor site is dressed as soon as the grafts are cut
- The skin graft can be used in its unmeshed state (most acceptable cosmesis) (if larger areas are to be covered the graft maybe meshed to expand it. To mesh the graft it is passed through a mesher.)
- Graft application and fixation:
  - The graft is placed on the recipient site and adjusted to conform to any irregularity of the bed.
  - The graft is tacked to the edges of the defect with a few well spaced sutures which can be left long and used to fix a 'tie-over' dressing
  - There are two ways of placing the graft:
    - Directly on the recipient site or
    - After first preparing it on a sheet of paraffin gauze spread on wooden board, the sheets of the graft skin are laid in a manner where their superficial surface lies in contact with the paraffin gauze.

  (*Meshing can also be done with a scalpel if no mesher is available*).

Q. What are the other surgeries done for pressure sore?

Surgical options:

A. Ischial sore—
- Gluteal thigh flap
- The inferior gluteus maximus myocutaneous flap.

B. Sacral—
- Inferiorly-based buttock rotation flaps
- Rhombic flaps
- Z-plasty-shaped transposition flaps
- Gluteus maximus myocutaneous flaps, (based on the superior and/or inferior gluteal arteries, as either v-y or island flaps, for deeper defects that require muscle-filling.)

C. Trochanteric—
- The tensor fascia lata myocutaneous flap (most common)
  a. Transposition flap,
  b. v-y advancement or island flap
- Rectus femoris or vastus lateralis myocutaneous flaps.

Hemostatic Forceps

Q. What is this?

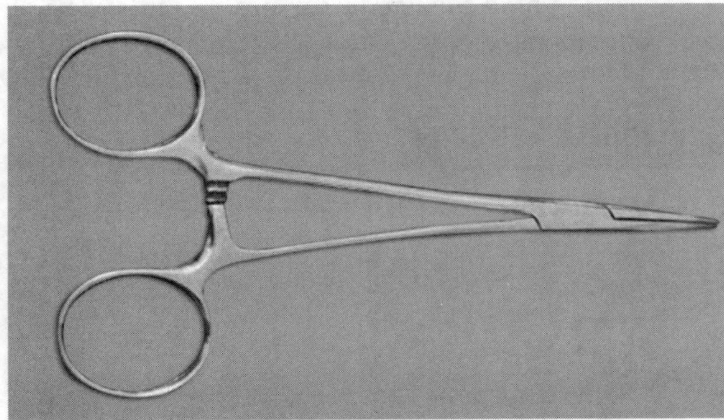

Figure 9.10: Hemostatic forceps

It is hemostatic forceps.

Q. What is its type?

A. Spencer Well's hemostatic forceps are provided with finger bows, a rachet, a pair of shaft and a pair of blades. Full length of blades are provided with transverse serrations. It may be curved or straight.

B. Kelly's hemostatic forceps are longer. The blades are comparatively smaller and the full length of the blades donot contain serrations.

Q. What are its uses?

- To grasp bleeding vessels during almost all operations to control hemorrhage.
- Used to dissect tissue plains while performing blunt dissection.
- Knot tying.

Q. Name one emergency operation related to rehabilitation where hemostatsis is very important?

Amputation surgery.

Q. What are the steps of below knee amputation surgeries?

- The longer posterior flap is marked out *(should be of length 1.5 times the diameter of the leg)*
- The anterior flap which has the poorer blood supply is cut down to bone at the level of bone division
- Elevation of the anterior flap of skin and muscle from the bone is kept to a minimum and 1 cm is adequate
- The tibia is then divided and bevelled anteriorly
- The fibula is divided 1 cm more proximally
- The posterior flap should retain deep fascia and some underlying muscle throughout its length to safeguard skin perfusion
- The posterior muscles are divided obliquely (*so that virtually all of the deep muscle is removed and distally only a thin remnant of the superficial gastrocnimeus remains)*
- Arteries are ligated as encountered and the nerves are divided so that they can retract.
- The muscles of the flap are apposed over the bone with sutures and the skin is closed over a suction drain.

Q. What are the important steps of above knee amputations?

Basic steps like BK

Special points regarding flap:

1. Either equal anterior and posterior myocutaneous flaps or unequal flaps with a longer anterior flap.
2. The quadriceps is sutured to the hamstring so that muscle action on the stump remains balanced.

If less than 10 cm of femur can be preserved then hip disarticulation may be preferred especially in younger patient.

Q. What are the steps of Ray's amputation surgery?

- *Anesthesia*: Regional or general anesthesia
  The limb is exsanguinated and a tourniquet is applied.
- *Incision*: A dorsal incision is made that extends along the shaft of the long finger ray dorsally.
  (*The distal ends of the incision are carried out over the proximal phalangeal skin to prevent sufficient skin for closure of the commissure between the index and ring fingers*).
- The extensor digitorum communis tendon to the long finger is divided proximally
- The long finger metacarpal is osteotomized at its base *(N:B before that subperiosteal dissection has been carried out and the intrinsic muscles have been reflected*)
- Volar dissection is carried out in the same subperiosteal plane and the digital vessels are ligated and the nerves transected as far distally as possible
- The flexor tendons are divided and allowed to retract proximally
- The deep intervolar plate ligaments are divided.
- The preosseous bands of palmar fascia are dissected out and the ray is removed.

- Transposition of the index metacarpal onto the base of the long finger metacarpal may or may not be done.

KOCHER'S HEMOSTATIC FORCEPS

Q. What is this?

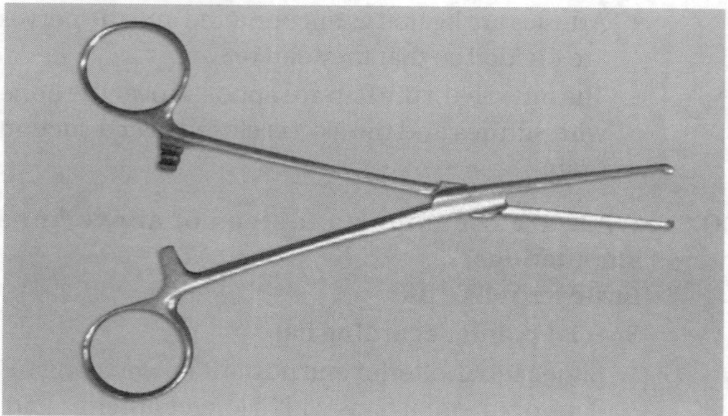

Figure 9.11: Kocher's hemostatic forceps

Figure 9.11 similar to Spencer Wells's forceps, except at the tip of the blades there is a tooth on one blade and a groove on the other where the tooth fits when the rachet is closed. So it is kocher's hemostatic forceps

Q. What are its uses?

1. Suitable for holding vessels in tough structures like palm, sole, scalp where the vessels tend to retract in the deep fascia.
2. To hold meniscus during menisectomy.

NEEDLE HOLDERS

Q. What is this?

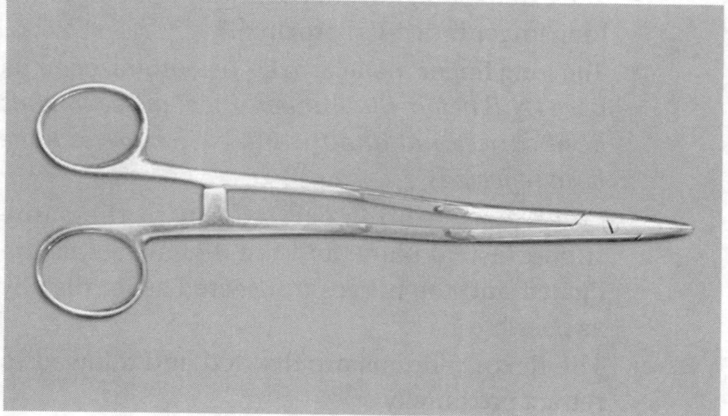

Figure 9.12: Needle holder

Here (Fig. 9.12) blades are smaller in comparison to shaft. Criss-cross serrations in the blades and a longitudinal groove in the center is present (may or may not be present). So it is needle holders (it may be straight or curved).

Q. What are its uses?

Used to hold the needle for suturing in almost all operations.

Langenbeck Retractor

Q. What is this?

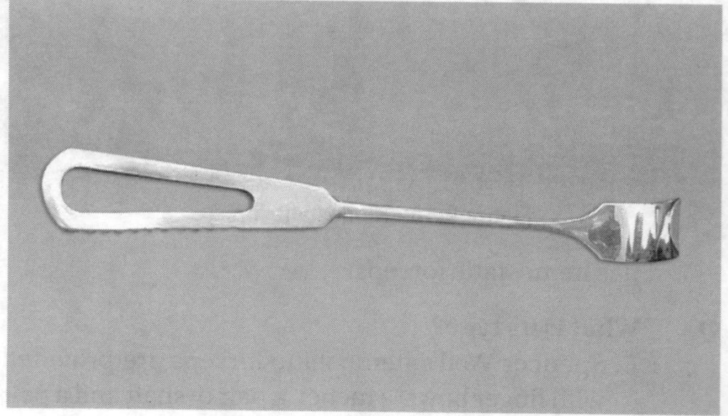

Figure 9.13: Langenbeck retractor

This is an instrument (Fig. 9.13) with the blades which are curved at right angles to the shaft and the shaft is long. So it is Langenbeck's rectractor.

ARMY NAVY RETRACTOR

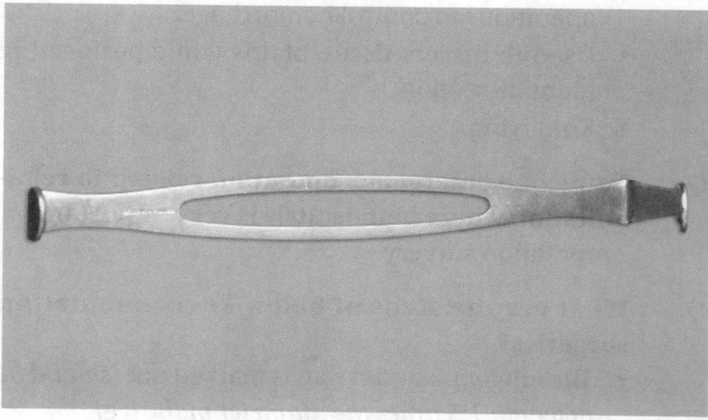

Figure 9.14: Army navy retractor

This is an instrument (Fig. 9.14) in which the blades are curved at right angle in both sides with spindle shape in the center. This is army navy retractor.

Q. What are the other types of retractors?

A. *Czerney's rectractor:* At one end there is a flat blade at right angles to the shaft and at the other end there is a biflanged hook.

B. *Morris retractor*: The handle is wider and the blade is also wider. The lower end of the blade is curved inwards at right angle.

C. *Hook retractors*: There is a shaft with a handle. There is a single or a double hook at the tip. The tip of the hook may be sharp or blunt.

D. *Cat's Paw or Volkman'sretractor*: There are multiple hooks with pointed edges. It may be used for retraction of skin flaps or fascia for surface surgeries.

E. *Deaver's retractor*: It is an S-shaped large curved retractor that comes in different sizes depending on its width.

F. *Joll's thyroid retractor*: There are two towel clip like forceps at either end. The two flanges can be adjusted by means of a screw mechanism.

Q. What are its uses?

- Used to retract skin fascia or muscle for better visualization
- Used in *vulipus operation.*

Q. What is Vulipus operation?

The Vulpius procedure is a simple and effective method for the release of gastrocnemius.

Q. What is the main advantage?

Long periods of immobilization of the foot and ankle is not needed.

Q. What is the procedure?

1. *Patient position*: Prone.
2. Extremity is fixed so that neither external nor internal rotation of the limb is present. (Mal positioned limb: Entrapment of the sural nerve).
3. The contralateral limb: Supported with a sandbag beneath the patient's hip.
4. *Incision*: The skin incision is 1.0–2.0 centimeters medial to midline and well below the heads of the gastrocnemius muscle. (No midline or lateral to midline incision as the sural nerve and its branches may be injured).
5. After the incision marking, it is usually infiltrated with bupivicaine with epinephrine for local hemostasis.
6. Blunt dissection with **metzenbaum scissors** is usually preferred as the inner layer is composed of adipose tissue (the lesser saphenous vein and nerve should be watched and if encountered they should be retracted, preferably laterally).
7. Additional hemostasis if required is achieved with electrocautery.
8. There is no adipose tissue beneath the deep fascia.
9. After the deep fascia is identified the subcutaneous layer is separated both medially and laterally along tissue plane.
10. Distinct separation of the skin and subcutaneous layer from the deep fascia also facilitates closure of the deeper tissues following tendon lengthening.
11. Next, the deep fascia and paratenon tissues are incised as a single layer. These two layers are intimately arranged.
12. Once the fascia and paratenon have been incised, they are separated from the underlying aponeurosis by taking the blunt back end of the scalpel handle and "sweeping" superiorly and then inferiorly both medially and laterally between the paratenon and the aponeurosis fibers. (The tendon itself should not be incised).
13. The skin, subcutaneous tissues, deep fascia and paratenon are now retracted medially and laterally with the deep end of the **army nary retractors.**
14. Tendon transaction is done.

TOWEL CLIP

Q. What is this?

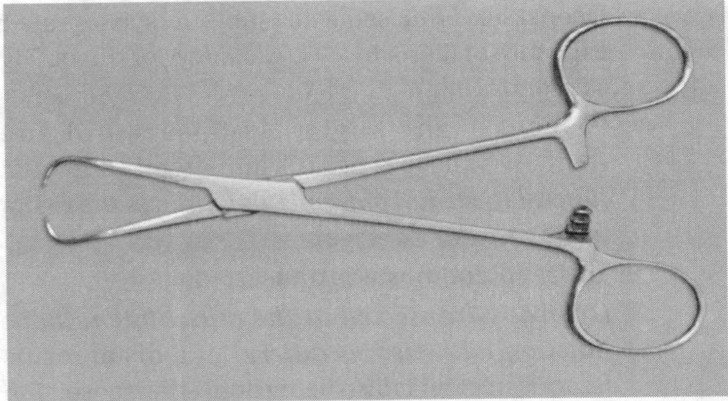

Figure 9.15: Towel clip

It (Fig. 9.15) has scissor action with ratchet fixation at the finger loops and sharp, incurving, needle-like blades. So it is towel clip.

Q. What are its uses?

1. Used to fix draping towels.
2. Used to fix electrosurgery, suction tubes , cables etc.
3. Used to hold ribs while elevating flail segment of chect.

DISSECTING SCISSORS

Q. What is this?

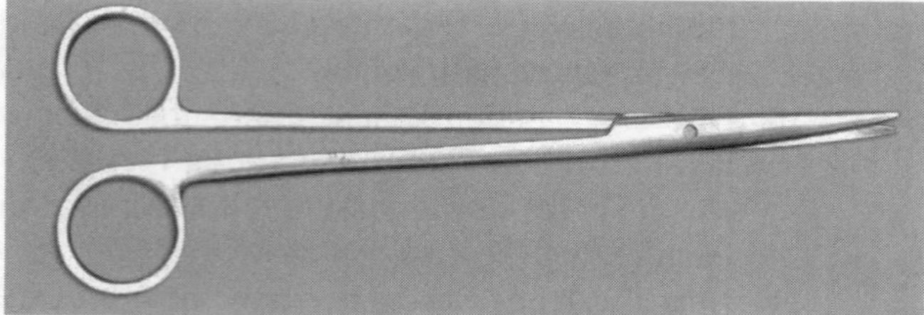

Figure 9.16: Dissecting scissors

This is dissecting scissors.

Q. What are the uses?

- Used in dissection of fascia
- Used in hamstring lengthening surgery.

Q. What are the steps of hamstring lengthening operation?

- Incision: 3–5 cm midline incision in the distal third of the posterior thigh.
- Dissection is carried out to expose the semitendinosus medially with electrocautery or **dissecting scissors.**
- Semitendinosus is isolated (the most superficial posteromedial structure and is tendinous distally) with electrocautery or dissecting scissors to expose the deep fascia.
- Deep fascia is incised with tenotomy scissors after exposure of fascia by electrocautery or dissecting scissors.
- Place a right angle clamp around the semitendinosus tendon from lateral to medial *(lateral to medial placement minimizes the risk of neurovascular damage).*
- The semitendinosus is transacted. *(typically transected at the musculotendinous junction with electrocautery)* [if a distal rectus femoris transfer is also being done, the transection is proximal to the musculotendinous junction (to allow enough tendon for the transfer)]
- Semimembranosus lengthening
  - Semimembranosus is isolated
  - Incision over the fascia over the semimembranosus with tenotomy scissors and the semimembranosus is isolated as far anteromedially as possible.
  - The aponeurosis is incised
  - Aponeurosis is cut transversely with a 15 blade at 1 or 2 levels
  - Underlying muscle is left undisturbed
  - Two cuts are made, the proximal cut is done first so that tissue is still on tension when the distal cut is made.
- Release is tested.
  - Knee is brought into full extension with the ipsilateral hip extended.
  - If the knee comes easily to full extension, lateral hamstring lengthening is not needed.

  Popliteal angle is not checked as this appears to increase the risk of postoperative peroneal neuropraxia.
- ***Biceps Femoris Lengthening***
  - Biceps femoris is isolated
  - Sharp dissection is done laterally (with electocautery or dissecting scissors) through the same midline incision and the deep fascia over the biceps femoris is exposed.
  - The deep fascia is incised with dissecting scissors to fully expose the biceps femoris.
  - Aponeurotic band is incised
  - The fascia over the biceps is incised with a 15 blade
  - The discreet apneurotic band is identified and isolated that is located laterally on the biceps
  - Transaction of this band at 1 or 2 levels is done while leaving the underlying muscle intact
  - Wound closure is done:
    - Sucbcutaneous closure is with simple sutures of 2-0 absorbable suture
    - Subcuticular closure is with an undyed, running 3-0 absorbable monofilament.

REVERSE CUTTING NEEDLE

Q. What is this?

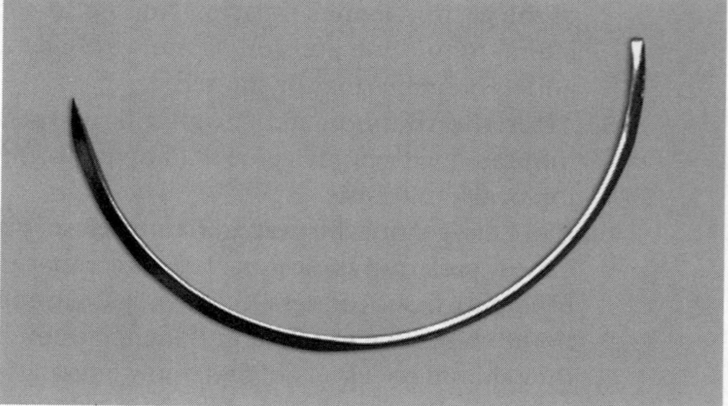

Figure 9.17: Reverse cutting needle

It (Fig. 9.17) is a needle, reverse cutting type, with the following parts—the tip (or point), the body and the shank.

Q. What are the types of tip?

Conventional cutting (sharp edge on the inside arc) or reverse cutting (sharp edge on the outside arc).

Q. What is the advantage and use of reverse cutting needles?

A reverse cutting needle provides less chance of the tissue tearing during suturing. A round needle with tapered tip is the least likely to cause tissue tearing, and is primarily used for suturing fascia, muscle and aponeuroses.

SURGICAL BLADE

Q. What is this?

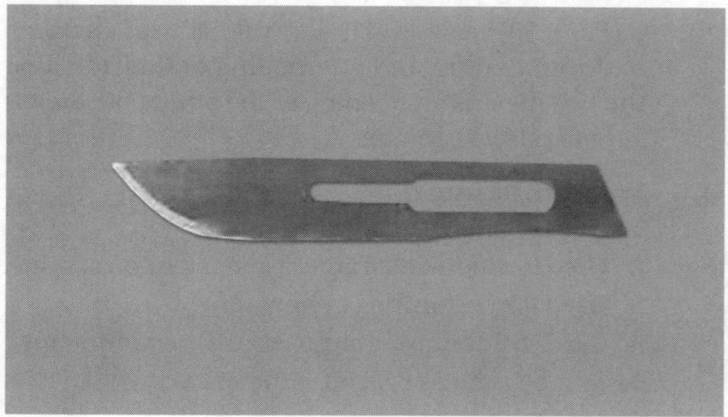

Figure 9.18: Surgical blade

This is surgical blade.

Q. What are the types and which type fits into which number of handle?

Blades number 10,11 and 12 fit in BP handle numbers 3, 5 and 7, respectively. Blade numbers 18–24 fit in BP handle number 4. The blades are detatchable.

The blade number 15 that fits in BP handle number 3 has a narrow shaft and is used for smaller incisions e.g. sebaceous cyst excision, venesection.

The blade number 11 is also known as the stab knife and is used for incision and drainage of abcess cavities.

Q. Name a rehab surgery which requires FOUR incisions?

SPOTT (posterior tibialis tendon transfers) technique for Tibialis Anterior Tibialis Posterior TRANSFER for varus deformity.

Q. What are the steps in SPOTT technique?

(Four separate incisions are used according to Green et al)

- **The first incision:** Two centimetres long, over the insertion of the posterior tibialis tendon on the navicular
  - The distal end of the tendon is identified and its sheath is opened
  - The tendon is then split longitudinally and the plantar half is dissected from its insertion
  - The free end is grasped and the tendon is split longitudinally as far proximally as possible
- **The second incision**: At the level of the medial malleolus and continued for approximately six centimetres
  - The free half of the tendon is transferred into the proximal incision and the longitudinal split in the tendon is continued to the musculotendinous junction
- **A third incision**: Posterior to the lateral malleolus beginning at the proximal tip of the malleolus and continuing proximally
  - The peroneus brevis is identified and its sheath is split longitudinally
  - The distal stump of the split posterior tibial tendon in the second incision is threaded into a tendon-passer that passed the split portion directly posterior to the tibia and fibula and anterior to all the neurovascular and tendinous structures so as to enter laterally to the opened sheath of peroneus brevis.
- **The fourth incision**: Along the peroneus brevis and distal to the lateral malleolus and continued distally just proximal to the insertion of the peroneus brevis on the base of the fifth metatarsal.
  - The distal part of the sheath is opened and the split posterior tibial tendon is sutured to the peroneal brevis tendon onto the cuboid by fish-mouth technique.

(*The tension should be adjusted so that the hind part of the foot will rest in neutral position, by holding the foot in neutral and pulling hard on the posterior tibial tendon and slightly reducing the pull.*)

- The heel-cord lengthening is usually performed prior to the procedure and a long cast was applied with the knee extended and the foot in neutral position.

Q. What is the postoperative care needed?

- The patient could bear weight on the cast as tolerated and four weeks later the cast was changed and a short walking cast was applied
- If the patient is able to dorsiflex the foot and ankle to neutral, no postoperative brace is used.

Q. What are the other techniques of TA TP transfer surgeries?

Splatt (Split tibialis anterior) technique.

Q. What are its step?

- First incision exposes the insertion of the tendon which was split longitudinally as far as through the musculotendinous junction
- The medial half of the tendon was left attached to the first metatarsal and first cuneiform, but the lateral half was detached from its insertion
- The split lateral half of the tendon is passed subcutaneously into the incision made over the cuboid
- Next it is inserted into the holes made in the bone and either sutured to itself under moderate tension or if the length of the stump was not sufficient, anchoring was carried out with any other technique (pull-out wire, anchoring to the periosteum, etc.).

Q. What is the goal of TA TP transfer surgery?

The goal of the semi-transfers is to affect the muscle-tendon complex in a way that it neither inverts nor everts the foot maintaining, thus its stability and flexibility.

(The splatt as described by Hoffer et al corrects supination and varus deformity of the midfoot secondary to spasticity of the anterior tibial muscle).

MISCELLANEOUS

Measuring Tape

Q. What is this?

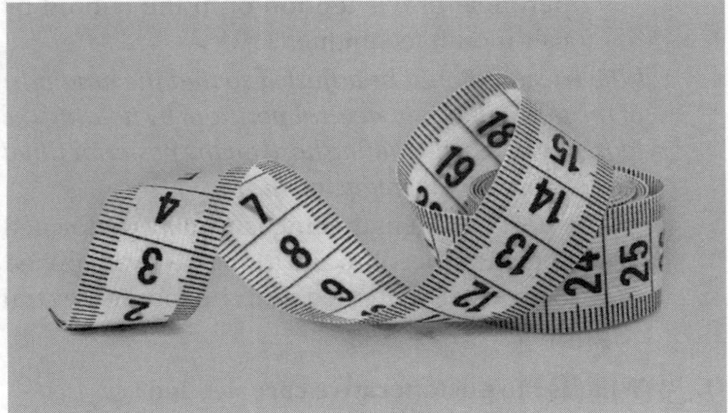

Figure 9.19: Measuring tape

It is a measuring tape.

Q. What are its uses?

1. Measuring girth of limbs.
2. Measuring distances from fixed bony points for surface marking of a specific point for percutaneous therapies.

Simple Rubber Catheter

Q. What is this?

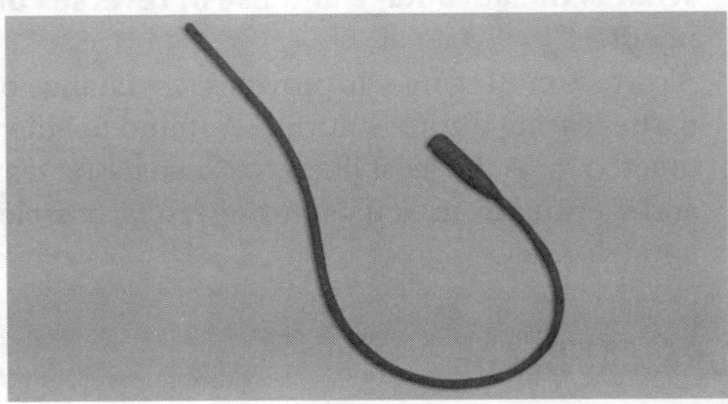

Figure 9.20: Simple rubber catheter

It (Fig. 9.20) is made of Indian rubber with a smooth and rounded tip and an opening at the side near the tip. There is an opening at the other end. So it is simple rubber catheter.

Q. What are its uses?

1. Used to relieve retention of urine.
2. Used to differentiate anuria and retention of urine.
3. Used for performing cystography.
4. Used to administer intravescical chemotherapy.
5. May be used as oxygen catheter.
6. May be used to irrigate an abcess cavity.
7. Used for CIC.

Antiseptic Solutions

Q. What is this?

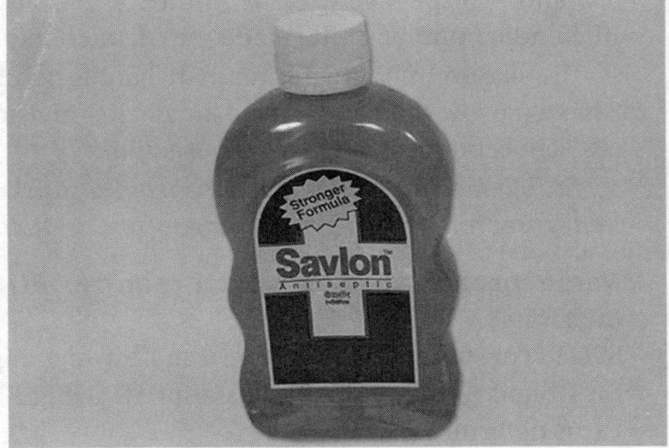

Figure 9.21: Antiseptic solutions

It (Fig. 9.21) is a bottle containing antiseptic solution.

Q. What is the composition?

Cetrimide 3.0% w/v, chlorhexidine gluconate 0.3% w/v. Also contains—Isopropyl alcohol, terpineol, liquid deodoriser, benzyl benzoate, d-gluconolactone, sodium hydroxide and purified water.

Q. What are the uses?

Used for skin cleansing, minor abrasions and burns, insect bites.

Q. What is this?

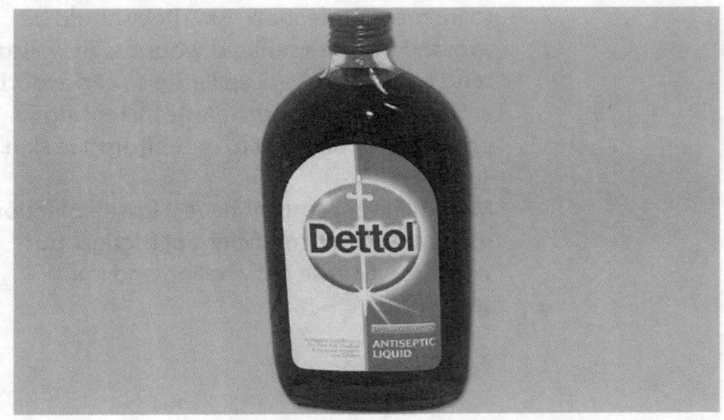

Figure 9.22: Antiseptic solutions

It (Fig. 9.22)is a bottle containing antiseptic solution.

Q. What is the composition?

- Chloroxylenol: 4.8% w/v
- Excipients: Castor oil soap 14.0–15.2% v/v.

Q. What are the uses?

As an antiseptic for prophylaxis of topical infection in intact and abraded skin and for skin preparation prior to surgical or diagnostic procedures.

Test Tube

Q. What is this?

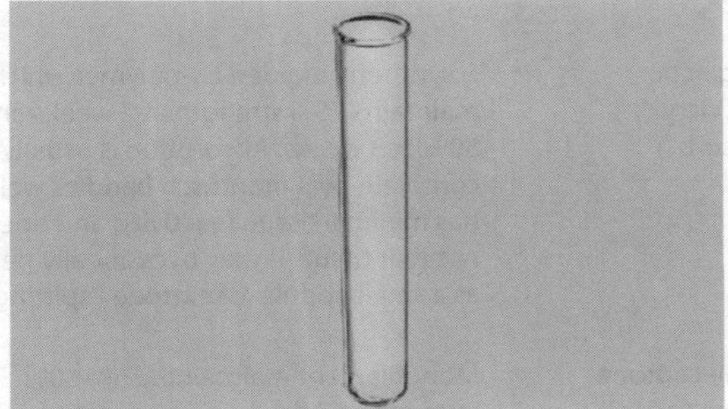

Figure 9.23: Test tube

This is a test tube.

Q. What are the uses?

1. Used to send wound swab culture, sputum culture, throat swab for culture, etc.
2. Used to check the mucosal integrity in an intestinal stoma.

Balloon Catheter

Q. What is this?

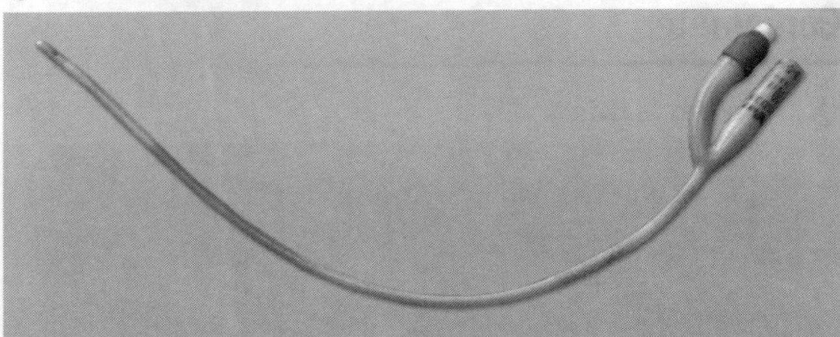

Figure 9.24: Foley's balloon catheter

It is a foley's balloon catheter.

Q. What are its type?

- In a two way Foley's catheter the side channel is used to inflate the balloon so that it is kept indwelling. There is a valve in the side channel. The main channel is for drainage of urine. The catheter number (ex 16 Fr) and the balloon capacity (30-50 mL) is mentioned on the main or side channel
- In a three way Foley's catheter an additional third channel for either irrigation or drainage is present.

Q. What are its uses?

1. Urethral cathetarization for planned operation, intake–output measurement or relief of retention of urine.
2. Used for suprapubic cystostomy.
3. Used for tube nephrostomy.
4. Used for feeding jejunostomy.

Tunning Fork

Q. What is this?

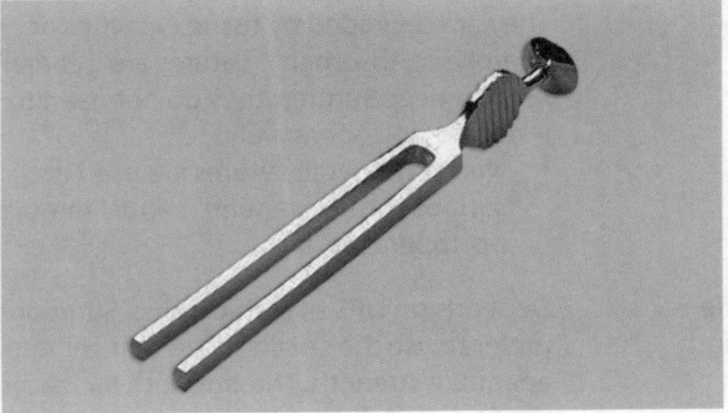

Figure 9.25: Tunning fork

This is 256 Hz tunning fork.

Q. What are the frequencies of tunning fork used commonly?

128 Hz: Vibration
512 Hz: Hearing
256 Hz: Both (Fig. 9.25).

Goniometer

Q. What is this?

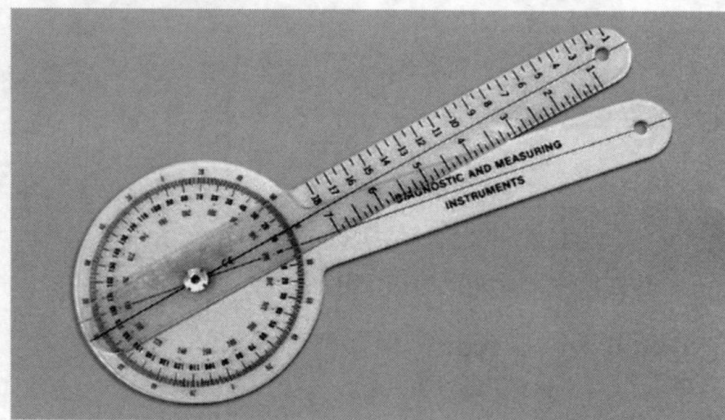

Figure 9.26: Goniometer

This is a goniometer

Q. What are the uses?

- Range of motions of joint
- Spasticity recordings (tardeu scale)
- Used to see cobbs angle measurement
- Q angle measurement.

Suture Material

Characteristics of suture material

The choice of suture is determined by a balance of the various characteristics of suture materials most appropriate for the specific wound closure situation.

Absorbable vs Non-absorbable	The major subdivision of sutures. Sutures that lose the majority of their tensile strength within 60 days are considered absorbable. They are degraded by tissue enzymes or hydrolysis. Absorbable sutures are generally used as deep sutures; they do not need to be removed postoperatively. • Non-absorbable sutures are used for surface sutures; require manual removal postoperatively.
Tensile strength	Depends on UPS size (thickness). Surgeons prefer to use the smallest size that will provide adequate strength. The strength increases as the first digit decreases. • 3-0 is a thick strong suture • 6-0 is a thin comparatively weak suture.
Plasticity and elasticity	The ability to retain length and strength after stretch, and the ability to regain its original length after stretch, respectively. This is important: • To accommodate postoperative oedema without cutting into the tissue • To maintain epidermal approximation once the edema has resolved.
Multifilament vs monofilament	• Multifilament braided sutures handle more easily and tie well, but can potentially harbor organisms between fibers leading to increased infection risk. They should be avoided in contaminated wounds. They also tend to have higher capillarity so can absorb and transfer fluid more easily increasing potential for bacteria to enter from the skin surface • Monofilament sutures have a lower infection risk and a lower coefficient of friction, but with a lower ease of handling and knot security.

Absorbable Sutures

Surgical Gut	• Plain gut loses its strength in 7–10 days and is completely digested by 60 days. It is seldom used now due to poor strength and high tissue reactivity (due to proteolytic enzyme degradation rather than hydrolysis) • Chronic gut has been manufactured with chromium salts to reduce enzyme digestion and therefore maintains strength for 10–14 days making it useful for mucosal closures. • Fast-absorbing gut is produced by pre-heating and can be used for attaching skin grafts, or in areas of low tension where the wound is well supported by deep sutures, and suture removal would be difficult. It maintains strength for 3–5 days.
Polyglactin 910 (Vicryl®, Polysorb®)	• A synthetic braided co-polymer which maintains 75% strength at 2 weeks and 50% at 3 weeks. Absorption is usually complete by 3 months. It handles well, has minimal tissue reactivity, and does not tear tissue. It may occasionally persist as a small nodule or extrude ('spitting').
Poliglecaprone 25 (Monocryl®)	• Monofilament maintaining 50–60% strength at 7 days with complete absorption by 3 months. It offers better handling and knot security than most other monofilament sutures, with even less tissue reaction than Vicryl® and is therefore useful where minimal tissue reaction is essential.

Polydioxanone (PDS II®)	• Monofilament polymer with prolonged tensile strength (70% at 2 weeks, 50% at 4 weeks) and may persist for more than 6 months. Good for high-tension areas or contaminated wounds, but being a monofilament it has poor handling and knot security. Its minimal tissue reaction makes it good for repair of cartilage where inflammation would lead to significant discomfort.
Polytrimethylene carbonate (Maxon®)	• A monofilament that combines the prolonged strength of PDS® and the good handling and knotting of Vicryl®. 80% strength at 2 weeks, 60% at 4 weeks, and complete absorption by 6 months. Minimal tissue reaction.
Glycomer 631 (Biosyn®)	• A monofilament similar to Monocryl® in characteristics but with prolonged strength akin to Maxon®.

Non-absorbable Sutures

Nylon (Ethilon®, Dermalon®, Surgilon®, Nurolon®, Nylene®)	• Inexpensive monofilament with good tensile strength, and minimal tissue reactivity. Disadvantages are its handling and knot security, but it remains one of the most popular non-absorbable sutures in dermatological surgery. Surgilon® and Nurolon® handle better but are more expensive.
Polybutester (Novafil®)	• A monofilament with good handling and excellent elasticity. It responds well to tissue edema, and is also suited to subcuticular running sutures.
Polypropylene (Prolene®, Surgilene®, Surgipro®)	• A monofilament polymer with a very low coefficient of friction making it the suture of choice for running subcuticular stitches. It has good plasticity but limited elasticity, poor knot security, and it is relatively expensive. Favored by some for facial repairs.
Silk (Dysilk)	• Braided natural protein with unsurpassed handling, knot security, and pliability (making it ideal for mucosal surfaces and intertriginous areas) but limited by its low tensile strength, and high coefficient of friction, capillarity, and tissue reactivity.
Polyester (Dacron, Mersilene, Ethibond)	• Braided multifilament suture with high strength, good handling, and low tissue reactivity. Ethibond is coated and has a low coefficient of friction. • Pliability makes these excellent for mucosal surfaces without the reactivity of silk.

10 Chapter

Miscellaneous

BASICS OF INTERVENTIONAL SPINAL PAIN MANAGEMENT

NEUROAXIAL PROCEDURES (TABLES 10.1 AND 10.2)

Table 10.1: Lumber neuraxial procedure

Procedure	*Caudal epidural*	*Transforaminal epidural (lumbar)*	*Interlaminar epidural (lumbar)*	*Facet joint injection*
Sedation	Not Required	Not Required	Not Required	Not Required
Needle	22–25 G	22–25 G	3 ½ in Tuohy needle	22–25 G
Drugs	2% Lignocaine 0.25% Bupivacaine 80 mg Depot methyl prednisolone N.S	2% Lignocaine 0.25% Bupivacaine 80 mg Depot Methyl prednisolone	2% Lignocaine 80 mg Triamcinolone	2% Lignocaine 3 mg Betamethasone
Patient positioning	Prone with pillow under abdomen, hips internal rotated	Prone	Prone	Prone
C arm positioning	Lateral	AP (Identify level) Squaring by tilting Ipsilateral oblique	AP (Identify level) Lateral Contralateral oblique	AP (Identify level) Squaring by tilting Ipsilateral oblique
Initial needle position	Sacral hiatus	Below the eye of the scotty dog	Interlaminar space	Facet joint (beside ear of scotty dog)
Final target	S3 segment	Within the foramen (lateral) 6 o' clock (AP)	Spinolaminar line	Between the ear of dog (same level) and forelimb of the dog (above)
Dye pattern	Christmas tree in AP view	In epidural space and along spinal nerve	Epidural spread	Straight line in oblique view
Volume to inject	15 mL	4 mL	10 mL	1 mL
Clinical confirmation	Relief of pain	Relief of pain	Immediate relief of pain	Relief of pain after provocative tests
Complication	See below	See below	See below	See below

Table 10.2: SI joint, cervical epidural and stellate ganglion block procedure

Procedure	*SI joint*	*Cervical epidural (Interlaminar)*	*Stellate ganglion*
Sedation	Not Required	Not Required	Not Required
Needle	22–25 G	3 ½ in Tuohy needle	22–25 G
Drugs	2% Lignocaine Triamcinolone	10 mg Dexamethasone Normal saline	2% Lignocaine 0.25% Bupivacaine, NS, Steroid
Patient positioning	Prone	Prone	Supine
C arm positioning	Ipsilateral oblique, Lateral, AP	AP Lateral Contralateral oblique	AP Lateral
Initial needle position	Lower 1/3 rd of joint	Interlaminar region	C7 transverse process
Final target	Lower 1/3 rd of joint	Spinolaminar line	C7 transverse process
Dye pattern	Spread in both medial and lateral joint surface	Epidural spread	Anterolateral of the vertebral bodies
Volume	4 mL	5 mL	6 – 9 mL
Clinical confirmation	Immediate relief of pain	Relief of pain	Horner syndrome
COMPLICATION	See below	See below	See below

Complications and Side Effects

From Local Anesthetics

- *Inadvertent puncture* of thecal sac while injecting local anesthetic causes possibility of prolonged paresthesia, pain in legs, transient paralysis (motor block).
- *Allergic reactions*: Vasomotor changes, hives/urticaria, bronchospasms.
- *Central nervous system toxicity*: Disorientation, lightheaded, nystagmus, tinnitus, muscle twitching, blurred vision, numbness of tongue, metallic taste, slurred speech, headache, seizures.
- *Cardiovascular vasoconstriction*: Increased heart rate, dysrhythmia, elevated blood pressure.

From Corticosteroids

- Intrathecal injection causes increased risk of *arachnoiditis.*
- *Fluid retention* (congestive heart failure, weight gain), steroid myopathy, irregular menstrual cycle, epidural lipomatosis, insomnia, osteoporosis.
- *Hyperglycemia* (maximum levels usually within 48 hours).
- *Facial flushing*: Possibly an immunoglobulin (IgE) mediated mechanism.
- *Less common*: Increase in temperature, euphoria, depression, mood swings (especially in patients with bipolar disorder), local fat atrophy, depigmentation of skin, headaches, pain flare, Cushing's syndrome, transient adrenal suppression (may take up to 2 weeks for hypothalamus-pituitary axis to resolve).

From Dye

- *Allergic reactions*: Urticaria, itching, bronchospasm, facial and laryngeal edema (usually occurs within 2 hours)
- Contrast induced nephropathy or thyrotoxicosis.

From Spinal Procedures

- Vasovagal reaction
- Meningitis: Bacterial or aseptic secondary to a dural puncture
- Epidural abscess/discitis/osteomyelitis
- Increased risk of bleeding in patients with hemophilia, Von Willebrand's disease, thrombocytopenia (>100K platelets is safe), anticoagulation therapy
- Injury to cauda equina, nerve roots, or spinal cord
- Paralysis: Usually secondary to radicular artery or Arteryof Adamkiewicz infarct, anterior spinal artery ischemia and cord infarct
- Postdural puncture headache ("spinal headache")
- Pneumothorax (during lower cervical or thoracic injections)
- Recurrent laryngeal nerve injury (during cervical injections)
- Urinary retention (local anesthetic effect on sacral roots).

APPROACH OF INTERVENTIONAL LUMBOSACRAL SPINAL PAIN MANAGEMENT

Q. What are the conventional rehabilitation management?

Bed rest: Absolutely not indicated

(Waddell et al : Bed rest may even delay recovery)

Pharmacological: Medicine cannot alter the disease course of radicular pain

- NSAID: Most important in facet joint pain.
- TRAMADOL: vomiting and sedation restricts its use.
- Oral steroid: Low level evidence about the role of steroid
- anti TNF: Still in experimental stage
- SSRI: Duloxetin is effective for reduction of radicular pain
- Pregabalin/ Gabapentin :- effective for radicular pain

Nonpharmacological:

- Exercise
  - By McKenzie centralization technique
    - Most useful and important
    - Change the location of pain to more central/ proximal position.

    (Decision regarding surgery for pain should be withhold until adequate centralization achieved.)
  - Stabilization and strengthening technique
- Modalities:
  - Cryotherapy can reduce pain
  - Heat
    - SWD and MWD: obsolete in current practice
    - UST: little role as per current evidence.
  - Electrotherapy—TENS: May be helpful in radicular pain
  - Traction—Controversial: Used to reduce intradiscal pressure (There are lots of contraindications See Chapter 8, Page no 226)
    - Reduce muscle spasm.
- Orthoses: S1 deficit- flexible post leaf spring AFO
  - L5 deficit–PPAFO (poly propelene ankle foot orthosis)
  - L3/4–knee extension orthoses.
- *Back school—very important.*

Q. How does LS Corset work?

Corset/ Brace: It can reduce intradiscal pressure by increasing intraabdominal pressure. Thus, it is helpful in reducing radicular pain.

Q. What should be the advices regarding travel walking and sports?

- **Travel**: Reduce time, drive in 45° reclined position
- **Walking**: May be acceptable in early stage
- **Swimming**: Crawl, breast stroke may be adviced
- **Sports:**
  - Asymptomatic for 3 weeks: High torque sports like golf, squash, tennis, bowling may be restarted
  - Asymptomatic for 6 weeks: Baseball, soccer, hockey may be restarted.

Q. What are the mimickers of PIVD?

- SI joint dysfunction
- Piriformis syndrome
- Intrinsic hip joint pathology
- Trochenteric bursitis.

(25% of referral to spine physician for radicular pain are mimickers).

Q. What should be the algorithmic approach for interventional management of lumbar pain?

I. **Radiculopathy secondary to herniated nucleosus pulposus (Flowcharts 10.1 to 10.4)**

Flowchart 10.1: Radiological differentiation

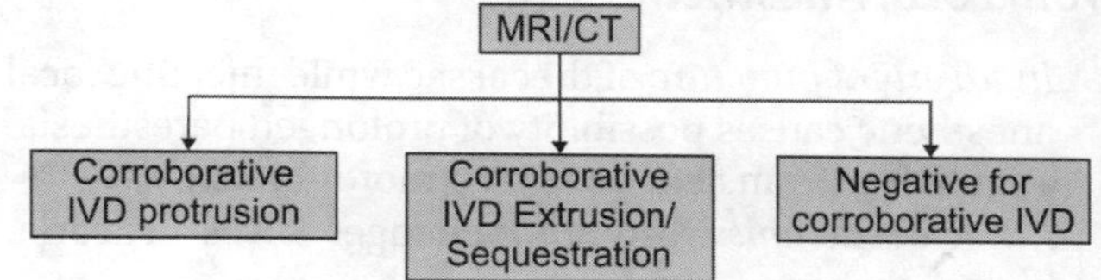

Flowchart 10.2: IVD protrusion

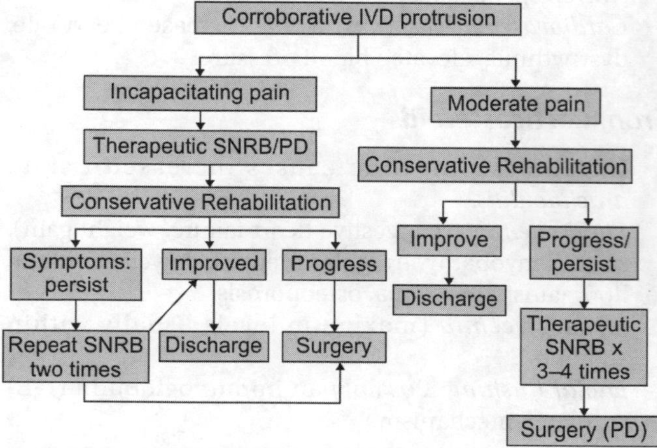

Abbreviation: PD, percutaneous disectomy

Flowchart 10.3: IVD extrusion/sequestration

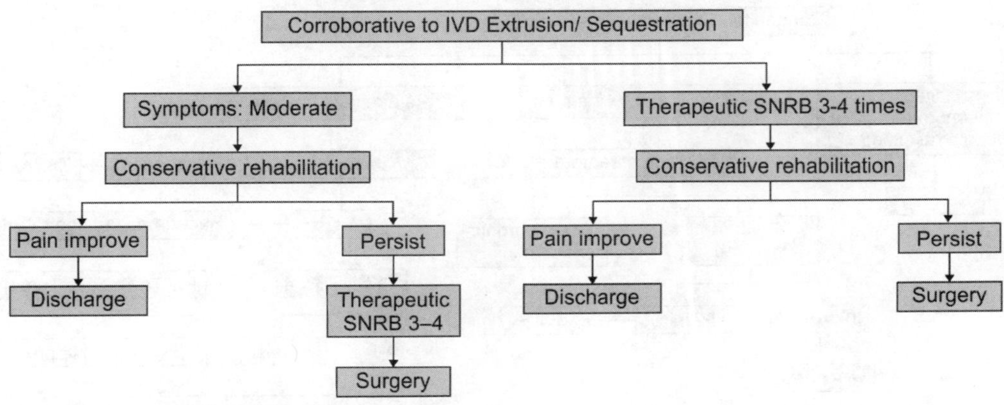

Flowchart 10.4: Negative for IVD

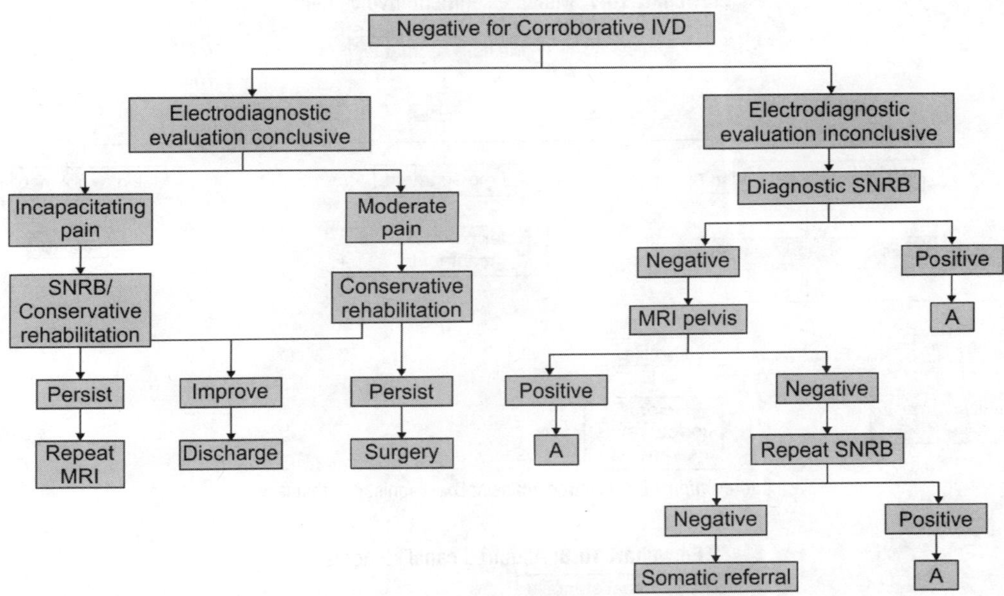

II. Neurogenic Claudication—congenital and acquired (Flowcharts 10.5 to 10.8)

Flowchart 10.5: Neurogenic claudication

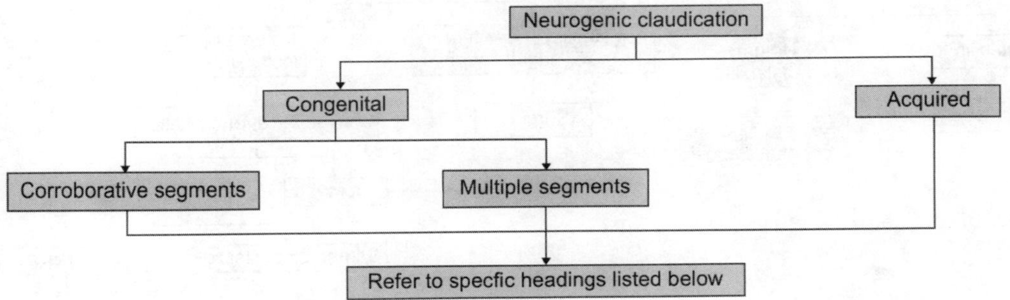

Flowchart 10.6: Congenital neurogenic claudication

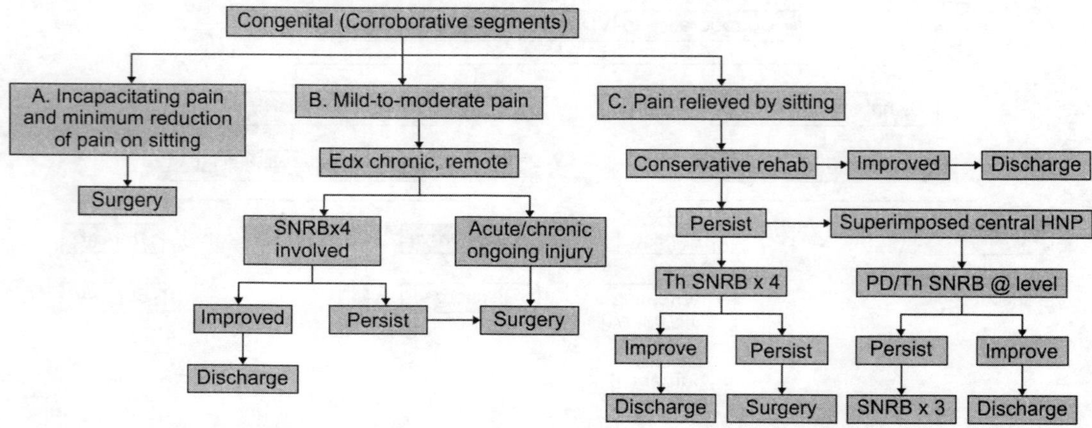

Abbreviation: EDX, electrodiagnosis; PD, percutaneus disectomy; Th SNRB, therapeutic selective nerve root block

Flowchart 10.7: Multiple segment involvement

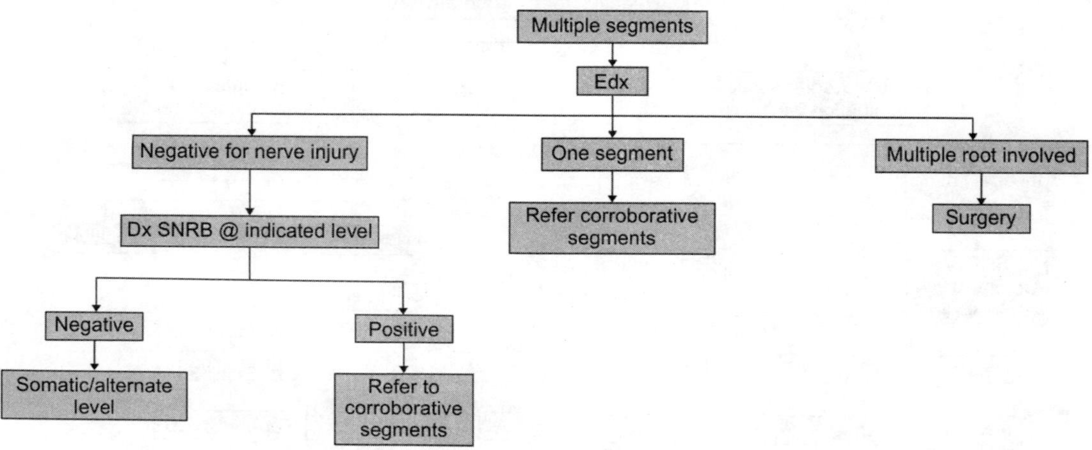

Abbreviation: EDX, electrodiagnosis; Dx, diagnistic at that level

Flowchart 10.8: Acquired canal stenosis

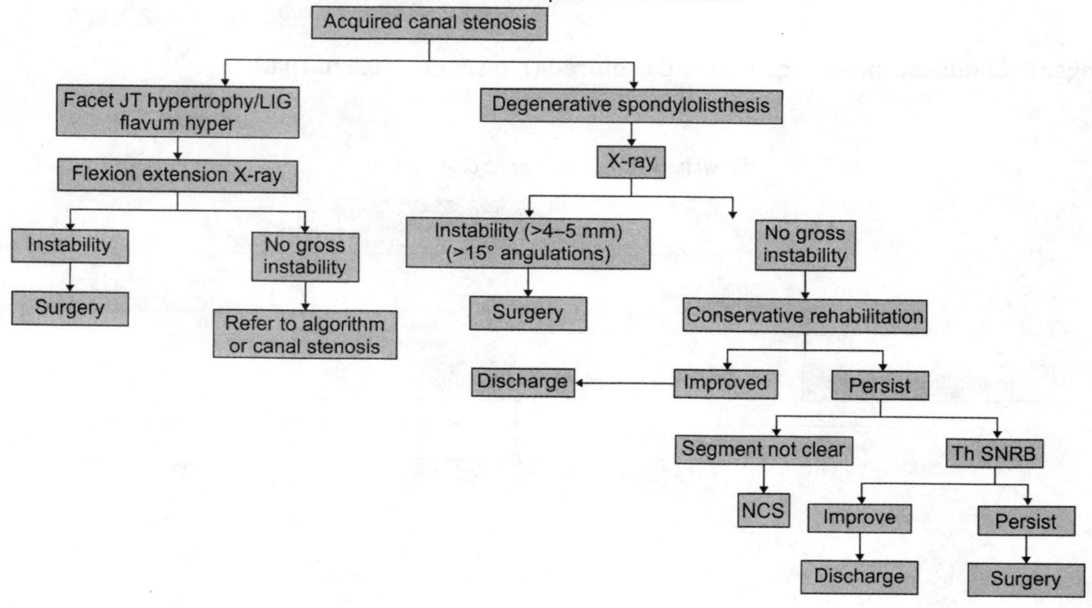

III. Radiculopathy due to lateral recess stenosis, foraminal stenosis, extraforaminal stenosis (Flowchart 10.9).

Flowchart 10.9: Lateral recess stenosis, foraminal stenosis, extraforaminal stenosis

Radiculopathy due to lateral recess stenosis, foraminal stenosis, extraforaminal stenosis
Rapid onset
1. Corroborative IVD protrusion-A
2. Corroborative IVD ext/seq-B
3. Negative for corroborative IVD-C
4. Intraspinal cyst
Intraspinal Cyst
Emanating from arthritic facet joint
X-ray
Stable
Unstable
Conservative rehabilitation
Surgery
Improve
Persist
Discharge
The SNRB x 3–4+PT
Cyst aspiration
Puncture
Surgery
Emanating from IVD, posterior longitudinal, spondylosis ligament
Moderate
Severe
Conservative rehabilitation
Th SNRB 3–4, PT
Improve
Persist
Discharge
Surgery
Gradual onset
Facet arthropathy/Lig flavum hypertrophy
Moderate
Severe
Flexion ex, core cond
Therapeutic SNRB 3–4/PT
Improve
Persist
Therapeutic SNRB 3–4/Cons.
Improve
Persist
Discharge
Surgery
Improve
Persist
Discharge
Surgery

Abbreviation: Pt, physical therapy; Ex, exercises cons conservative

IV. Postoperative radiculopathy (Flowchart 10.10)

Flowchart 10.10: Postoperative radiculopathy

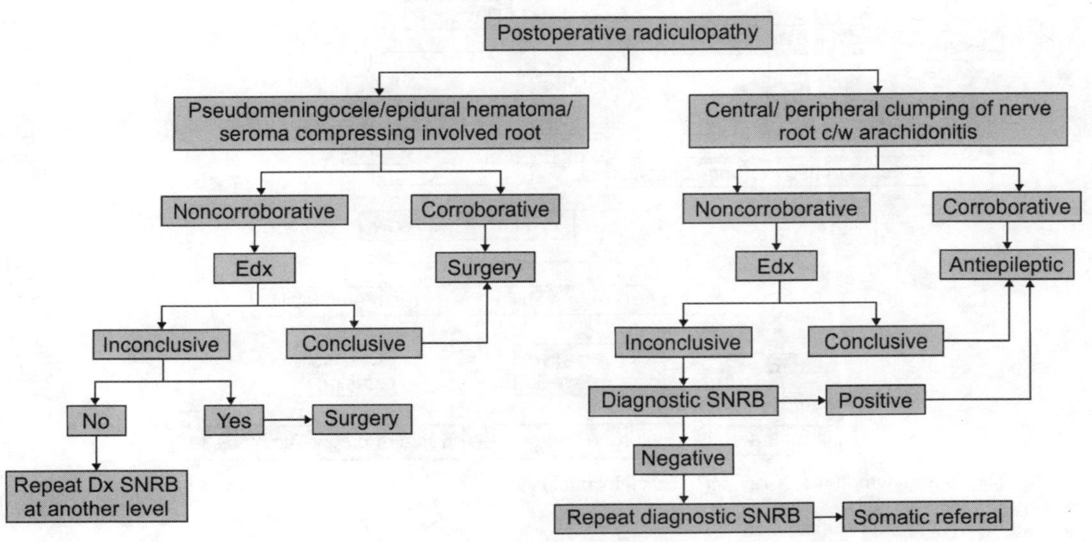

Abbreviation: EDX, electrodiagnosis; Dx, diagnosis

Q. Most important thing to consider in management of cervical radicular pain?

Which pain is more: Neck pain > arm pain or arm pain > neck pain.

Q. What is the difference between cervical radicular pain and facet pain?

The difference between cervical facet pain and radicular pain is given in Table 10.3.

Table 10.3: Difference between cervical facet pain and radicular pain

	Cervical facet pain	*Radicular pain*
Axial neck pain	More severe than extremity	More pain in extremity
Pain distal to elbow	Usually not present	Present usually

Q. How to approach a patient with neck pain greater than arm pain?

The approach is as follows (Flowchart 10.11, 10.12 and Table 10.4):

INTERVENTIONAL APPROACH TO CERVICAL RADICULOPATHY

Q. What is cervical radicular pain?

- It should follow cervical myotomal/ dermatomal distribution
- NCS should be corroborative
- It may/may not coexist with radiculopathy.

Q. What is the diagnostic approach?

A. Spondylotic:

- Atraumatic:
  - It is exceedingly common
  - Only minority cases are symptomatic
  - Axial pain
  - If severe weakness then surgery is required
- Traumatic:
  - Cervical spondylosis misleading
  - Discogenic, muscle, appophseal joint pain
  - It is complex clinically
  - If compression then surgery is required

Flowchart 10.11: Approach of Neck pain greater than Arm pain

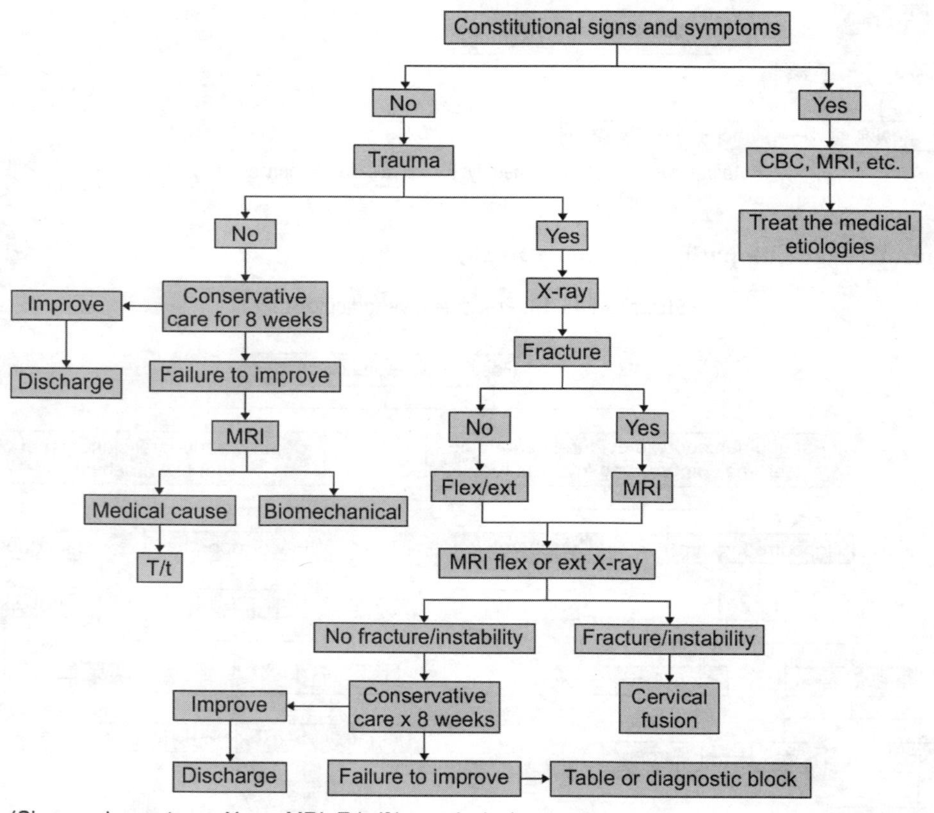

(Signs and symptoms, X-ray, MRI, Edx if inconclusive)
t/t : Treatment
Flex/ext : Flexion/ extension

Table 10.4: Table of diagnostic block

Posterior neck and upper trapezius		***Scapular***		***Chest***	***Deltoid***		***Upper arm***			***Forearm***		
Posterior upper trapezius	Anterior upper trapezius	Superior	Middle/ inferior		Anterior	Posterior	Postero-lateral	Antero-lateral	Antero-medial	Ventral	Radial dorsal	Ulnar dorsal
Dx	Dx	Dx	Dx	Dx	Dx	Dx	Dx	Dx	Dx	Dx	Dx	Dx
C4 ↓ C7 ↓ C6 ↓ C8	C6 ↓ C5 ↓ C4 ↓ C7	C6 ↓ C7 ↓ C8 ↓ C5 ↓ C4	C8 ↓ C7 ↓ C6 ↓ C5	C7 ↓ C8 ↓ C4	C6 ↓ C5 ↓ C7 ↓ C8 ↓ C4	C7 ↓ C5 ↓ C4 ↓ C6 ↓ C8	C6 ↓ C7 ↓ C5 ↓ C8	C6 ↓ C7 ↓ C5 ↓ C8	C8 ↓ C6 ↓ C5	C6 ↓ C7 ↓ C5 ↓ C8	C6 ↓ C7 ↓ C8	C8 ↓ C7 ↓ C6

B. Nonspondylotic:
- Atraumatic
  - Brachial plexopathy
  - Shoulder joint pain
  - Demyelinating disease
  - CRPS.
- Traumatic
  - Diagnostic challenge
  - Discogenic/ facet syndrome
  - *MRI/NCS most often negative.*

Flowchart 10.12: Result of diagnostic block

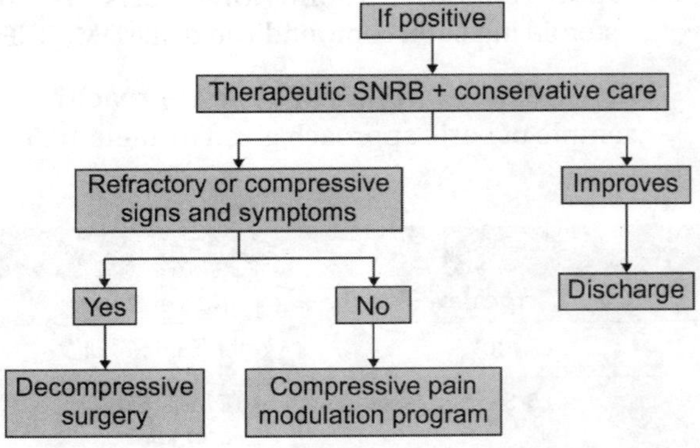

Q. How to approach if arm pain > neck pain?

Approach given in Flowchart 10.13 and 10.14.

Flowchart 10.13: Approach of arm pain greater than neck pain

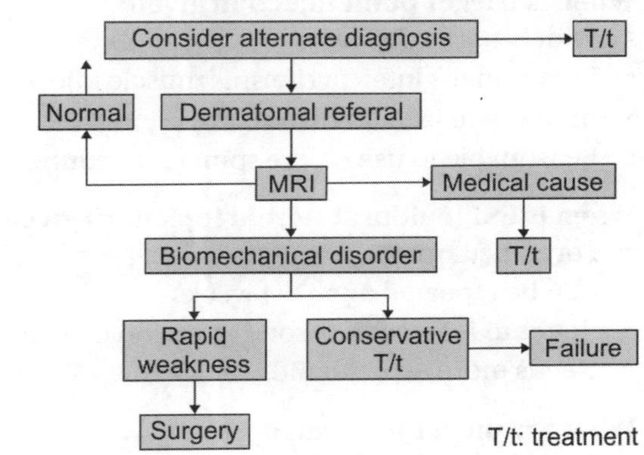

Flowchart 10.14: After MRI correlation

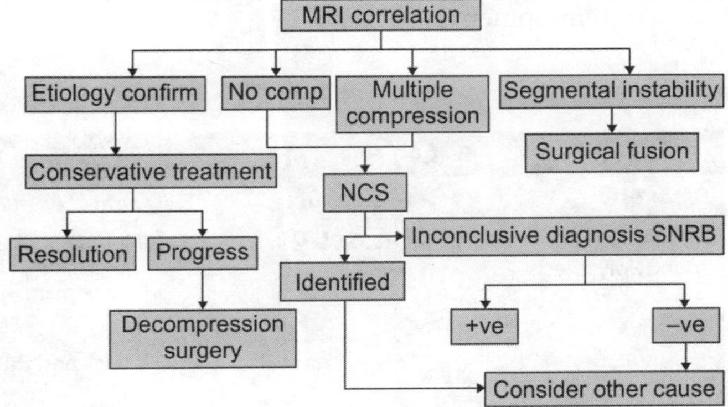

INTERVENTIONAL APPROACH TO SPONDYLOLISTHESIS

Basic Approach (Flowchart 10.15)

Flowchart 10.15: Basic interventional approach

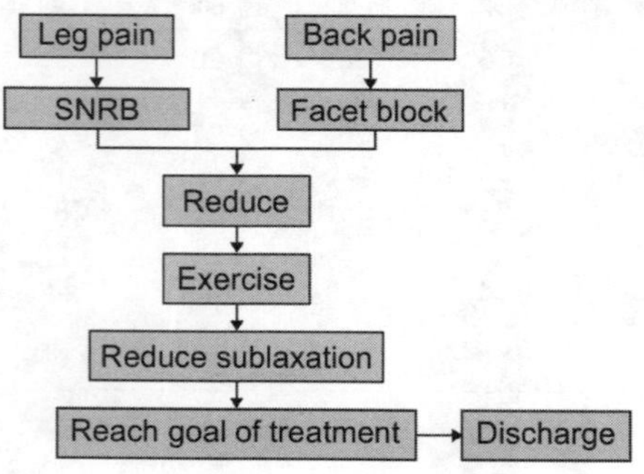

Q. When is trigger point injection given?
- Widely used over years
- Para spinal/glutei/pyriformis muscle injection
- Infiltrate to facet joint/bursa
- Reasonable to use before spinal procedures.

Q. When is ESI (epidural steroid injection) given?
- For radiculopathy
- Can be repeated after 1-4 weeks
- Better to reassess if second injection one failed
- Needs more expert hand.

Q. What are the target levels?
- **Transiting root**—in degenerative spondylolysthesis (canal stenosis)
- **Exiting root**—in ischemic spondylolysthesis (entrapment)

Transforaminal approach is the best option in degenerative spondylolysthesis/ischemic spondylolysthesis.

Q. When is intralaminar approach preferred ?
- Difficult technique
- Tough to control injection flow
- Risk of dural puncture
- Frequently unilateral
- Good way in multilevel stenosis.

Q. What is role of caudal epidural steroid injection?
- Safe
- Easy to perform
- Useful for L5 and sacral roots

Q. What are the role of facet joint intervention?
- Treatment of choice in degenerative spondylolysthesis with back , buttock and thigh pain
- Difficult to perform in degenerative spine.
- Level—same level of spondylolysthesis
- Dubious role in ischemic spondylolysthesis

Q. What are the role of injection in pars defect?
- In ischemic spondylolysthesis
- Rationale unclear
- Some pain generator within the fibrous union are present due to neural element in pars (As per nonconclusive study).

Q. What are the role of radio frequency denervation?
- Facet joints
- In degenerative spondylolysthesis for whom steroid injection contraindicated like DM, CCF etc.

Q. What are the examples of basic approach?
Example of basic approach given in Table 10.5.

Table 10.5: Examples of basic approach

Diagnosis	*Subtype*	*Clinical features*	*Target level*	*Intervention*
Degenerative spondylolysthesis	L5S1 Level	If leg pain > back pain	L5 root	IL/TF L5 S1 ESI
		If back pain > leg pain	L5/S1 root, facet joint	TF L5/S! ESI, Facet joint block
	L4L5 radiculopathy	If back and thigh pain> leg pain	Facet joint	Facet L4/5 Intralaminar ESI
		If thigh and leg pain> back	L4 root	Trans-foraminal ESI L4/5
Ischemic spondylolysthesis	L5S1 radiculopathy	Unilateral leg	L5 root	Trans-foraminal ESI
		Back pain	?structure	Caudal ESI

Abbreviation: IL, intra lamellar; ESI, epidural steroid injection; TF, transforaminal

Q. What are the surgical options?

- Pars repair
  - Buck screw fixation
  - Scott's transverse process wiring
- Neural decompression with or without stabilization
- Spinal fusion.

Q. What are the surgical approach for patients with spondylolysthesis of adult?

The surgical approach for patients with spondylolysthesis of adult is given in Flowchart 10.16.

Flowchart 10.16: Approach of surgeries

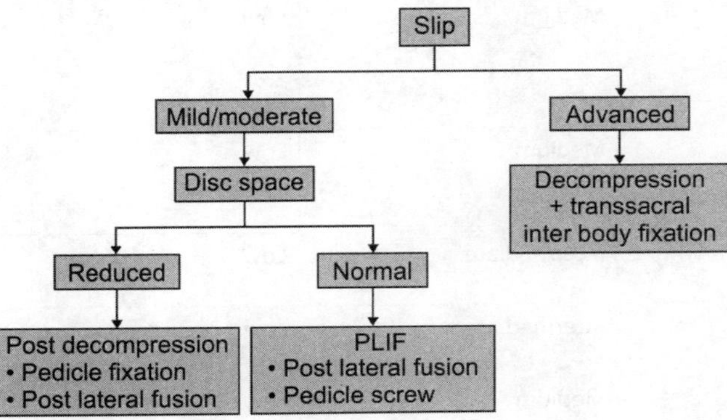

N:B Grade IV – post grafting with extensive correction.
Post: Posterior

Q. What are the indications for surgery in childhood and adolesence?

- Symptomatic—grade II
- Grade III and IV—even asymptomatic
- Slip angle> 45°
- Mandatory to prevent progression.

Q. What is the approach for spondyloptosis?

- Reduction is essential as significant stretching of nerve root occurs
- L5/S1 disectomy and sacral osteotomy are done then followed by L4/S1 fixation and posterolateral fusion.

BASIC PRINCIPLES OF THERAPEUTIC EXERCISE

Q. What are therapeutic exercises?

Exercises for therapeutic benefits of the patient are called therapeutic exercises.

Q. What are the properties of skeletal muscle?

Skeletal muscle tissue has four properties related to its ability to produce force and movement about joints

- Irritability or excitability
- Contractility
- Extensibility
- Elasticity.

Q. What are the different types of therapeutic exercises?

- Postural correction exercises
- Strengthening exercises
- Mobilization exercises
- Coordination exercises
- Balance training
- Gait training
- Endurance training
- Relaxation exercises
- Re-education exercises
- Ergonomic exercises
- Hydrotherapy
- Suspension therapy.

Q. What is oxygen debt?

After a period of strenuous exercise, a person continues to breathe hard and to consume large amounts of oxygen for at least a few minutes and sometimes for as long as 1 hour thereafter. This additional oxygen is used:

1. To reconvert the lactic acid that has accumulated during exercise back into glucose.
2. To reconvert adenosine monophosphate and ADP to ATP.
3. To reconvert creatine and phosphate to phosphocreatine.
4. To re-establish normal concentrations of oxygen bound with hemoglobin and myoglobin.
5. To raise the concentration of oxygen in the lungs to its normal level.

This extra consumption of oxygen after exercise is over is called repaying the *oxygen debt.*

Q. What are the energy sources of a muscle?

- Stored ATP: 3 sec
- Creatinine Phosphokinase system: 5–8 sec
- Glycolytic pathway: 1.3–1.6 minutes
- Aerobic pathway: As long as "fuel" lasts!

Q. What are the determinants of muscle strength?

- Cross-sectional area
- Muscle shape: Pennate > Parallel
- Insertion: Distal insertion dives more strength
- Recruitment
- Rate of firing.

Q. What are the different types of muscle contraction?

- Isometric
- Isotonic
  - Concentric
  - Eccentric.

Q. What are the different types of muscle fibers?

Table 10.6: Types of muscle fibers

Fiber Type	*Type I fibers*	*Type II A fibers*	*Type II B fibers*
Contraction speed (milliseconds)	Slow (90–140 ms)	Fast (50–100 ms)	Very Fast (40–90 ms)
Size of motor neuron (bigger motor neurons allow nerve impulses to operate more quickly)	Small	Large	Very large
Resistance to fatigue	High	Intermediate	Low
Activity used for	Endurance type activities	Short (less than 2 minutes) high intensity activities	Very short (1–30 seconds max) maximal intensity activities
Force production	Low	High	Very high
Efficiency (think fuel consumption here—high efficiency is like a scooter—doesn't burn much fuel or produce much force. A V8 produces heaps of force but is definitely not 'efficient')	High	Medium	Low
Number of mitochondria [mitochondria are located in muscle fibers and produce energy aerobically (with oxygen)]	High	Medium	Low
Capillary density (Capillaries transport oxygen and nutrients to muscles and remove waste products)	High	Intermediate	Low
Oxidative capacity (This refers to the capacity of the muscle fiber to use oxygen for the production of energy)	High	Intermediate	Low
Myoglobin content (Myoglobin is a pigment that binds to oxygen giving the fiber a red color)	High	Medium	Low
Glycolytic capacity (refers to the fibres capacity to store and breakdown glycogen for use as a high intensity energy source)	Low	High	High
ATPase levels (this is an enzyme that controls the breakdown and synthesis of ATP for energy)	Low	Intermediate	High

Q. What is isometric contraction?

- Tension is developed within muscle but joint angles remain constant
- Static contractions
- Significant amount of tension may be developed in muscle to maintain joint angle in relatively static or stable position
- May be used to prevent a body segment from being moved by external forces
- E.g. Pushing a wall.

Q. What is isotonic contraction?

- Isotonic contractions involve muscle developing tension to either cause or control joint movement
- Dynamic contractions
- The varying degrees of tension in muscles result in joint angles changing
- Isotonic contractions are either concentric or eccentric on basis of whether shortening or lengthening occurs.

Q. What is eccentric contraction?

- Muscle lengthens under tension
- Occurs when muscle gradually lessens in tension to control the descent of resistance
- Weight or resistance overcomes muscle contraction but not to the point that muscle cannot control descending movement
- Controls movement with gravity or resistance
- Force developed by the muscle is less than that of the resistance
- Results in the joint angle changing in the direction of the resistance or external force
- Causes body part to move with gravity or external forces (resistance)
- Used to decelerate body segment movement

Q. What is concentric contraction?

- Muscle develops tension as it shortens
- Occurs when muscle develops enough force to overcome applied resistance

- Causes movement against gravity or resistance
- Described as being a positive contraction
- Results in joint angle changing in the direction of the applied muscle force.

Q. What is isokinetic exercise?

It is a type of dynamic exercise using concentric and/or eccentric muscle contractions.

- *Speed (or velocity) of movement is constant*
- Muscular contraction (ideally maximum contraction) occurs throughout movement
- E.g. Biodex, cybex.

Q. What is progressive resisted exercise?

The progressive increase in resistance (overload) in training to increase muscle strength is called as progressive resisted exercise.

Q. What is DeLorme regimen?

It is one form of progressive resistive exercise (Flowchart 10.17).

Flowchart 10.17: Steps of DeLorme regimen

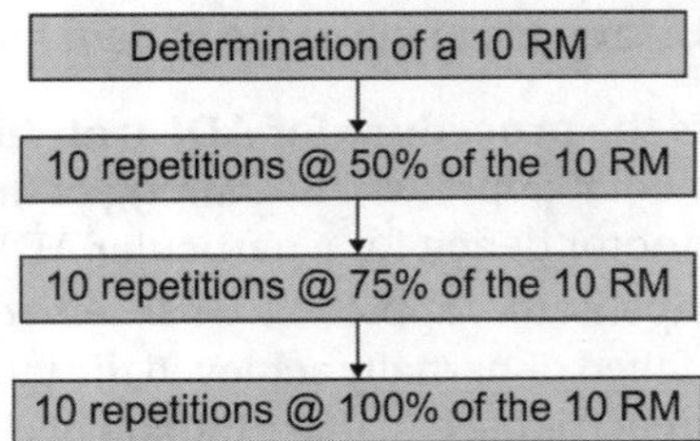

Q. What is Oxford regimen?

It is a regressive resisted exercise regimen (Flowchart 10.18).

Flowchart 10.18: Steps of oxford regimen

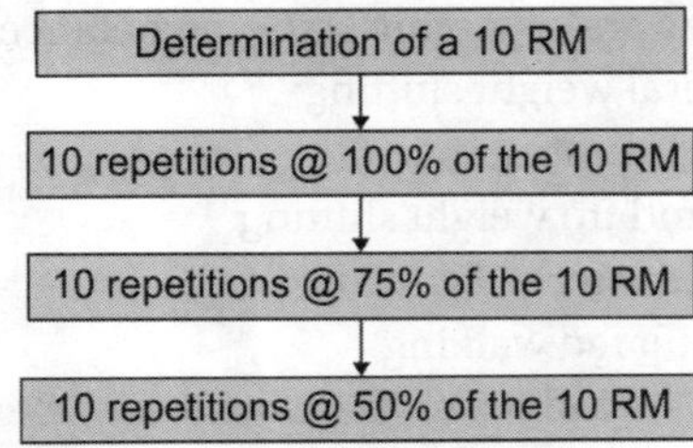

Q. What is active and passive insufficiency?

- *Active insufficiency* is reached when the muscle becomes shortened to the point that it can not generate or maintain active tension
  E.g. Rectus femoris contracts concentrically to both flex the hip and extend the knee—can completely perform either action one at a time but actively insufficient to obtain full range at both joints simultaneously.
- *Passively insufficiency* is reached when the opposing muscle becomes stretched to the point where it can no longer lengthen and allow movement.
  Hence, hamstrings cannot usually stretch enough to allow both maximal hip flexion and maximal knee extension due passive insufficiency.

Q. What is open chain and closed chain exercise?

- When distal segment is fixed or stabilized or weight bearing, it is considered closed and involves fixed joints with mobile joints in between. E.g. squatting
- When distal segment is free and mobile it is open chain. E.g. seated leg extension.

Q. What is concurrent shift?

When concentric and eccentric contractions occur at opposite ends of a muscle during closed kinetic chain movement, e.g. during squat to stand the hip and knee both extend and the rectus femoris shortens at the distal end and lengthens at the proximal end

Q. What is plyometric exercise?

These exercises use the principle of brief stretch followed by contraction. The preceeding stretch facilitates the subsequent contraction. E.g. jumping over boxes.

Q. What is mobilization exercise? Its indications and contraindications?

It is a method to restore and maintain joint movement, performed in such a manner that the patient can voluntarily stop the movement.

Indications:

- Pain and muscle spasms
- Progressive limitation of joint ROM Restricted ROM.

Contraindications:

- Hypermobile joints
- Joint effusion/infection
- Articular surface fracture
- Acute inflamed joints
- Neoplasm
- Bleeding disorder.

Q. What is Frenkel's exercise?

This uses sensation of sight, touch and sound to improve balance by compensating the kinesthetic sensory loss.

Q. What are the relaxation techniques?

- *Jacobson's progressive relaxation technique*: Sequence of tensing and relaxing group of muscles sequentially while focusing on the contraction and relaxation

- *Mitchell's relaxation technique*: Based on reciprocal innervation where contraction of agonists causes reflex relaxation of antagonist
- *Progressive relaxation training*: Contraction of a muscle for 5–7 s and concentrate on the feeling and then relaxed
- *Alexander technique*: Reeducates the body to perform and conserve energy
- *Feldenkrais technique*: Awareness through movement.

Q. What are the re-education exercises?

- Bobath neurodevelopmental technique
- Proprioceptive nuromuscular facilitation

Q. How does hydrotherapy work?

- **Buoyancy** provides the patient with relative weightlessness and joint unloading, allowing performance of active motion with increased ease
- **Hydrostatic pressure** reduces or limits effusion, assists venous return, induces bradycardia, and centralizes peripheral blood flow
- Water's **viscosity** creates resistance with all active movements
- An extremity that moves through the surface performs more work than if kept under water due to **surface tension** and so using equipment at the surface of the water increases the resistance
- As the speed of movement through water increases, resistance to motion increases due to **drag**.
- Water retains **heat** 1000 times more than air and **conducts** temperature 25 times faster than air.

NOTE: In the vertical position, the human center is located at the sternum.

BASIC PRINCIPLES OF OCCUPATIONAL THERAPY

Q. What are the frame of references of occupational therapy?

A. **Biomechanical frame of reference.**
The treatment protocol that is used to develop structural stability, endurance, decrease edema, straight path under biomechanical frame of reference. E.g. Fracture, amputation.

B. **Neurodevelopmental frame of reference.**
The treatment protocol that is used to develop normal reflex, evaluation and normalization of synergy, normalization of muscle tone. E.g. treatment of CVA, cerebral palsy.

C. **Cognitive disability frame of reference.**
This frame of reference helps the patients to develop cognitive functions which otherwise affects activities of daily living and daily functioning.

D. **Sensory integration frame of reference.**
This frame helps in treatment of sensory processing disorders.

E. **Rehabilitation frame of reference.**
This frame of reference includes all the upper extremity orthosis, environmental modification, wheel chair modification, adaptive devices, adaptive procedure

F. **Model of human occupation frame of reference.**
This frame of reference helps the person to participate in various activities and occupation in the environment.
It is a correlation of volition → habituation → performance → environment

Q. How does occupational therapy work?

Occupational therapy uses purposeful activities for therapeutic interventions.

- Activity analysis is done to identify individual activity for particular patient
- Activity modification and grading is done as per need
- Main target is to make the patient independent.

Q. What is the procedure for ADL training?

- Remedial approach: Retraining of the patient for the motor deficit for a particular ADL activity
- Compensatory approach: Once remedial approach has failed or partially achieved the target, then this approach is used to make the subject independent. E.g. Adaptive device, assistive device.

Q. What are the steps of gait training?

- Core body strengthening
- Static and dynamic sitting balance
- Supported standing
- Static and dynamic standing balance
- Lateral weight shifting
- Single limb stance
- To and fro weight shifting
- Assessment of gait aids
- Simulated walking
- Initiate indoor mobility with or without gait aid
- Specific gait pattern according to condition and gait aid
- Obstacle crossing
- Sideways walking
- Walking in a specific demarked area
- Staircase ascending and descending
- Outdoor/community mobility

Q. What are the transfer techniques?

- **Independent:**
  a. Stand pivot transfer.

b. Transfer board transfer.
c. Transfer without use of transfer board.

- **Independent with device: Transfer and bed mobility with:**
a. Bed Ladder Pull up.
b. Leg lifter.
c. Over-head trapeze bar.
- **Dependent transfer:**
a. Stand pivot transfer.
b. Lift transfer.
c. Transfer belt transfer.

TILT TABLE

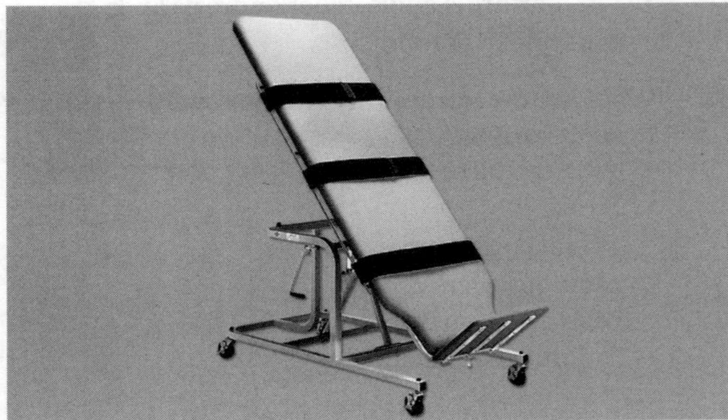

Figure 10.1: Tilt table

Q. What is tilt table?

- It is a padded table with a top capable of being rotated on its transverse axis so that a patient lying on it can be brought into the erect position (Fig. 10.1).
- Initially used as a diagnostic tools 'Tilt Table Test' for assessment of syncope.
- Serves as an integral part of therapy for physiological accommodation to an upright position.
- It also provides an opportunity for early weight bearing in lower limbs.

Q. What are the types of tilt table?

- Manual tilt table
- Electric tilt table
- Pediatric tilt table
- W/H accessible Hi-lo tilt table.

Q. What are the procedures for tilt table training?

- Before transferring to tilt table, measure the baseline resting BP and pulse rate
- Transfer the patient to the tilt table
- The patient lies supine on top of the table with foot flat on the foot board
- Therapist secures the safety straps over the knee, pelvic and chest
- Secure abdominal binder and antiembolism stocking/elastic stocking.
- Then gradually elevate the tilt table to upright position.

Raising and lowering the patient:

- Slowly elevate to 20°
- Take BP/HR
- Elevate the patient to 45°—repeat vitals.
- Elevate the patient to 85°—repeat vitals
- Check the BP and HR of the patient every 3-5 minutes
- Gradually to return to horizontal position and check vital signs
- Transfer the patient back.

Q. What should be the duration of tilt table training?

- Perform once/twice a day regime for up to 10-30 min each session.
- One level below where the fainting starts.
- Up to 4 weeks, then try a higher level

Q. What are the contraindications of Tilt Table training?

- Bone tumors
- Fresh fracture
- Fresh implant
- Neoplastic disease of spine
- Pregnancy
- Acute inflammatory condition in pelvis or lower limb
- Patient refusal
- Acute spinal or pelvic fractures
- Acute cardiac infarctions.

STEM CELL IN PMR

Q. What is a stem cell?

Stem cells are undifferentiated biological cells that can differentiate into specialized cells and can divide to produce more stem cells.

Q. What are the properties of a stem cell?

- Self-renewal: The ability to go through numerous cycles of cell division while maintaining the undifferentiated state
- Potency: The capacity to differentiate into specialized cell types.

Q. What are the different types of potency?

- *Totipotent stem cells* can differentiate into embryonic and extraembryonic cell types and can construct a complete, viable organism. These

cells are produced from the fusion of an egg and sperm cell.
- *Pluripotent stem cells* are the descendants of totipotent cells and can differentiate into nearly all cells.
- *Multipotent stem cells* can differentiate into a number of cell types.
- *Oligopotent stem cells* can differentiate into only a few cell types.
- *Unipotent cells* can produce only one cell type, their own.

Q. What are the types of stem cell?
- Embryonic stem cell
- Adult stem cell.

Q. What are the sources of stem cell?
- Fetal tissues
- Placenta
- Amniotic fluid
- Blood
- Bone marrow
- Adipose tissue
- Muscle
- Brain tissue
- Joint fluid
- Menstrual blood.

Q. How does stem cell work?
- Providing an anti-inflammatory effect
- Homing to damaged tissues and recruiting other cells, such as endothelial progenitor cells, that are necessary for tissue growth
- Supporting tissue remodeling over scar formation
- Inhibiting apoptosis
- Differentiating into bone, cartilage, tendon and ligament tissue.

Q. What are the evidences of efficacy as per animal studies?
- Myocardial infarction
- Stroke
- Tendon and ligament damage
- Osteoarthritis and osteochondrosis and
- Muscular dystrophy.

Q. What are the minimum evidence of efficacy as per human studies?
- Pressure ulcer
- Stroke
- Spinal cord injury
- Multiple sclerosis
- Motor neuron disease
- Traumatic brain injury.

Chapter 11

Scales of PMR

SCALES ON CONSCIOUSNESS

Glasgow Coma Scale

- **Eyes**
  - Open spontaneously **4**
  - Open to verbal command **3**
  - Open to painful stimuli **2**
  - No response **1**
- **Verbal response**
  - Oriented and converses **5**
  - Disoriented and converses **4**
  - Inappropriate words **3**
  - Incomprehensible sounds **2**
  - No response **1**
- **Motor response**
  - Obeys verbal commands **6**
  - Responds to painful stimuli by: purposeful localization **5**
  - Withdrawal **4**
  - Flexor posturing **3**
  - Extensor posturing **2**
  - No response **1**

Score **3–15**

SCALES ON COGNITION

Rancho Los Amigos Levels of Cognitive Functioning (Table 11.1)

Table 11.1: Rancho Los Amigos levels of cognitive functioning

I. No response	Unresponsive to any stimuli and there is no evidence of language processing
II. Generalized response	Reacts inconsistently and unpurposefully to stimuli in nonspecific manner. Receptively and expressively there is no evidence of processing or verbal or gestural expression
III. Localized response	Reacts specifically, but inconsistently, to stimuli. May follow simple commands in an inconsistent, delayed manner. Language begins to emerge (e.g. automatic verbal and gestural responses, yes/no head nodding, single words, limited reading)
IV. Confused, agitated	Behavior may appear bizarre and outbursts may be common. Attention to environment is very short and recall is limited. Disinhibition is common with inability to self-monitor behavior. Literal paraphasia may be present and incomplete expression of thoughts. Marked disruptions in auditory and visual processing may be apparent
V. Confused, inappropriate, nonagitated	Able to respond to simple commands with consistency. Disoriented/Confused with limited short-term recall. May be able to sustain short bursts of appropriate automatic social behavior. Verbalizations may be bizarre with many confabulatory statements. Semantic and syntactic confusion may be impaired
VI. Confused, appropriate	Shows goal-directed behavior, follows simple commands, and demonstrates some increases in short-term memory. Processing of receptive language is delayed with some difficulty in retaining and synthesizing information. Difficulty with new learning is evident. Speech may be characterized by monopitch, monostress and monoloudness
VII. Automatic, appropriate	Appropriate and oriented to immediate environment, able to follow daily routine with structure/support. Ability to process and retain receptive language improves for simple/concrete information. Expressive language may be tangential, concrete, and self-oriented. Judgment remains impaired
VIII. Purposeful and appropriate	Increasing memory/recall and ability to learn and retain new information. May demonstrate higher level cognitive-language deficits that become more apparent under new or stressful situations

Mini Mental Scale (Table 11.2)

Table 11.2: Mini mental scale

Category	*Possible points*	*Description*
Orientation to time	5	From broadest to most narrow. Orientation to time has been correlated with future decline
Orientation to place	5	From broadest to most narrow. This is sometimes narrowed down to streets and sometimes to floor
Registration	3	Repeating named prompts
Attention and calculation	5	Serial sevens, or spelling "world" backwards. It has been suggested that serial sevens may be more appropriate in a population where English is not the first language
Recall	3	Registration recall
Language	2	Naming a pencil and a watch
Repetition	1	Speaking back a phrase
Complex commands	6	Varies. Can involve drawing shown figure

IQ Assessment (Table 11.3)

Table 11.3: IQ assessment

IQ Range	*Classification*
110–120	Superior intelligence
90–110	Normal or average intelligence
80–90	Dullness
70–80	Borderline deficiency

Agitated Behavior Scale

1. Short attention span, easy distractibility, inability to concentrate.
2. Impulsive, impatient, low tolerance for pain or frustration.
3. Uncooperative, resistant to care, demanding.
4. Violent or threatening violence toward people or property.
5. Explosive and/or unpredictable behavior.
6. Rocking, rubbing, moaning, or other self-stimulating behavior.
7. Pulling at tubes, restraints and so on.
8. Wandering from treatment areas.
9. Restlessness, pacing, excessive movement.
10. Repetitive behaviors, motor and/or verbal.
11. Rapid, loud or excessive talking.
12. Sudden changes of mood.
13. Easily initiated or excessive talking.
14. Self-abusive physically and/or verbally.

Total score

1 = Absent: The behavior is not present.

2 = Present to a slight degree: The behavior is present but does not prevent the conduct of other, contextually appropriate behavior (the individual may redirect spontaneously, or the continuation of the agitated behavior does not disrupt appropriate behavior).

3 = Present to a moderate degree: The individual needs to be redirected from an agitated to an appropriate behavior, but benefits from such cueing.

4 = Present to an extreme degree: The individual is not able to engage in appropriate behavior because of the interference of the agitated behavior, even when the external cueing or redirection is provided.

SCALES ON FUNCTIONAL ASSESSMENT

FIM Score (Table 11.4)

Table 11.4: FIM score

LEVELS	Independence 7—Complete independence (no helper, no setup, no device) 6—Modified independence (device, extra time, safety)	No Helper	DOMAINS **Self-care:** Eating Grooming Bathing Dressing: Upper body Dressing: Lower body Toileting **Sphincter control** Bladder management Bowel management **Transfers:** Bed, chair, wheelchair toilet tub, shower Locomotion: Walk/wheelchair Stairs **Motor Subtotal Rating** **Communication** Comprehension Expression **Social cognition** Social interaction Problem solving Memory **Cognitive Subtotal Rating**
	Modified dependence 5—Supervision (standby assist, setup) 4—Minimal assist (patient = 75%+) 3—Moderate assist (patient = 50–74%)	Helper Needed	
	Complete dependence 2—Maximal assist (patient = 25– 49%) 1—Total assist (patient = less than 25%)		

GMFCS, MACS and CFCS (Table 11.5)

Table 11.5: GMFCS, MACS, and CFCS

Level	*GMFCS*	*MACS*	*CFCS*
I	Walks without limitations	Handles objects easily and successfully	Sends and receives information with familiar and unfamiliar partners effectively and efficiently
II	Walks with limitations	Handles most objects but with somewhat reduced quality and/or speed of achievement	Sends and receives information with familiar and unfamiliar partners but may need extra time
III	Walks using a hand-held mobility device	Handles objects with difficulty; needs help to prepare and/or modify activities	Sends and receives information with familiar partners effectively, but not with unfamiliar partners
IV	Self-mobility with limitations; may use powered mobility	Handles a limited selection of easily managed objects in adapted situations	Inconsistently sends and / or receives information even with familiar partners
V	Transported in a manual wheelchair	Does not handle objects with severely limited ability to perform even simple actions	Seldom effectively sends and receives information even with familiar partners

Medicare Functional Classification Level (MFCL) (Table 11.6)

Table 11.6: Medicare functional classification level (MFCL)

K0	No ability or potential to ambulate or transfer with use of a prosthesis and prosthesis does not enhance the quality of life
K1	Ability or potential to transfer or ambulate with a prosthesis for household distances on level surfaces at a fixed cadence
K2	Ability or potential to ambulate limited community distances and traverse low-level environmental barriers. Ambulation at a fixed cadence
K3	Ability or potential to ambulate unlimited community distances and traverse most environmental barriers. Ambulation with variable cadence
K4	Ability or potential to ambulate exceeding basic ambulation skill exhibiting high impact, stress or energy level—typical of active adult or child

MANUAL MUSCLE TESTING

Modified Oxford Scale Used to Grade Internal Manual Muscle Testing of the Pelvic Floor Muscles (Table 11.7)

Table 11.7: Modified oxford scale

Grading	*Contraction*	*Lift or tighten*
0/5	No	No
1/5	Flicker	No
2/5	Weak	No
3/5	Moderate	Some lifting/ tightening, contraction visible
4/5	Good	Holds for 5+ seconds
5/5	Strong	Holds for 10+ seconds

Sensory System

A 3-point scale is used to score light touch and pinprick sensation separately:

Score: **0** Absent
1 Impaired
2 Normal

Pinprick testing: Using the sharp edge of a *safety pin,* sensation is compared to that of the face. The patient must be able to differentiate the sharp and dull edge of a safety pin.

Score: **0** No sensation at all or unable to differentiate between the sharp and dull edge
1 The pin is not felt as sharp as on the face, but able to differentiate sharp from dull
2 Pin is felt as sharp as on the face

Light touch testing: A cotton tip applicator is used and sensation is compared to the face.

Scores: **0** Absent sensation
1 Impaired—light touch is felt but less than that on the face
2 Normal—Same as on face

Muscle Power

Manual Muscle Testing Grading System

Score	**Description**
0	No movement
1	Palpable or visible contraction but no movement

2	Active movement through full range of motion with gravity eliminated
3	Active movement through full range of motion against gravity
4	Active movement against moderate resistance through full range of motion
5	Normal strength based on age, sex and body habitus

SCALES ON SPASTICITY

Modified Ashworth Scale

Score	Description
0	No increase in muscle tone
1	Slight increase in muscle tone manifested by a catch and release at end range of motion
1+	Slight increase in muscle tone, manifested by a catch followed by minimal resistance throughout the remainder of the range of motion
2	More marked increase in tone, through most of the range of motion but joint easily moved
3	Considerable increase in muscle tone, passive movement is difficult
4	Affected part is rigid in flexion or extension

Bilateral Adductor Spasticity Scale

- No increase in muscle tone ---------------- 0
- Increased tone, hips easily abducted to 45° by one person ---------------- 1
- Hips abducted to 45° by one person with mild effort ---------------- 2
- Hips abducted to 45° by one person with moderate effort ---------------- 3
- Two peopled are required to abduct the hips to 45° ---------------- 4

Spasm Frequency Score

How many spasm has the patient had in last 24 hours in the affected extremity is recorded.

	SCORE
No spasm	0
1/day	1
2–5/day	2
5–9/day	3
>10/day	4

Note: As far as possible the action of each muscle should be observed separately.

Tardieu Scale

No resistance throughout the course of passive movement --------- 0

Slight resistance throughout the course of passive movement with no clear catch at precise angle --------- 1

Clear catch at precise angle, interrupting the passive movement followed by release --------- 2

Fatigable clonus, less than 10 seconds when maintaining pressure appearing at precise angle --------- 3

Nonfatigable clonus more than 10 seconds when maintaining pressure, at precise angle --------- 4

SCALES ON STROKE

Grades of Intraventricular Hemorrhage in the Premature Brain

Grade	Hemorrhage
1	Isolated to the germinal matrix
2	With normal ventricular size
3	With ventricular dilation
4	With parenchymal hemorrhage

Barthel Index

FEEDING
- 0 = Unable
- 5 = Needs help cutting, spreading butter, etc. or requires modified diet
- 10 = Independent

BATHING
- 0 = Dependent
- 5 = Independent (or in shower)

GROOMING
- 0 = Needs to help with personal care
- 5 = Independent face/hair/teeth/shaving (implements provided)

DRESSING
- 0 = Dependent
- 5 = Needs help but can do about half unaided
- 10 = Independent (including buttons, zips, laces, etc.)

BOWELS
- 0 = Incontinent (or needs to be given enemas)
- 5 = Occasional accident
- 10 = Continent

BLADDER
0 = Incontinent, or catheterized and unable to manage alone
5 = Occasional accident
10 = Continent

TOILET USE
0 = Dependent
5 = Needs some help, but can do something alone
10 = Independent (on and off, dressing, wiping)

TRANSFERS (BED TO CHAIR AND BACK)
0 = Unable, no sitting balance
5 = Major help (one or two people, physical), can sit
10 = Minor help (verbal or physical)
15 = Independent

MOBILITY (ON LEVEL SURFACES)
0 = Immobile or <50 yards
5 = Wheelchair independent, including corners, >50 yards
10 = Walks with help of one person (verbal or physical) >50 yards
15 = Independent (but may use any aid; for example, stick) > 50 yards

STAIRS
0 = Unable
5 = Needs help (verbal, physical, carrying aid)
10 = Independent

Brunnstrom Stages of Stroke Recovery

1. Flaccidity.
2. Spasticity appears.
3. Increased spasticity, basic synergy pattern appears, minimal voluntary movements.
4. Decreased spasticity, some movements out of synergy patterns.
5. Further decrease in spasticity, more complex movement combinations, synergy patterns no longer dominate.
6. Disappearance of spasticity, able to move individual joints, coordination near normal.
7. Normal function is returned.

Concussion Grading Scales (Table 11.8)

Table 11.8: Concussion grading scales

	Grade 1	*Grade 2*	*Grade 3*
Colorado	1. Confusion without amnesia 2. No loss of consciousness	1. Confusion with amnesia 2. No loss of consciousness	Loss of consciousness (of any duration)
AAN	1. Transient confusion 2. No loss of consciousness 3. Concussion symptoms or mental status changes resolve in less than 5 minutes	1. Transient confusion 2. No loss of consciousness 3. Concussion symptoms or mental status changes last longer than 15 minutes	1. Loss of consciousness (brief or prolonged)
CANTU	1. No loss of consciousness OR 2. Posttraumatic amnesia or signs/ symptoms last longer than 30 minutes	1. Loss of consciousness lasts less than 1 minute OR 2. Posttraumatic amnesia lasts longer than 30 minutes but less than 24 hours	1. Loss of consciousness lasts >1 minute OR 2. Posttraumatic amnesia lasts longer than 24 hours OR 3. Postconcussion signs/symptoms last longer than 7 days

Scales on SCI

AIS Impairment Scale

A. **Complete:** No motor or sensory function in the lowest sacral segment (S4–S5).
B. **Incomplete:** Sensory function below neurologic level and in S4–S5, no motor function below neurologic level.
C. **Incomplete:** Motor function is preserved below neurologic level and more than half of the key muscle groups below neurologic level have a muscle grade less than 3.
D. **Incomplete:** Motor function is preserved below neurologic level and at least half of the key muscle groups below neurologic level have a muscle grade 3.
E. **Normal:** Sensory and motor function is normal.

Pressure Sore Grading (Table 11.9)

Table 11.9: Pressure sore grading

Pressure ulcer categories	*Stages description*
Suspected deep tissue injury	Purple or maroon localized area of discolored intact skin or blood-filled blister resulting from damage of underlying soft tissue from pressure and/ or shear
Category/Stage I	Intact skin with nonblanchable redness of a localized area usually over a bony prominence
Category/Stage II	Partial thickness loss of dermis presenting as a shallow open ulcer with a red pink wound bed, without slough

Contd...

Pressure ulcer categories	*Stages description*
Category/Stage III	Full-thickness tissue loss. Subcutaneous fat may be visible, but bone, tendon, or muscle is not exposed
Category/Stage IV	Full-thickness tissue loss with exposed bone, tendon, or muscle
Unstageable/ Unclassified	Full-thickness tissue loss in which the base of the ulcer is covered by slough (yellow, tan, gray, green, or brown) and/or eschar (tan, brown, or black) in the wound bed

Scales on Sexuality

ALLOW, PLISSIT, and BETTER Models for Facilitating Communication About Sexuality

- A **Ask** the patient about sexual function and activity.
- L **Legitimize** the patient's problem and acknowledge that sexual dysfunction is a relevant clinical issue.
- L **Limitations** in the evaluation of the sexual dysfunction should be identified.
- O **Open up** the discussion: Potentially refer the patient to a subspecialist.
- W **Work together** to develop goals and a treatment plan.
- P **Permission** should be obtained from the patient to discuss sexuality.
- LI **Limited information** should be given (e.g., about normal sexual functioning and effects of disability).
- SS **Specific suggestions** should be given about the patient's particular complaint.
- IT **Intensive therapy** may be required, including referral to a subspecialist or therapist.
- B **Bring up** the topic of sexuality.
- E **Explain** that sexuality is important and that you are open to discussion of it with your patient.
- T **Tell** your patient about resources that you will use to assist them.
- T **Time** the discussion to the patient's preference.
- E **Educate** the patient about the side effects of treatment medications and the disability itself.
- R **Record** that you had a conversation about sexuality in the patient's medical record.

Scales on Diabetic Foot Ulcer

Wagner Grade

1. A Wagner designation is retained as long as a wound persists. For instance, if toe gangrene occurs and the toe is amputated and the incision does not "durably" heal, the Wagner IV designation continues. When durable healing occurs, the foot reverts to Wagner 0.
2. Wagner II is to some degree an archaic designation. This is because of improved imaging methods. When the scale was first published in 1980, magnetic resonance imaging was not available for clinical use.

Wagner I	Is an uncomplicated neuropathic ulcer through skin and subcutaneous tissue (discussed earlier).
Wagner II	Through fascial plane but no infection by clinical appearance.
Wagner III	In general, diabetic foot ulcer with "hospital level infection": Cellulitis beneath fascial plane, osteomyelitis, septic arthritis, or tendonitis.
Wagner IV	Localized gangrene (likely to involve deep soft tissue or bone).
Wagner V	Extensive gangrene.

Wagner–Meggitt Classification of Diabetic Foot

Grade 0	Foot symptoms like pain only
Grade 1	Superficial ulcers
Grade 2	Deep ulcers
Grade 3	Ulcer with bone involvement
Grade 4	Forefoot gangrene
Grade 5	Full foot gangrene.

Scales on COPD (Table 11.10)

Table 11.10: Classification scheme for chronic obstructive pulmonary disease severity: National Heart, Lung, and Blood Institute—World Health Organization Global Initiative for Chronic Obstructive Lung Disease Criteria

Stage *	*Criterion*
0	Normal lung function
1 (Mild)	FEV1 ≥80% of predicted
2 (Moderate)	50–79% of predicted
3 (Severe)	30–49% of predicted
4 (Very severe)	FEV1 <30% of predicted or presence of respiratory failure or clinical signs of right-sided heart failure

Scales on OA Knee

Kellgren–Lawrence Radiographic Grading Scale for Osteoarthritis of the Tibiofemoral Joint (Table 11.11)

Table 11.11: Kellgren–lawrence radiographic grading scale

Grade of Osteoarthritis	*Description*
0	No radiographic findings of osteoarthritis
1	Doubtful narrowing of joint space and possible osteophytic lipping
2	Definite osteophytes with possible narrowed joint space
3	Definite osteophytes with moderate joint space narrowing and some sclerosis
4	Definite osteophytes with severe joint space narrowing, subchondral sclerosis, and definite deformity of bone contour

WOMAC

- None = 0
- Minimal = 1
- Moderate = 2
- Severe = 3
- Very severe = 4

Pain

1. Walking on flat surface.
2. Going up/down stairs.
3. At night.
4. Sitting/lying.
5. Standing upright.

Physical function

1. Descending stairs.
2. Ascending stairs.
3. Getting out of chair.
4. Remaining in standing position.
5. Bending.
6. Walking on flat surface.
7. In/Out of car
8. Shopping.
9. Socks/Stockings on.
10. Getting out of bed.
11. Socks/Stockings off.
12. Lying in bed.
13. In/Out bath.
14. Sitting.
15. Toileting.
16. Heavy domestic duties.
17. Light domestic duties Stiffness.

Knee stiffness?

1. After first wakening in the morning?
2. After sitting, lying or resting later in the day?

Subtotal: **Total:**

Scales on AS

Radiograph Grading of Sacroiliitis

Grade 0: Normal
Grade 1: Suspicious changes
Grade 2: Minimal abnormality—small localized areas with erosions or sclerosis, without alteration in the joint width
Grade 3: Unequivocal abnormality—moderate or advanced sacroiliitis with erosions, sclerosis, widening, narrowing, or partial ankylosis
Grade 4: Total ankylosis

Bath Ankylosing Spondylitis Metrology Index (BASMI)

Table 11.12: Bath ankylosing spondylitis metrology index

Function	*For*
S=(21.1 cm-A)/2.1 cm	Lateral lumbar flexion (mean right/left)
S=(A-8 cm)/3 cm	Tragus to wall distance (mean right/left)
S=(7.4 cm-A)/0.7 cm	Lumbar flexion (modified Schober)
S=(124.5 cm-A)/10 cm	Maximal intermalleolar distance
S=(89.3u - A)/8.5u	Cervical rotation angle (mean right/left)

The average score of the five assessments gives the BASMI linear result. The additional condition 0<S<10 is always applied. A—result of assessment.

Bath Ankylosing Spondylitis Disease Activity Index (BASDI)

Patient is asked to place a mark on each line below to indicate the answer to each question relating to **the past week.**

1. How would you describe the overall level of **fatigue/ tiredness you have experienced?**
   NONE ____________________ VERY SEVERE
2. How would you describe the overall level of AS **neck, back or hip pain you have had?**
   NONE ____________________ VERY SEVERE
3. How would you describe the overall level of **pain/ swelling in joints other than neck, back, hips you have had?**
   NONE ____________________ VERY SEVERE

4. How would you describe the overall level of **discomfort you have had from any areas tender to touch or pressure?**
   NONE ________________________ VERY SEVERE
5. How would you describe the overall level of **morning stiffness you have had from the time you wake up?**
   NONE ________________________ VERY SEVERE
6. How long does your **morning stiffness last** from the time you wake up?

   ____

   0 hrs ½ 1 1½ 2 or more hours

Ankylosing Spondylitis Disease Activity Score (ASDAS) (Table 11.13)

Table 11.13: Ankylosing spondylitis disease activity score

Disease activity states	
Inactive disease	<1.3
Moderate disease activity	1.3 – 2.1
High disease activity	2.1 – 3.5
Very high disease activity	>3.5
Cut off scores for improvement	
Clinically important	> 1.1
Major	> 2.0

- Calculated from ASDAS–CRP and ASDAS – ESR formulae

Bath Ankylosing Spondylitis Functionality Index BASFI

1. Putting on your socks or tights without help or aids.
2. Bending from the waist to pick up a pen from the floor without aid.
3. Reaching up to a high shelf without help or aids (helping hand).
4. Getting up from an armless chair without your hands or any other help.
5. Getting up off the floor without help from lying on your back.
6. Standing unsupported for 10 mins without discomfort.
7. Climbing 12–15 steps without using a handrail or walking aid.
8. Looking over your shoulder without turning your body.
9. Doing physically demanding activities (physiotherapy exercises, gardening, sports).
10. Doing a full days activities whether it be at home or at work.

The average score out of 10 is considered as the BASFI score.

Bath Ankylosing Spondylitis Radiology Index (BASRI)

AP view of both SI joints are scored according to NY criteria 1979 as

0 No disease
1 Suspicious for disease
2 Minimal disease
3 Moderate disease
4 Severe disease

Scales on Spine

Meyerding Grading System for Spondylolisthesis (Table 11.14)

Table 11.14: Meyerding grading system

Grade	*Percentage slip*
1	<25
2	25–49
3	50–74
4	75–99
5	≥100 (spondyloptosis)

Grading Lumbar Stenosis on Magnetic Resonance Imaging (Table 11.15)

Table 11.15: Grading lumbar stenosis on magnetic resonance imaging

Grade	*Percentage of the anteroposterior canal dimensions at a normal level*
Mild	75–99
Moderate	50–74
Severe	<50

Scales on Shoulder

Stages of Adhesive Capsulitis (Table 11.16)

Table 11.16: Stages of adhesive capsulitis

Stage	*Symptom duration*	*Signs and symptoms*
1	1–3 months	Painful shoulder movement, minimal restriction in motion
2	3–9 months	Painful shoulder movement, progressive loss of glenohumeral joint motion
3	9–15 months	Reduced pain with shoulder movement, severely restricted glenohumeral joint motion
4	15–24 months	Minimal pain, progressive normalization of glenohumeral joint motion

Shoulder Pain and Disability Index (SPADI)

Pain scale: No pain at all
0 1 2 3 4 5 6 7 8 9 10
Worst pain imaginable

How severe is your pain?

1. At its worst? 0 1 2 3 4 5 6 7 8 9 10
2. When lying on the involved side? 0 1 2 3 4 5 6 7 8 9 10
3. Reaching for something on a high shelf? 0 1 2 3 4 5 6 7 8 9 10
4. Touching the back of your neck? 0 1 2 3 4 5 6 7 8 9 10
5. Pushing with the involved arm? 0 1 2 3 4 5 6 7 8 9 10

Disability scale: No difficulty
0 1 2 3 4 5 6 7 8 9 10
So difficult it requires help

How much difficulty do you have?

1. Washing your hair? 0 1 2 3 4 5 6 7 8 9 10
2. Washing your back? 0 1 2 3 4 5 6 7 8 9 10
3. Putting on an undershirt or pullover sweater? 0 1 2 3 4 5 6 7 8 9 10
4. Putting on a shirt that buttons down the front? 0 1 2 3 4 5 6 7 8 9 10
5. Putting on your pants? 0 1 2 3 4 5 6 7 8 9 10
6. Placing an object on a high shelf? 0 1 2 3 4 5 6 7 8 9 10
7. Carrying a heavy object of 10 pounds? 0 1 2 3 4 5 6 7 8 9 10
8. Removing something from your back pocket? 0 1 2 3 4 5 6 7 8 9 10

Scales on Ligament Injury

Ligamentous Injury Grading Scale (Table 11.17)

Table 11.17: Ligamentous injury grading scale

Grade	*Signs*
1	Tenderness to palpation without joint laxity
2	Tenderness to palpation with joint laxity but a good end point
3	Tenderness to palpation with significant joint laxity and no end point

Scales on Nerve Injury

Classification of Nerve Injury

Table 11.18: Seddon and sunderland systems

Seddon	*Sunderland*	*Description*
Neurapraxia	First-degree	Focal conduction block without axonal damage
Axonotmesis	Second-degree	Axon damage with Wallerian degeneration, supporting structures intact
Neurotmesis	Third-degree	Damage to axon and endoneurium
	Fourth-degree	Damage to perineurium and endoneurium
	Fifth-degree	Damage to axon and all supporting structures

Scales on NCS

Electrodiagnostic Criteria for Demyelinating Peripheral Neuropathy

- Conduction velocity slowed to <80% of the lower limit of normal (LLN) if the compound muscle activated potential (CMAP) is >80% of LLN and <70% if CMAP is <70% of lower limit of normal (LLN)
- Distal latency is prolonged more than 125% of the upper limit of normal (ULN) if CMAP is >80% of LLN and more than 150% of ULN if CMAP is <80% of LLN
- F wave latency more than 120% of ULN if CMAP amplitude was >80% of LLN and more than 150% of ULN if CMAP is <80% of LLN, or absence of F wave response
- Partial conduction block with a >30% decrease in amplitude between stimulation of proximal and distal sites.

Scales on Hypermobility

The Beighton score

- One point is assigned for the ability to accomplish each of the following movements:
- Bending your small finger back further than 90 degrees (1 point each side)
- Bending your thumb forward to touch your forearm (1 point each side)
- Hyperextending your elbows and knees, that is bending them beyond a straight line (1 point each joint, each side)
- Putting your palms flat on the floor without bending your knees (1 point).

Scales on Myasthenia Gravis

Severity: (Osserman Classification)

- I: Ocular myasthenia
- IIA: Mild generalized myasthenia with slow progression: No crises, responsive to drugs
- IIB. : Moderately severe generalized myasthenia: Severe skeletal and bulbar involvement but no crises; drug response less than satisfactory
- III: Acute fulminating myasthenia, rapid progression of severe symptoms, with respiratory crises and poor drug response
- IV: Late severe myasthenia, same as III but progression over 2 years from class I to II.

BIBLIOGRAPHY

1. Abrams P. Urodynamics. 3rd ed. Springer London Ltd.1997.
2. David Cifu. Braddom's physical medicine and rehabilitation. Fifth Edition. Elseviers;2015.
3. Walter R, Frontera. Delisa's physical medicine and rehabilitation: Principles and practice. Fifth Edition. Lippincott Willium and Wilkins;2010.
4. Kasper DL, Hauser SL, et al. Harrison's principles of internal medicine. 19th ed. USA. The McGraw-Hill Company; 2015.
5. Preston DC, Saphiro BE. Electromyography and neuromuscular disorders. 2nd ed. Philadelphia: Elsvier; 2005.
6. Sara Cuccurullo. Physical medicine and rehabilitation board Review. Second Edition. DesmoMedical;2009.

Index

Page numbers followed by *f* refer to figure and *t* refer to table